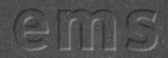

Prehospital Behavioral Emergencies and Crisis Response

AAOS
AMERICAN ACADEMY OF ORTHOPAEDIC SURGEONS

Dwight A. Polk, MSW, NREMT-P
Paramedic Program Director
University of Maryland Baltimore County (UMBC)
Department of Emergency Health Services
Baltimore, Maryland

Jeffrey T. Mitchell, PhD
Clinical Professor
University of Maryland Baltimore County (UMBC)
Department of Emergency Health Services
Baltimore, Maryland

Benjamin Gulli, MD
Medical Editor

JONES AND BARTLETT PUBLISHERS
Sudbury, Massachusetts
BOSTON   TORONTO   LONDON   SINGAPORE

Handwritten inscription, left: Marion – It was great meeting you at the Congress. Best wishes in all that you do with ICISF. Dwight 2/28/09

Handwritten inscription, right: Marion, Thanks for all your support and the gifts you have given to so many – Jeff Mitchell

Library of Congress Cataloging-in-Publication Data
Prehospital behavioral emergencies and crisis response / AAOS, Dwight Polk, Jeffrey T. Mitchell.
     p. ; cm.
  Includes bibliographical references.
  ISBN-13: 978-0-7637-5120-3
  ISBN-10: 0-7637-5120-0
  1. Psychiatric emergencies. 2. Crisis intervention (Mental health services) 3. Emergency medical services. I. Polk, Dwight A. II. Mitchell, Jeffrey T. III. American Academy of Orthopaedic Surgeons.
  [DNLM: 1. Crisis Intervention—methods. 2. Emergency Treatment—psychology. WM 401 P923 2008]
  RC480.6.P73 2008
  616.89'025—dc22
                    2008039027

6048
Printed in the United States of America
12 11 10 09 08   10 9 8 7 6 5 4 3 2 1

Special Thanks

Our appreciation goes out to the following UMBC Paramedic students—without your drive, talent, and dedication to the field of EMS, this book never would have been possible. Thanks for devoting your time and talent by assisting in the research and writing of chapters for this book. You are indeed the best of the best!

Ali Aledhaim
Brian Boone
Victor Carrio-Vazquez
Blakeslee Davis
Benjamin Dunn
Wendi Florio
Jessica Johnston
Marie Lee
Alon Manela
Malgorzata Nowaczyk
Theresa Schmitz
Garrett Snyder

Contents

About the Authors

Dwight A. Polk, NSW, NREMT-P – Paramedic Program Director, University of Maryland Baltimore County

Involved in EMS since 1975, and a paramedic since 1982, Dwight Polk has held the position of Paramedic Program Director at the University of Maryland Baltimore County (UMBC) since 1990. Prior to arriving at UMBC, Mr. Polk was a field paramedic and Education Coordinator at Acadian Ambulance Service in Lafayette, Louisiana. He is also currently employed by the Grassroots Crisis Intervention Center in Columbia, Maryland as a Mobile Crisis Team Counselor and serves as a mental health professional for two CISM teams in the Baltimore area.

Jeffrey T. Mitchell, PhD, CTS – Clinical Professor of Emergency Health Services at the University of Maryland and President Emeritus of the International Critical Incident Stress Foundation

After serving as a firefighter/paramedic, Dr. Mitchell developed a comprehensive, integrated, systematic, and multi-component crisis intervention program called Critical Incident Stress Management. He has authored over 250 articles and 10 books in the stress and crisis intervention fields. He serves as an adjunct faculty member of the Emergency Management Institute of the Federal Emergency Management Agency.

Acknowledgments

Jones and Bartlett Publishers would like to thank the following individuals for their review of the manuscript.

Reviewers

David Leven, EMT-B
University of Rochester Medical Center
Rochester, New York

Dave Foster, CEO, AAS, EMT-P
Emergency Medical Solutions Training Center
Fleming Island, Florida

Robert Mauch, BS, NREMT-P
Sussex County (DE) EMS, Paramedic
Supervisor, and Christiana Care Health
Systems, LifeNet, Flight Paramedic
Milford, Delaware

Kenneth L. Pardoe, MS, PA-C, NREMT-P
Retired Battalion Chief, Anne Arundel County
Fire Department, Millersville, Maryland;
Emergency Medicine Physician Assistant,
Anne Arundel County, Maryland; Former
Academic Coordinator: Physician Assistant
Program, Anne Arundel Community College;
Former Instructor, Emergency Health Services
Program at University of Maryland Baltimore
County
Arnold, Maryland

Victor Welzant, PsyD
International Critical Incident Stress
Foundation and Sheppard Pratt Health Systems
Towson, Maryland

Resource Preview

Prehospital Behavioral Emergencies and Crisis Response

This textbook is designed to give prehospital providers the knowledge and skills they need to manage behavioral emergencies and respond to crisis situations in the field. Features that reinforce and expand on essential information include:

In the Field

Important tips for applying concepts to real-life situations prehospital responders encounter in the field, including step-by-step recommendations for conducting assessments.

---

in Hurricane Katrina. The prominent emotions typically are anxiety, relief, emotional numbness, fear, apprehension, and confusion. Emotional breakdowns are more likely to show up in this stage. More people who were not physically wounded will now be seeking evaluation by medics and treatment in emergency departments. Information, reassurance, and guidance, often provided by large-group Crisis Management Briefings (CMB), are going to be most helpful to the population.

The final stage of a disaster, *reconstruction*, is one in which a surprising array of negative feelings might arise. This is the rebuilding stage, and it is the longest. Even 3 to 4 years after Hurricane Katrina, rebuilding is still going on. People who are caught up in what appears to be an endless process of disappointments and frustrations lose patience and become depressed. Common feelings during the reconstruction period include frustration, grief, anger, disappointment, and feeling emotionally and physically overwhelmed. Although things are being rebuilt, there are delays, shortages, frustrations over unfulfilled government promises, disputes with insurance companies, and a host of other problems. People become distracted by their emotions. Injuries increase, as do illnesses. In the Texas City incident previously mentioned, blood pressure climbed and stayed elevated in most patients for almost a year after the explosion.

In the aftermath of disasters that have caused great losses, some people contemplate suicide. It is not unusual to find somewhat elevated suicide rates after tornadoes, hurricanes, floods, and earthquakes. People have lost almost everything they owned and the cost is far beyond what can be measured by means of a price tag. There are the emotional costs as well. Eventually, as things slowly progress, hope for a resolution of the disastrous situation may finally arise.

Psychological Reactions to Disaster

The psychological reactions to a disaster are many and varied. They can usually be sorted into five main categories: cognitive, physical, emotional, behavioral, and spiritual. Some reactions, such as agitation and distractedness during a disastrous event, are short-term and generally resolve with the passage of time or with a limited amount of emotional support. Some reactions and stress symptoms, however, do not resolve easily and eventually become manifestations of long-term psychological conditions.

Short-Term Reactions

- Worry and fear
- Bad memories
- Gastrointestinal symptoms (upset stomach and diarrhea)
- Sadness
- Mental confusion (feeling lost and disoriented)
- Feeling overwhelmed
- Acute emotional discharge or tirade
- Brief psychotic reactions
- Shock

In the Field

Psychological Stages of a Disaster

- Warning
- Alarm
- Impact
- Inventory
- Rescue
- Recovery
- Reconstruction

In the Field

Five Categories of Psychological Reaction to Disaster

- Cognitive
- Physical
- Emotional
- Behavioral
- Spiritual

Vital Views: The Importance of Crisis and Behavioral Emergencies Training   **Chapter 1**   7

Prep Kit

Ready for Review

- It is important for emergency service providers to be trained in dealing with behavioral emergencies. Knowledge of crisis intervention and management will help personnel function safely in the field while making a positive impact on the lives of others.
- Many organizations provide only minimal attention to training in the area of behavioral emergencies. In reality, emergency services providers need more education and practice in dealing with those in crisis. Without exception, all police, fire, and EMS calls contain some behavioral aspects.
- Behaviors are activities and reactions in response to either internal or external stimuli. In most situations, people respond appropriately to those stimuli. However, in the field of emergency services, patients often present behaviors that appear unusual, extreme, or threatening. Those patients frequently are in severe distress and need support and assistance.
- A crisis is an acute emotional reaction to a powerful stimulus. In most cases, crises are normal reactions of normal people to abnormal circumstances.
- Crisis reactions come from four main sources. Reactions can be self-contained, can overlap with each other, and can sometimes contribute to one another. The four crisis reactions are: developmental or maturational stages of life; distressing situations; severe traumatic events; and severe mental illness.
- The emergency services provider will use crisis intervention in an effort to mitigate the patient's distress. Crisis intervention is a temporary, active, and supportive entry into the life of someone during acute distress.

Vital Vocabulary

behavior Any organism's activities and reactions in response to either internal or external stimuli.

crisis An acute emotional reaction to a powerful stimulus (plural: crises).

crisis intervention A temporary, active, and supportive entry into the life situation of a person or a group during a period of acute distress.

emergency A life-threatening situation that requires an immediate response.

Assessment in Action

Answer key is located in the back of the book.

1. Generally speaking, it is safe to say that nearly all EMS calls will require the emergency service provider to use some crisis intervention skills.
   - A. True
   - B. False

2. Upon arriving at the side of a patient whose wife has just died, you witness that he is pacing back and forth and repeating, "I can't believe she's gone." This activity is best described as the patient's:
   - A. mental status.
   - B. neurological condition.
   - C. behavior.
   - D. stage of life.

3. "Normal reactions of normal, healthy individuals" best defines:
   - A. emotional turmoil.
   - B. stress.
   - C. traumatic event.
   - D. crisis.

4. From the following list, select the one that is NOT a goal of crisis intervention.
   - A. Assist the patient in using his or her normal recovery process.
   - B. Return the patient to his or her adaptive functions.
   - C. Conduct deep exploration of the individual's social and mental health history to discover what caused the crisis.
   - D. Help the patient to mitigate the crisis.

5. There is no such thing as a "behavioral emergency," because emergencies only exist as medical or trauma events.
   - A. True
   - B. False

Prep Kit

Provides the student with the tools necessary to understanding and using the information presented in the chapter. **Ready for Review** offers quick summary points of the chapter's key concepts, **Vital Vocabulary** emphasizes crucial terms that first responders should know when responding to behavioral emergencies, and **Assessment in Action** quiz questions evaluate students' understanding of the material.

---

146   Prehospital Behavioral Emergencies and Crisis Response

OPQRST

- **Onset:** When did the symptoms begin? Sudden onset or chronic condition?
- **Provocation:** What happened today to trigger someone to call EMS?
- **Quality:** How pervasive or significant are the patient's feelings and emotions at the time of assessment?
- **Radiation:** Is the state of confusion being experienced by the patient radiating out to family members, neighbors, or others? Has it affected important components of the patient's life, such as employment, or simply the ability to live alone?
- **Severity:** On a scale of 0–10, how severe is the distress today for the patient? For family or others involved?
- **Time:** How long have the symptoms lasted since the time of onset? Is there a need for the patient to be transported for lifesaving intervention? Has the time arrived for family members to request that a symptomatic family member be evaluated for some complication of an organic brain syndrome?

strangely and may not recognize familiar faces or things. You will have to rule out many causes of this altered mental status, based on your other medical training. It is always important to remember that no matter how confusing a scene may be, the management of life-threatening illness and injury takes precedence over psychological presentations.

Alcohol Withdrawal and Delirium Tremens

One specific type of delirium that is common in the prehospital environment is delirium tremens or simply "the DTs." Alcohol withdrawal syndromes can range from mild symptoms to full-blown DTs. The DTs are the result of withdrawal in a person who is chronically and chemically dependent on alcohol. Because of the nature of the addiction, alcohol withdrawal can be life threatening and the patient may experience seizures, coma, and death.

Alcohol is a central nervous system depressant. For the person who is addicted to alcohol, the brain's neurotransmitters have worked for years to compensate and maintain a normal level of stimulation. When the person stops drinking, the sympathetic nervous system is no longer being suppressed. As a result, numerous neurotransmitters in the brain that have worked against the depressive agent now overload the brain (**Table 11-2**). Seizures can occur as a result (**Figure 11-3**). Aggressive advanced life support care must be provided to stop the seizures and maintain the patient's airway and cardiovascular status.

Patients presenting with acute DTs might develop seizures due to alcohol or chemical withdrawal. Emergency responders should be knowledgable about local protocols, which may include the pharmacologic sedation of the patient to prevent or treat seizures.

Dementia

Dementia presents as a gradual decline in mentation and cognitive function (**Table 11-3**). Generally speaking, there is a loss of alertness and a decline in memory, particularly recent memory. Thorough questioning of the patient can investigate events of the far, intermediate, and recent past.

Prehospital providers should resist the notion that dementia is strictly a disease of the elderly; although dementia is more common after the age of 65 years and the incidence increases greatly after the age of 75 years, the condition may be seen in younger patients, particularly those with chronic conditions. Human immunodeficiency virus (HIV) disease, cerebral trauma, Alzheimer's disease (AD), and Parkinson's disease are all possible causes of dementia.

Dementia patients often present with some unusual characteristics not generally seen in the delirium patient (**Table 11-4**). Patients with chronic changes in mentation, such as Alzheimer's disease, will often invent

SEA-3 for Delirium, Dementia, and Amnesia

Speech: Able to speak; however, note any confusion.

Emotion: May present with a normal affect, or anxiety or anger may be present.

Appearance: Varies depending on the degree of confusion. May present as normal or altered. Patients may be wearing inappropriate clothing for the seasonal temperature.

Alertness: Generally alert but commonly confused. May not be oriented to person, place, or event.

Activity: Activity varies for patients with dementia or delirium. The range of sedation to agitation may be exhibited. Note that medications can alter activity levels.

SAMPLE, OPQRST, SEA-3, and SAFER-R Boxes

Provide easy-to-follow methods for quickly evaluating behavioral emergencies using familiar information-gathering tools.

Vital Views: The Importance of Crisis and Behavioral Emergencies Training

Without exception, every emergency call has some behavioral elements. Emergency personnel are involved almost daily in the most difficult situations in other people's lives. Some of these calls may appear routine, but a crisis is anything but routine to the person in the midst of it. More than likely, it is among one of the worst moments in that person's life. You will be better able to handle these crises well and offer aid to the people experiencing these crises if you have received proper training (**Figure 1-1**).

Some situations present a clear and imminent threat to the people involved. In a few cases, the threat may extend to emergency personnel. Having knowledge of crisis intervention and knowing how to manage behavioral emergencies will help emergency personnel function safely in the field while making a positive impact on the lives of others.

It may be difficult for people who recently joined the field of emergency services systems to believe, but prior to 1970, many ambulance personnel had no formal training in first aid. Some managed to get by with only minimal training that emphasized bleeding control, bandaging, and the use of splints. Only a small percentage of ambulance personnel actually had substantial prehospital training and well-developed skills. Almost everyone in that last category had functioned as a medic for the military, and many had refined their medical skills on the battlefields of Vietnam. In contrast, today's

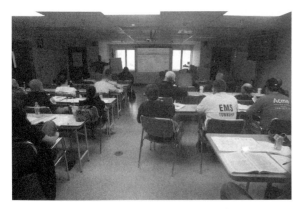

Figure 1-1 Preparing for the behavioral aspects of an emergency keeps you and your patients safe.

emergency personnel participate in extensive prehospital technical training and skills development, and the hiring organization likely requires certification of some type.

Although there have been impressive developments in the technical aspects of prehospital emergency medical care, the human elements of patient care generally have lagged far behind. Many training facilities still give only cursory attention to training in behavioral emergencies. Some instructors believe it is more efficient to use course time to conduct practical sessions on the management of acute physical illnesses and injuries rather than on the management of behavioral emergencies.

Emergency personnel participating in training programs also may be reluctant to discuss behavioral emergencies. Trainees have often said things like:

- "Oh, not this stuff again!"
- "We're never going to use it. Why are we wasting our time when we could be practicing skills to help the people who really need us?"
- "I didn't sign up to deal with crazy people. Leave that to the psych people."

These attitudes and statements indicate a significant misinterpretation of both the nature of behavioral emergencies and the pressing need for emergency personnel to possess crisis intervention knowledge and skills. It is important to remember that all police, fire and EMS runs contain behavioral aspects. Therefore, it is unacceptable and potentially dangerous for emergency personnel to engage in fieldwork without proper education, skills training, and appropriate motivation to handle behavioral emergencies.

Human Behavior

Behaviors are activities and reactions in response to either internal or external stimuli. In its broadest definition, behavior includes both observable activities and inferred activities such as imagination and other thinking processes that are impossible for an observer to see or otherwise sense directly.

Most human behavior is appropriate to the circumstances that triggered it. For instance, when emergency personnel ask a patient a question about a medical condition, the patient answers and provides important information. If an emergency medical technician (EMT) or a paramedic instructs the patient to assume a certain position to alleviate pain or to protect an injury site, the patient attempts to comply with the instructions.

If a situation or stimulus is highly unusual, extreme, or threatening, it may cause a person to experience a state of crisis. That is, the situation produces significant distress for the person or people involved, resulting in a state of emotional turmoil. However, emotional turmoil, including but not limited to intense feelings of anxiety, confusion, and feeling overwhelmed, does *not* indicate mental illness. It is a typical, healthy, and expected behavioral response to a powerful negative stimulus.

Intense loss, fear, threat, illness, injury, and pain may distress people beyond their ability to cope and may change their behaviors in such a way as to complicate the overall management of an emergency medical call (**Figure 1-2**). In some cases, altered behaviors may even make the management of emergency medical situations more dangerous to responding personnel.

We All Have Crises

Every human being has crises. In fact, most people encounter multiple situations that produce a crisis reaction during their lifetimes. From a psychological point of view, a <u>crisis</u> is an acute emotional reaction to a powerful stimulus. In most cases, crises are normal reactions of normal, healthy people to unusual or abnormal circumstances. For example, when a person is robbed on the street by a man holding a gun, it is perfectly natural for that person to feel intense anxiety and fear. Normal people may feel nauseous, have a dry mouth, experience uncontrollable shaking, and be unable to think clearly. The person in a state of crisis is normal and experiencing normal reactions to a highly disturbing event.

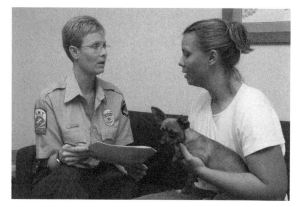

Figure 1-2 Human behaviors change during a crisis.

Human behaviors change during a crisis reaction. In fact, people must alter their behaviors to adapt to the situation. If managed well, however, crises resolve relatively quickly, and people recover and continue to live and function. They may always have a memory of the event or circumstances that caused their crisis reaction, but even when they have experienced significant losses, such as the death of a loved one, the vast majority of people eventually resume normal life functions.

Sources of Crisis Reactions

There are four main sources of crisis reactions. They may overlap each other and sometimes may contribute to one another.

> ### In the Field
>
> It is a normal reaction for a person to change or alter his or her behavior in response to a crisis. This may help the person resolve the crisis and prevent it from progressing into a behavioral emergency.

1. **Developmental or maturational stages of life.** Births, adolescence, marriage, midlife, retirement, growing old, and approaching death are typical crises that arise in the course of a lifespan.
2. **Distressing situations.** Events such as the loss of a job, property destruction, accident, burglary, illness, conflict, and the loss and grief caused by a death, marital separation, or divorce are other sources of crises.
3. **Severe traumatic events.** Such events may include violent actions against one's person, disasters, terrorism, torture, sexual assault, and life-threatening accidents; these are the third source of crisis reactions (**Figure 1-3**).
4. **Severe mental illness.** Some mental illnesses may make a person more susceptible to crisis reactions. A circumstance that would not cause most people to experience acute emotional distress can produce a significant crisis for a person with mental illness; persons with mental illness may have more crises; and a crisis may agitate a person with mental illness in such a way as to cause or exacerbate a more severe crisis reaction.

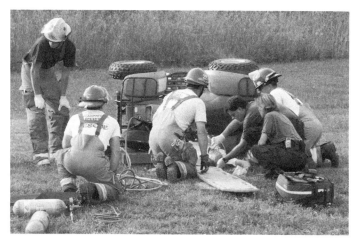

Figure 1-3 Traumatic events are a common source of crisis reactions.

Crisis Intervention

If a person, a family, or even an organization does not manage a crisis efficiently and quickly, it often escalates to more severe, but less controllable, levels of intensity. Sometimes a person or a group is not able to handle a crisis alone, and outside support is required. Family members, friends, and, on occasion, a specially trained crisis support person or a crisis team may then enter into the situation and provide crisis intervention services. Crisis intervention is a temporary, active, and supportive entry into the life of an individual, a family, or an organization during a period of acute distress. Individuals providing crisis intervention services are actually providing psychological first aid. The main goals of crisis intervention are to:

- Mitigate the impact of a crisis on the people involved,
- Facilitate normal recovery processes, and
- Restore people to adaptive functions, such as making simple decisions, caring for themselves or family members, or managing their affairs.

The focus in crisis intervention is *not* treatment or cure. Instead, the focus is on support, information, and guidance toward the three goals outlined above. When trained crisis team members provide skillful crisis support services, the overwhelming majority of people will not need formal psychological services. In fact, good crisis intervention may be just enough support in many cases to prevent a crisis from becoming an emergency. However, crisis intervention is not a clinical psychotherapy process or a substitute for psychotherapy. It is a support service only. A trained crisis intervention team establishes a referral system for people who exhibit signs and symptoms of behavioral emergencies and who need professional evaluation and more intensive care.

Some Crises Turn Into Emergencies

If a state of emotional turmoil is excessive and/or prolonged, certain negative consequences may appear, and some crises may turn into emergencies. An emergency is a life-threatening situation that requires an immediate response. Suicide attempts, substance abuse behaviors that lead to an overdose, and the escalation of a crisis to a point of a violent outburst are examples of crises that became emergencies (**Figure 1-4**).

The crisis intervention procedures discussed in this and subsequent chapters can be applied for both crises and behavioral emergencies. Crisis intervention in behavioral emergencies has a greater sense of urgency because and the life-threatening aspect of the situation. The focus of crisis intervention services for a behavioral emergency is on preserving life. A prehospital responder must concentrate his or her efforts on:

- Securing physical safety
- Removing the person from danger
- Reducing disturbing stimuli
- Lowering tension
- Preventing physical violence

Early crisis intervention efforts should emphasize crisis assessment and immediate support. Furthermore, every effort must be made to neutralize stress and reduce interpersonal conflict. It is important for emergency personnel who are managing a behavioral crisis to call for additional resources when the patient's behavior suggests that the crisis is turning into an emergency. Calling for help should never be seen as an admission of weakness or incompetence. Instead, it should

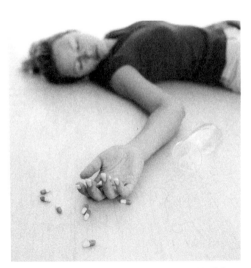

Figure 1-4 Most suicides could be preventable if the right help is available early enough.

be viewed as the mature decision of a knowledge-able and skilled provider who is doing the very best to reduce the potential that a crisis could explode into a complex and dangerous behavioral emergency.

> ### In the Field
>
> The prehospital provider must always remember that the acute crisis environment can escalate to an emergency at any time. Maintaining a controlled and safe environment is important to everyone.

Benefits of Crisis Intervention and Behavioral Emergencies Training

Training in behavioral emergencies management and crisis response has many important benefits for emergency service providers. Consider these six benefits:

1. **Safer work environment.** Providers trained in the prehospital management of crises and behavioral emergencies can work in a safer manner. They may recognize early danger signals in their patients, and they can respond quickly to mitigate distress and resolve problems.

2. **Better communication.** Crisis training can help emergency medical services (EMS) providers improve their communications with all of their patients, not just with the patients experiencing a behavioral crisis.

3. **Saves lives.** Training in the management of behavioral emergencies may ultimately help to save human lives. For example, suicide experts tell us that most suicides are preventable if the right help is available early enough.

4. **More effective assistance.** Crisis-response training conditions emergency personnel to assist distressed people more effectively. Communications may be more precise and easier to achieve. As a result, providers are less prone to inadvertently trigger negative reactions in their patients.

5. **Positive psychological and physiological effects.** There are huge health benefits for patients who receive care from EMS providers who understand the behavioral reactions to illness and injury and treat their patients with respect, concern, and human dignity. Studies conducted during the last 50 years clearly demonstrate that when emergency medical and hospital staff manage people who are in a state of emotional crisis with patience, kindness, and gentleness, patients experience positive psychological and physiological changes such as lowered anxiety, decreased blood pressure, and a slower pulse rate.

6. **Personal benefits from care and compassion.** Emergency service providers who are trained in behavioral emergencies and crisis intervention that enhances their personal care and compassion toward suffering people also may gain a great deal personally (**Figure 1-5**). Providing excellent care for others often simultaneously generates strong feelings of self-confidence and job satisfaction. The confidence that providers develop when they have adequate knowledge and skills to manage a crisis or a behavioral emergency may stimulate them to reach out to others in ways not previously imagined. Therefore, they can achieve their own personal best in the field of EMS and may experience even greater satisfaction.

Final Thoughts

The overwhelming majority of people who experience a crisis do not need formal psychological care. Some behavioral emergencies can even be managed and mitigated in the prehospital environment if providers

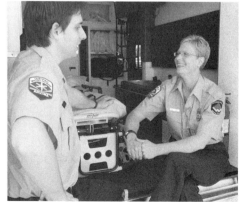

Figure 1-5 Adequate knowledge provides the confidence to reach out with compassion in a crisis.

In the Field

The emergency service provider who is educated in techniques of crisis response will present with a calm, controlled demeanor that will instill trust in most patients.

have been adequately trained in crisis intervention principles and procedures. If emotional distress is prolonged and/or severe, EMS providers should transport the patient to a hospital and inform the medical staff of the difficulties the patient is experiencing.

No one should underestimate the power of well-timed, simple, and supportive crisis intervention tactics to mitigate a disruptive and potentially threatening experience. The majority of patients respond positively to the support provided by crisis-trained emergency personnel. Tension, anxiety, and symptoms of emotional turmoil generally subside when providers supply crisis intervention services during emergencies. Without a doubt, front-line providers make a huge difference in the reduction of human distress.

Selected References

International Federation of Red Cross and Red Crescent Societies: *Community-Based Psychological Support: A Training Manual.* Geneva, Switzerland, IFRC, 2003.

Mitchell JT: *Group Crisis Support: Why It Works; When and How to Provide It.* Ellicott City, MD, Chevron Publishing Corporation, 2007.

Rosen A: Crisis management in the community. Available at: http://www.mja.com.au/public/mentalhealth/articles/rosen/rosen.html. Accessed August 12, 2008.

Sherwood DA: *Crisis Theory and Intervention: A Handout.* Waco, TX, School of Social Work, Baylor University, 1996.

Vandenbos GR (ed): *American Psychological Association Dictionary of Psychology.* Washington, DC, American Psychological Association, 2007.

Prep Kit

Ready for Review

- It is important for emergency service providers to be trained in dealing with behavioral emergencies. Knowledge of crisis intervention and management will help personnel function safely in the field while making a positive impact on the lives of others.

- Many organizations provide only minimal attention to training in the area of behavioral emergencies. In reality, emergency services providers need more education and practice in dealing with those in crisis. Without exception, all police, fire, and EMS calls contain some behavioral aspects.

- Behaviors are activities and reactions in response to either internal or external stimuli. In most situations, people respond appropriately to those stimuli. However, in the field of emergency services, patients often present behaviors that appear unusual, extreme, or threatening. Those patients frequently are in severe distress and need support and assistance.

- A crisis is an acute emotional reaction to a powerful stimulus. In most cases, crises are normal reactions of normal people to abnormal circumstances.

- Crisis reactions come from four main sources. Reactions can be self-contained, can overlap with each other, and can sometimes contribute to one another. The four crisis reactions are: developmental or maturational stages of life; distressing situations; severe traumatic events; and severe mental illness.

- The emergency services provider will use crisis intervention in an effort to mitigate the patient's distress. Crisis intervention is a temporary, active, and supportive entry into the life of someone during acute distress.

Vital Vocabulary

behavior Any organism's activities and reactions in response to either internal or external stimuli.

crisis An acute emotional reaction to a powerful stimulus (plural: crises).

crisis intervention A temporary, active, and supportive entry into the life situation of a person or a group during a period of acute distress.

emergency A life-threatening situation that requires an immediate response.

Assessment in Action

Answer key is located in the back of the book.

1. Generally speaking, it is safe to say that nearly all EMS calls will require the emergency service provider to use some crisis intervention skills.

   A. True
   B. False

2. Upon arriving at the side of a patient whose wife has just died, you witness that he is pacing back and forth and repeating, "I can't believe she's gone." This activity is best described as the patient's:

   A. mental status.
   B. neurological condition.
   C. behavior.
   D. stage of life.

3. "Normal reactions of normal, healthy individuals" best defines:

   A. emotional turmoil.
   B. stress.
   C. traumatic event.
   D. crisis.

4. From the following list, select the one that is NOT a goal of crisis intervention.

   A. Assist the patient in using his or her normal recovery process.
   B. Return the patient to his or her adaptive functions.
   C. Conduct deep exploration of the individual's social and mental health history to discover what caused the crisis.
   D. Help the patient to mitigate the crisis.

5. There is no such thing as a "behavioral emergency," because emergencies only exist as medical or trauma events.

   A. True
   B. False

Chapter 2

Crisis Intervention Principles for Prehospital Personnel

At first glance, assisting patients in the midst of an emotional crisis or a behavioral emergency may appear to be an overwhelming task to an emergency service provider. This is especially so if you have limited training in dealing with behavioral emergencies and little actual crisis intervention experience. An old adage in psychology notes that a good theoretical base is the foundation of good practice. In this chapter, we will establish the basic crisis intervention principles that will serve as guidelines for you throughout this book. They will also serve you well when you are providing support to the distressed people that you meet under real-world field conditions. The essential principles of crisis intervention make the job of providing prehospital crisis intervention a much easier process than the task initially appears.

Starting Points

Crisis states and behavioral emergencies do not appear spontaneously or without a cause. Some internal or external stimulus has to be present for a crisis reaction to begin. Internal stimuli are perceptions, feelings, thoughts, memories, and possibly some bodily reactions. Common external stimuli, such as financial difficulties, illness, grief, and minor property losses, are usually called crisis events or situations. The most powerful of them are given the name <u>critical incidents</u>. They are significant, severe events that can overwhelm a person's or a group's ability to cope and that disrupt normal functions. People experiencing a critical incident may find it to be overwhelming, threatening, frightening, disgusting, dangerous, or grotesque, or some combination. Examples of critical incidents are serious accidents, crimes, disasters, deaths of loved ones, violence against one's person, significant threats, unwanted pregnancies, drug overdoses, major changes in financial circumstances (losses or gains), public humiliations, personal rejections, life-threatening diseases, and major changes in property (again, losses or gains). Both internal and external stimuli can cause a person to enter a state of acute emotional turmoil or crisis (**Figure 2-1**).

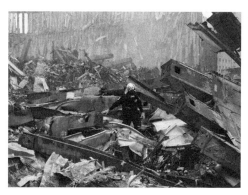

Figure 2-1 Critical incidents can cause severe emotional turmoil.

Criteria for a Crisis

A crisis is not the event itself, but it is the patient's perception of and response to the situation that is the essence of a crisis. Every emotional crisis has three central conditions:

1. *There is a substantial internal or external stimulus that starts the crisis reaction.* The sudden death of a loved one, for example, may be the event that triggers the state of crisis for an individual or a family.

2. *The person senses that the disturbing stimulus or situation can lead to considerable disruption or emotional upset in his or her life.* In fact, the patient in a state of crisis always experiences significant distress, impairment, or dysfunction. People are often in a state of shock and disbelief when a loved one dies. In severe crisis states, a family member might be unable to care for himself or might lock herself in a room and stop communicating with others.

3. *The person is unable to use his or her usual means of coping to resolve the problem, or those means are ineffective.* For instance, a person who experienced less-severe losses in the past and managed the grief by talking to a friend might find that, in the case of the death of a loved one, talking to a friend is not immediately helpful. The person's capacity to think clearly may decline, and he or she may be so overwhelmed by grief that he or she is unable to eat, sleep, think clearly, or organize appropriate responses. In situations in which a patient's thinking is impaired by a crisis reaction and feelings are uncontrolled, outside crisis intervention, also known as psychological first aid, may be required.

The Nature of Crisis Intervention

Remember from the first chapter, <u>crisis intervention</u> is defined as a temporary, active, and supportive entry into the life situation of a person or a group during a period of acute distress. Crisis intervention is not one thing, but a collection of supportive

In the Field

A crisis is not the event itself; it is the patient's perception of and response to the situation that is the essence of a crisis.

helping processes that are linked and blended together and applied during circumstances of extreme distress. Crisis intervention procedures aim primarily at:

- **Stabilization.** Crisis intervention works toward stabilizing both the event and the patient's reaction to the event.
- **Mitigation.** Crisis intervention works toward reducing or modifying the impact of the critical incident.
- **Facilitation.** The person performing crisis intervention procedures helps the person experiencing the emotional crisis utilize normal recovery processes.
- **Restoration.** The goal of crisis intervention is to help the patient return to acceptable, healthy levels of adaptive functioning.
- **Identification.** Crisis intervention also includes determining whether there are people who may need additional support or referral for professional mental health intervention.

Crisis intervention has proven to be helpful, especially in the most acute phases of a state of emotional turmoil, but it is neither psychotherapy nor a substitute for psychotherapy. Prehospital personnel using crisis intervention do not attempt to eliminate all of the symptoms of distress that a patient may be experiencing. Emergency service providers' psychological first aid skills are not capable of curing any physical disease or psychopathology.

Crisis intervention procedures work best when emergency personnel apply them to alleviate the impact of a crisis experience and to assist patients in mobilizing appropriate resources to manage both the disturbing situation and their emotional reactions to it. Providers may contribute to lessening the effects of psychological trauma, but in reality, crisis intervention's greatest benefit is that it provides practical methods through which patients may resume normal daily functions while they work their way through a crisis.

Brief Historical Overview

It is impossible to find the exact origins of crisis intervention. All recorded human history relates stories of people helping others. The structured framework for modern crisis intervention services, however, is only about 100 years old. The earliest applications of crisis intervention theory can be traced to the beginning of the 1900s, when crisis intervention principles were applied to the family members and friends of over a thousand miners who were killed in a coal mine explosion in the Courrieres mine in northern France in 1906. Many of the miners were children. Crisis intervention procedures also became part of suicide prevention programs in the United States around the same time. In the subsequent century, warfare, disasters, law enforcement programs, and EMS all influenced the development of today's crisis support programs.

The great world wars and several horrific disasters brought about many developments in the field of crisis intervention (**Figure 2-2**). Of particular note is the Cocoanut Grove fire in Boston, Massachusetts, in 1942, in which 492 people lost their lives. After that tragedy, crisis intervention programs expanded around the world, and over time, they have become more sophisticated. Crisis intervention programs now are comprehensive, integrated, systematic, and multi-tactic. From around the time of World War II, the use of trained paraprofessionals, such as police officers, fire fighters, and emergency medical personnel, has been an integral part of crisis support.

During the first 30 years of its existence, crisis intervention services focused predominantly on individuals in distress. In the 1930s, Kurt Lewin, a noted expert on groups, initiated group applications of crisis intervention. The success of these early efforts set the stage for further developments, in the mid 1970s, of methods for crisis intervention such as Dr. Jeffrey T. Mitchell's Critical Incident Stress Debriefing (CISD) for emergency services groups.

Today, emergency personnel and first responders routinely apply crisis intervention procedures to individuals and groups in hospitals, the military services, law enforcement agencies, fire services, EMS programs, alcohol and other substance abuse treatment centers, school systems, businesses, and communities. It is estimated that if every conceivable type of crisis intervention service were counted, between 35 and 40 million people per year receive organized crisis support. In just one century, crisis intervention theory and practice has grown into a formal body of knowledge and become a part of everyday life.

Crisis Intervention Concepts and Principles

Basic Concepts

Every field of human endeavor has basic concepts that underlie its operations. Likewise, crisis intervention has some core concepts that form its foundation.

Every person is vulnerable to experiencing a crisis at almost any time. No one can claim an exemption from either maturational or situational crises during an entire lifetime. Maturational crises are those that occur as part of the growth process. They include such issues as becoming a teenager, developing independence from one's parents, turning 30 (or 50 or 60) years old, growing older, and retiring. Situational crises are those that are associated with events or circumstances such as accidents, illness, financial losses, marital problems, and being exposed to a disaster.

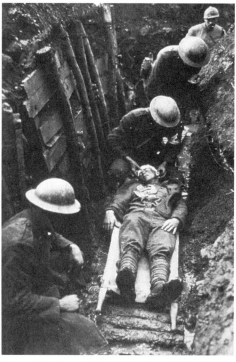

Figure 2-2 The great World Wars brought about many developments in the field of crisis intervention.

A crisis reaction is always distressing to the person involved in it. Other people may not see the same event as upsetting, because people experience the same event differently and have different responses to it.

Most crises are sudden. Part of what makes a crisis situation difficult is that it is unexpected. People may not be adequately prepared to manage the event. The majority of crises are temporary. Most acute crisis reactions subside in 24 to 72 hours.

During a crisis the usual coping methods fail. People ordinarily use multiple tools and strategies to help themselves cope on a day-to-day basis. A person's inability to control the critical event makes it seem much worse, heightens the state of emotional turmoil, and turns the distressing event into a crisis.

Crisis events produce at least a potential for dangerous or unacceptable behaviors in those who are suffering through them. When thinking ability becomes impaired, as it does in a crisis event, people are prone to make decisions that can actually make the situation worse.

Most distressed patients react positively to crisis intervention efforts. Most people who are experiencing a crisis reaction will respond positively to support services provided by others. Crisis support lowers tension and helps people to gain control of themselves and the situation, which reduces the distress of the situation.

Multiple strategies are necessary. Emergency medical personnel should provide various types of crisis intervention services according to the needs of the people in the crisis. One technique will not work equally well for all situations. In most cases, your goal as an emergency provider is to transport a distressed patient to a hospital. Appropriate crisis intervention procedures help you to achieve that aim safely.

Crisis reactions tend to occur relatively soon after the critical event. Most crisis interventions occur within 3 to 4 weeks of the stimulus that initiated the crisis reaction, although there are many exceptions to this general rule. A good rule of thumb is to apply crisis intervention procedures when patients are in a state of emotional turmoil, even if a long time has passed since the critical incident. This approach means you will be less likely to underestimate the need for crisis intervention strategies.

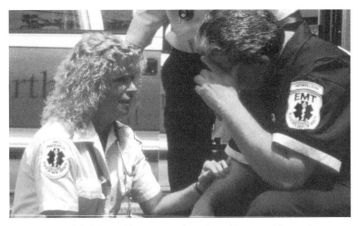

Figure 2-3 Crisis intervention personnel must provide support in a safe zone.

The amount of time required for crisis intervention may vary, and may be longer than you initially think will be necessary. In a field situation, provide crisis support until the person shows signs of recovery, until appropriate resources are obtained, or until any necessary referrals are made.

Crisis intervention often involves multiple contacts. It is typical to have between one and three brief contacts with a person in a crisis before resolution of the crisis is evident. If four to six contacts are necessary, there is a greater chance that a referral for further evaluation and possible professional services will be required. If seven or more contacts are required, then further evaluation and a referral for professional services is strongly indicated.

Primary Principles of Crisis Intervention

Experts have developed seven important principles of crisis intervention. These basic principles are extremely important for prehospital personnel who are working within a chaotic situation that is producing emotional disturbance for those involved. Every crisis-oriented decision and every action should be made in concert with these primary principles. The seven core principles of crisis intervention are:

1. **Simplicity.** Keep it simple. People cannot do complex things in a crisis. Simple procedures have the best chance of producing a positive effect.
2. **Brevity.** Keep it short. No one has the luxury of abundant time in a crisis. Remember you are only providing psychological first aid.
3. **Innovation.** Be willing to use novel ideas to help. Sometimes, you just have to be a little creative because specific instructions do not exist for every single case or circumstance.
4. **Practicality.** Keep it practical. If what you suggest is not practical, the person will not be able to do it and will then feel more frustrated and out of control. The person will also lose confidence in you.
5. **Proximity.** Offer support services close to the person's normal area of function, for instance, at home, in the workplace, or close to where the distressing situation occurred. The most important thing about proximity is that support must be given in a safe zone (**Figure 2-3**).
6. **Immediacy.** Provide services right away. Start crisis support as soon after the beginning of the crisis as possible. Delays in offering crisis intervention make such services less effective.
7. **Expectancy.** The person or group in crisis is encouraged to recognize that help is present and believe that there is hope and that the situation is manageable. If appropriate, it may be helpful to let the person know that, although it is overwhelming right now, most people can and do recover from crisis experiences.

In the Field

There are seven principles of crisis intervention: simplicity, brevity, innovation, practicality, proximity, immediacy, and expectancy.

Important Guidelines for Prehospital Personnel

Always keep the seven basic principles of crisis intervention in mind. These principles will help you streamline and focus your support services for patients in crises. There are also a few important guidelines for you to remember. These can enhance your ability to provide psychological first aid. These guidelines will also help you avoid serious mistakes or possibly dangerous conditions.

Stay within your training levels at all times. Never attempt to do things in crisis intervention work unless you have proper training. Do not hesitate to call for assistance if you lack either appropriate training or the necessary experience for a specific crisis intervention task. For example, it is not advisable to allow a very new EMT to work alone with an extremely distraught patient.

Always take care of the biological, safety, and security needs of a person before doing anything else. Managing the immediate needs of an individual in distress is the primary step in all crisis intervention. In fact, it is the most obvious form of psychological or emotional first aid. Acknowledge and relieve the pressures for a person's physical needs; assure safety, privacy, and security; and provide information and guidance. Do these things as quickly as possible or you run the risk that the overall crisis intervention process may fail.

Provide limited, targeted assistance. Prehospital crisis support personnel should avoid "unboxing" any topic that cannot be "re-boxed" in the time available to work with the patient who is experiencing the crisis. In other words, do not encourage people to discuss deep and complex personal issues, because there is insufficient time to hear everything the person has to say. In addition, discussions of painful personal material may stir powerful emotional reactions that will be difficult to manage in the field.

Always remember that crisis intervention does not constitute psychotherapy, nor is it a substitute for psychotherapy. Do not use crisis intervention to attempt to treat deep-seated psychological problems (**Figure 2-4A,B**). Emergency personnel providers should do what they can to manage a patient in the field who is experiencing mental disturbances, but that patient will need evaluation and treatment in professional mental health settings, that is, treatment that is beyond the scope of crisis intervention personnel or settings.

Do not encourage discussions of excessive details of old psychological material when dealing with a crisis. Like the previous guideline, this guidelines requires that crisis intervention personnel focus predominantly on the "here and now" issues. If you encounter someone who obviously

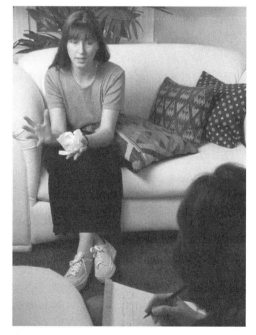
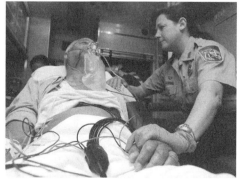

Figure 2-4 Crisis intervention is not the same as psychotherapy. A. Therapeutic counseling. B. Crisis intervention in an emergency setting.

needs more extensive assistance, suggest to the hospital staff that they make a referral for the patient to a mental health professional.

Never be the only one helping in a suicidal crisis. Call for help from the other members of your crew or from other resources. Make sure you inform the hospital staff of the potential threat to life. Remaining the only person active in helping a suicidal patient is extremely dangerous for you and the patient you are trying to help. Keep in mind that a suicidal patient can also become homicidal if the pressures continue to rise and you are viewed as an obstacle to the suicide attempt.

Do not promise anything that you cannot control or deliver. For example, never promise someone that he or she will not be arrested even if the patient broke the law. Just because the patient is emotionally upset does not mean that authorities will not hold the patient responsible for his or her actions. Also, do not promise that you will not tell other helping resources that the patient expressed a desire to either commit suicide or kill someone. There are certain things that must be reported to appropriate authorities (eg, police and hospital emergency room staff) in all cases. That includes threats to self or others.

Expect quick improvement. Once emergency personnel begin to assist a person in crisis, that person's emotional condition usually improves in about 15 to 20 minutes. If at least minimal signs of improvement do not appear in a relatively short time after prehospital personnel begin crisis intervention, the patient most likely needs further evaluation and possibly professional care. Crisis intervention should continue until the situation is resolved or until a referral for additional assistance is made. Attempting to help a person when your help is no longer needed or desired will be interpreted as an unnecessary intrusion into a person's life. Avoid the temptation to stay involved in a crisis if the person indicates that he or she can handle the situation or that he or she has located preferable resources. Bring the patient to a hospital if the distress is extreme, if no calming or recovery is evident, or if serious impairment persists beyond a reasonable time. If the person is emotionally out of control, irrational, or incoherent, or if every effort to help has failed and no improvement is noted within 30 minutes, further evaluation is required by medical personnel and should be provided in a contained environment like a hospital emergency department.

Stages of Crisis Intervention

Several crisis intervention models may be useful for prehospital personnel. This section will provide an overview of one of the most common crisis intervention models. The next chapter of this book provides other crisis models. Dr. Albert Roberts, a well-known crisis intervention specialist, developed the model provided here. Dr. Jeffrey T. Mitchell, the author of this chapter, developed many of the questions included in this chapter.

Crisis Assessment

Crisis assessment covers two important features. A *situational assessment* is essential. What has just happened or is happening now? If you do not know what is going on, it is impossible to develop an adequate crisis intervention plan. The *severity of emotional distress* is the second important feature. Assessment of the level of severity of emotional distress gives us insight into how assertively and how quickly we need to act to assist the person in a state of crisis.

Begin by obtaining basic information. What is the situation? It might be an auto accident, overdose, sexual assault, sudden death of a loved one, suicidal threat, violent act, other criminal acts, severe illness, fire, flood, property loss, terrorist act, loss of job, physical injury, or psychiatric breakdown. Is alcohol or another drug involved? Does the patient have a history of psychiatric disturbance? Can witnesses inform you if the patient is impaired?

Are there any life-threatening conditions present (drug overdose, suicidal threat, or a weapon)? Again, information from witnesses may help answer this question.

Is the impact on those involved mild, moderate, or severe? Examples of mild symptoms would be dry mouth, feeling hyper-alert, anxiety, or difficulties in decision making and problem solving. Moderate signals of distress include mental confusion, disorientation to place and time, fine motor muscle tremors, and fear. Signs of a severe psychological impact include fainting, shock, large muscle tremors or general body shaking, uncontrollable weeping, shouting, rage reactions or violence, unconsciousness, chest pain, and sudden severe headaches.

Are the patient's symptoms expected or very unusual? Expected symptoms are increased heart rate and breathing rate. Unusual symptoms would be hallucinations and chest pain. The more out of the ordinary the symptoms are, the more likely a patient needs immediate professional assistance from medical or psychiatric resources.

Who needs help? Is just one individual involved or are there several? Are children or family members involved? Is a whole group, community, or organization experiencing a crisis reaction? If multiple people are involved, everyone may not display the same symptoms or have similarly severe or mild reactions.

What type of assistance is required? Do you need police support, additional emergency medical assistance, hospitalization, family involvement, or crisis-worker support only? What resources are necessary to provide the right help?

Does the person with whom you are working require immediate or intensive assistance? Are there other patients whose needs are greater? Are there people around who can provide additional assistance to the persons who need it most?

Additional specific information on assessment will be provided in the next chapter. Assessment is mentioned here only because it is part of an overall crisis intervention approach.

Establish Rapport

Establishing <u>rapport</u> is often accomplished simultaneously with assessment. To establish rapport, you can:

- Make contact and introduce yourself (**Figure 2-5**).
- Convey respect for and acceptance of the patient.
- Assure the patient that you are there to help and that other resources are available.
- Listen carefully to the patient.
- Avoid being judgmental.
- Do not rush the patient.
- Be friendly, kind, and concerned, but also professional.
- Use appropriate body posture and try to get on the same eye level.
- Speak calmly, with confidence and in a controlled manner.

Explore the Crisis Problem

Getting a person to talk about the crisis is important for two reasons. First, it lowers tension levels, because the crisis conversation helps the person feel that he or she is being heard. Second, the exploration helps the crisis worker develop some intervention alternatives as the worker acquires more information about the situation.

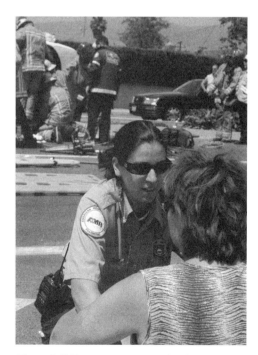

Figure 2-5 The emergency responder should always introduce himself or herself to the patient and establish a rapport as quickly as possible.

- Was there some event that just occurred that started the crisis reaction?
- Ask if this is the first time this happened. Is there some previous experience of such an event? What is the recent and past history for this patient?
- Ask how the patient has coped with stressful experiences in the past.
- Discuss any dangerous or possibly lethal aspects of the current crisis experience.
- A series of open-ended questions is most helpful to gain information from a distressed person; ask the patient to tell his or her own story of the current situation.
- Listen carefully and empathetically; do not rush the patient.
- Reflect emotional content and paraphrase what the patient says to ensure you are hearing accurately and communicating with the patient.

Explore Feelings and Emotions

Once the discussion of the situation begins, typically emotions connected to the situation start to arise. Discussions of emotional content further reduce the patient's tension. The best alternatives can be chosen if all aspects of the situation and the patient's reaction are taken into consideration.

A person may have spontaneously discussed some emotional distress in the previous stage. If the individual did not discuss emotional material then, it is important to bring up the main emotional features of the situation in this stage. Active and intense listening coupled with concern and support for the person is the best technique to generate expressions of emotionally laden content.

Try to imagine yourself in the patient's situation. Ask yourself, "What would help me?" If you cannot relate to a patient's particular situation, you might ask, "If this patient was someone I loved, what would help my loved one through the situation?" In most cases, you will pick something that is supportive and helpful. In addition, the patient's responses will help you determine whether you are going in the right direction.

Generate and Explore Alternatives

When the crisis worker has formed a relatively complete picture of the situation and the reactions of the individual, the crisis worker then can help the distressed person develop a list of potential solutions to the problem. If solutions can be applied, then the crisis is well on the way to resolution.

The patient even may be able to provide guidance about which solutions will be helpful. In order to guide the patient toward potential solutions, you the crisis worker can ask questions about the patient's coping methods during previous crises, ask the patient if he or she knows what would be most helpful right now, or ask the individual if he or she has already tried the suggestions.

The crisis worker can encourage the person to try some helpful things if the patient has not tried them yet. Be prepared to offer some suggestions about managing the crisis, event if the patient is unable to generate any practical options.

Develop and Implement a Crisis Action Plan

When the crisis worker and the patient have explored a set of possible alternatives, then an action plan must be developed and implemented as quickly as possible. The crisis intervention process is moving toward a conclusion.

The crisis worker should formulate a list of options based on his or her assessment of the crisis and the patient's reaction. The list is likely to be a mental one, because there is rarely time to write such lists. The crisis worker should include any possible solutions to the crisis, even options that he or she suspects the patient will reject. This helps to avoid overlooking potential helpful solutions. It also helps to identify any potential failure points before going too far along in developing a crisis action plan.

With the feedback of the patient, pick out the very best options and develop a crisis action plan. Implement the chosen crisis action plan immediately. Delays often allow complications to creep in, which then inhibit a successful resolution of the crisis. Provide whatever assistance appears necessary to ensure that the crisis action plan is implemented as quickly as possible.

Check on the Plan's Success and Follow Up

Getting an action plan implemented immediately is not enough. The crisis worker must monitor the progress of the plan and make sure that it is working. Alter a course of action when necessary. Never be so caught up in a specific plan that you rigidly adhere to it even when it is failing.

> ## In the Field
>
> **Stages of Crisis Intervention**
>
> 1. Assess the crisis.
> 2. Establish rapport.
> 3. Explore the crisis problem.
> 4. Explore the feelings and emotions.
> 5. Generate and explore alternatives.
> 6. Develop and implement a crisis action plan.
> 7. Check on the plan's success and follow up to make sure it is working.

Check to see that the plan is successful, and change or refine the plan if it is necessary; this is another time when the mental list of options can be useful. Maintain a successful plan until resolution of the crisis reaction is achieved. Provide follow-up services with the patient or group members involved in the crisis.

If the crisis is resolved, the plan can be abandoned and crisis intervention is closed out. If significant and continued impairment is evident, the crisis worker should make referrals for further assessment and possible professional care.

A Formula for Strategic Crisis Planning

It is crucial for prehospital personnel to provide crisis intervention or psychological first aid strategically. Strategic crisis planning means that EMS personnel select the right tactics, apply them at the most appropriate time, and utilize the best available resources. A simple model—one that is easy to remember, even in an emergency—can help a crisis worker organize his or her thinking and develop a strategic plan for crisis intervention quickly. All of the components of the strategic planning formula must be bundled together if the crisis intervention plan is to make sense.

One such model offers five Ts: target, type, timing, theme, and team. The *target* is specific individuals or groups who need some assistance. The *type* represents an evaluation of the situation to identify a combination of crisis interventions that are likely to be helpful in a given situation. The interventions are frequently referred to as tactics. It is rare for a single crisis tactic to appear in isolation. Typically, one supportive crisis intervention tactic is attached to other tactics so that a package of supportive interventions is developed. The *timing* of any intervention is very important. If the timing of crisis help is wrong, that is, if the help comes too early or too late, it will be essentially unhelpful. In addition, people have to be psychologically ready to accept help. Sometimes that is the most difficult issue to determine in crisis work. It would certainly be appropriate to ask people if they are willing and ready to accept assistance, although the crisis worker may not receive an adequate or clear answer.

The *theme* refers to anything that influences the patient's reaction or specific needs. Themes are any issues, concerns, considerations, or circumstances that influence the selection of targets or the types and timing of the interventions. Once we have determined the *target, type, timing,* and *theme,* we need to make sure the right *team* or resources are available to intervene. Sometimes a team is made up of several specially trained people on a Critical Incident Stress Management (CISM) team. At other times, a collection of several resources are combined to assist a person in crisis. For example, an EMS unit begins the crisis intervention and then hospital personnel take over the emotional care. Finally, others, such as psychological professionals, may enter the picture to complete the care.

The Effective Crisis Plan

To be effective, strategic crisis intervention plans need to have the following characteristics:

- Simple
- Practical
- Designed for the short term
- Immediately implemented
- Provided close to one's comfort zone or close to the distressing situation
- Action oriented
- Innovative if necessary
- A source of calm, a sense of control and hope
- Well thought out and organized
- Flexible and adaptable to change if required
- Within the capabilities of the person(s) involved in the crisis situation
- Within the capabilities of the crisis worker
- Coordinated with other agencies that have a role in the crisis event
- Developed with referrals in mind, should the crisis intervention not be sufficient to resolve the crisis

Final Thoughts

A century of thought and work in crisis intervention has generated practical and useful crisis management guidelines, stages, and models. If emergency medical personnel understand crisis intervention and appropriately apply its guidelines, prehospital psychological first aid will be successful.

Selected References

American Psychiatric Association: *First Aid for Psychological Reactions in Disasters.* Washington, DC, American Psychiatric Association, 1954.

Antonellis PJ, Mitchell SG: *Posttraumatic Stress Disorder in Firefighters: The Calls That Stick With You.* Ellicott City, MD, Chevron Publishing Corporation, 2005.

Caplan G: *An Approach to Community Mental Health.* New York, NY, Grune & Stratton, 1961.

Caplan G: *Principles of Preventive Psychiatry.* New York, NY, Basic Books, 1964.

Caplan G: Opportunities for school psychologists in the primary prevention of mental health disorders in children, in Bindman A, Spiegel A (eds): *Perspectives in Community Mental Health.* Chicago, IL, Aldine, 1969, pp 420–436.

Everly GS Jr: Emergency mental health: an overview. *Int J Emerg Ment Health,* 1999: 1–37.

Everly GS Jr, Mitchell JT: *Critical Incident Stress Management: A New Era and Standard of Care in Crisis Intervention.* Ellicott City, MD, Chevron Publishing Corporation, 1999.

Kardiner A, Spiegel H: *War, Stress, and Neurotic Illness.* New York, NY, Hoeber, 1947.

Lewin K: *Resolving Social Conflicts: Selected Papers on Group Dynamics.* New York, NY, Harper & Row, 1948.

Lindemann E: Symptomatology and management of acute grief. *Am J Psychiatry,* 1944;101:141–148.

Mitchell JT: Crisis management, in Coombs RH (ed): *Addiction Counseling Review: Preparing for Comprehensive, Certification and Licensing Examinations.* Mahwah, NJ, Lawrence Erlbaum Associates Inc, 2005, pp 401–422.

Mitchell JT: *The Quick Series Guide to Crisis Intervention for Emergency Personnel.* Fort Lauderdale, FL, Luxart Communications, 2005.

Mitchell JT: *Group Crisis Support: Why It Works, When and How to Provide It.* Ellicott City, MD, Chevron Publishing Corporation, 2008.

Mitchell JT, Bray G: *Emergency Services Stress: Guidelines for Preserving the Health and Careers of Emergency Service Personnel.* Englewood Cliffs, NJ, Prentice Hall, 1990.

Mitchell JT, Resnik HLP: *Emergency Response to Crisis.* Ellicott City, MD, Chevron Publishing Corporation, 1986. Reprinted from original.

Neil T, Oney J, DiFonso L, Thacker B, Reichart W: *Emotional First Aid.* Louisville, KY, Kemper-Behavioral Science Associates, 1974.

North CS, Pfefferbaum B: Research on the mental health effects of terrorism, *JAMA,* 2002;288:633–636.

Parad HJ: Crisis intervention, in Morris R (ed): *Encyclopedia of Social Work.* 1971, pp 196–202.

Reese JT: *A History of Police Psychological Services.* Washington, DC, US Department of Justice, Federal Bureau of Investigation, 1987.

Reese JT, Horn JM, Dunning C (eds): *Critical Incidents in Policing.* Revised. Washington, DC, US Government Printing Office, 1991.

Roberts AR: An overview of crisis theory and crisis intervention, in Roberts A (ed): *Crisis Intervention Handbook: Assessment, Treatment, and Research,* ed2. New York, NY, Oxford University Press, 2000, pp 3–30.

Roberts A: Bridging the past and present to the future of crisis intervention and crisis management, in Roberts A (ed): *Crisis Intervention Handbook: Assessment, Treatment, and Research,* ed5. New York, NY, Oxford University Press, 2005, pp 3–34.

Salmon TS: War neuroses and their lesson. *NY Med J,* 1919;108:993–994.

Slaikeu KA: *Crisis Intervention: A Handbook for Practice and Research.* Boston, MA, Allyn & Bacon, 1984.

Stierlin E: *Psycho-neuropathology as a Result of a Mining Disaster March 10, 1906.* Zurich: University of Zurich; 1909.

Solomon Z, Benbenishty R: The role of proximity, immediacy, and expectancy in frontline treatment of combat stress reaction among Israelis in the Lebanon War. *Am J Psychiatry,* 1986;143:613–617.

Stedman's Medical Dictionary for the Health Professions and Nursing, ed5. Baltimore, MD, Lippincott Williams & Wilkens, 2005.

Prep Kit

Ready for Review

The most powerful of crisis states and behavioral emergencies are known as critical incidents. These situations are significant, severe events that can overwhelm one's ability to cope. Critical incidents are always perceived as one or more of the following: overwhelming, threatening, frightening, disgusting, dangerous, or grotesque. These incidents will generally disrupt a person's normal functioning.

Every emotional crisis has three central conditions in that there is a substantial internal or external stimulus that starts the reaction; the patient senses that the disturbing situation can disrupt his or her life; and the patient will be unable to resolve the presenting problem by his or her usual means.

Crisis intervention aims primarily at stabilizing the situation, mitigating the impact of the critical incident, facilitating a normal recovery process, restoring acceptable levels of adaptive function, and identifying those who will need additional support or referral.

Everyone is vulnerable to experiencing a crisis at some point in his or her life. Most crises are sudden and unexpected, so we are not prepared to adequately manage them. Generally speaking, the majority of crises are temporary and reactions tend to subside within 24 to 72 hours.

The goal of the emergency responder during a patient's behavioral emergency is to provide appropriate crisis intervention and safe transport to a hospital for evaluation.

Vital Vocabulary

crisis intervention A temporary, active, and supportive entry into the life situation of a person or a group during a period of acute distress.

critical incident Significant, severe events that can overwhelm a person's or even a group's ability to cope; these events disrupt normal functions.

maturational crises Crises that occur as part of the growth process.

rapport A feeling of relationship, especially when characterized by emotional affinity or bonding.

situational crises Crises that are associated with events or circumstances such as accidents, illness, financial losses, marital problems, and being exposed to a disaster.

Assessment in Action

Answer key is located in the back of the book.

1. From the following list, select the one that is NOT representative of a critical incident.

   A. A train crash with multiple casualties
   B. Accidentally grabbing a snake while rock climbing and then developing hyperventilation syndrome
   C. The sudden, unexpected death of a sibling
   D. Being the victim of a violent attack or sexual assault

2. Crisis intervention is designed as a tool for the responder to immediately mitigate the patient's distress and then start the investigation of the patient's history to determine why the patient reacted in the manner that he or she did at the time.

   A. True
   B. False

3. "Keep it short, simple, and practical" are key tenets of successful crisis intervention.

   A. True
   B. False

4. You are dispatched to a scene of a patient who has attempted suicide by slicing her wrist with a razor blade. Which of the following statements best exemplifies a good rapport-building technique?

A. "Can you tell me why you did this to your-self today?"

B. "Your mother is going to be very upset with you."

C. "Hi there, I'm a paramedic with the city EMS. I'd like to help you today. Would it be ok if I look at your arm?"

D. "After we get you bandaged, we're going to take you to the hospital."

5. When exploring a person's crisis event, which of the following techniques would be most helpful to the responder in gathering infor-mation about the emotional status of the patient?

A. A checklist of questions, symptoms, and history to be completed by the patient

B. Open-ended questions

C. Yes-or-no questions

D. Have the patient write down his or her feelings while en route to the hospital

3

Assessment in the Prehospital Environment

Francis Bacon (1561–1626), the English philosopher, statesman, and essayist said, "Knowledge is power." When you know what something is, you can usually figure out how to deal with it. The opposite is also quite true. What you do not know in a crisis can be very disruptive to your crisis management efforts, and, sometimes, not knowing something actually might hurt the patients you are trying to help. In a worst-case scenario, you could get hurt as well. Therefore, knowledge of appropriate assessment technique is crucial for the survival and performance of emergency personnel.

Simply knowing that assessment is important is not enough. Prehospital personnel need to know what to assess and how to proceed through the assessment. Assessment means that we appraise and evaluate a person's safety and physical and emotional condition, as well as his or her words and behaviors. Emergency personnel review and measure words and behaviors in a crisis and compare and contrast them to certain typical or normal behaviors and common standards.

Assessment procedures typically employ direct observations and questions (**Figure 3-1**). To some degree, an assessment also may utilize information provided by family members, friends, neighbors, and, sometimes, strangers. The most essential task for emergency medical personnel is to collate and organize the information from all of the sources. Emergency service providers then must make patient-care decisions and provide appropriate crisis interventions that match the needs of the patients they are attempting to help.

Several simple field assessment models make the assessment task easier and more efficient. This chapter includes descriptions of some practical field assessment tools along with a brief overview of the more sophisticated assessment procedures that mental health professionals use in hospitals and psychiatric facilities.

The multi-axial assessment and the mental status examination, described below, are both rather complex assessment procedures and they will have little application under field conditions. To be used properly, the multi-axial assessment and the mental status examination require a substantial amount of training, extensive knowledge of mental disorders, and considerable experience with the procedures. These assessment tools are presented in this chapter only to alert prehospital personnel that there are standardized procedures that mental health facilities apply routinely.

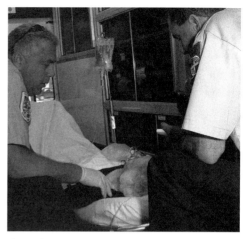

Figure 3-1 Assessment procedures typically employ direct observations and questions.

Key Assessment Concerns

To be effective in the field environment, assessment tools must have three essential conditions.

1. **Safety.** Both the provider and the patient should be safer because of the assessment. An assessment should indicate if there are signs of danger to the patient or to those providing care.

2. **Simplicity.** Assessment tools must be easy to remember and easy to apply. They should not require extensive mental health knowledge on the part of emergency personnel in the midst of an emergency.

3. **Speed.** Emergency personnel must be able to utilize field assessments quickly. In emergencies, speed of application of the assessment tool is crucial. Slow, cumbersome assessment tools may be assessing more than prehospital personnel can actually use during patient care and transportation of the patient to the hospital; more important, slow, cumbersome tools delay emergency care.

Safety First

Responding personnel should be able to assess both medical and psychological crises. There are three reasons for this.

The first task of responders is to ensure the safety of responding personnel and the safety of people involved in the emergency. Assessment of the people involved in the crisis provides critical information and will guide all subsequent action. It is very important to ensure that the patient or patients involved in a distressing event are not in a life-threatening medical crisis and that they do not present a danger to themselves or others.

Second, once medical or psychological personnel are able to confirm a patient's safety and survivability, assessment helps health care personnel select the most appropriate medical and/or psychological interventions or treatments.

Third, the ability to assess both medical and psychological crises will enable responders to determine an appropriate action plan. A good assessment helps everyone decide on an action plan to assist those in the crisis, even if the people experiencing the crisis do not need specific medical or psychological treatment.

Without doubt, safety should always be the most important consideration regardless of the procedures selected to assess both the situation and the patient. Every provider faced with patients in crisis should ask: Is there any danger to myself, my crew, the patient involved in the crisis, or anyone else? Does the situation constitute a significant medical emergency that requires immediate prehospital care and transport to a hospital? Do I have sufficient help on hand to manage the situation?

Responding personnel should also avoid taking unnecessary risks. If the assessment suggests that there is considerable danger to a responder or others, then the choices of action are simple and focused on immediate safety.

- **Withdraw from contact** until the situation calms.
- **Contain the situation** and try not to let it spread to other places or to involve other people.
- **Keep the patient at the scene** if you can do so safely.
- **Call for adequate help** to be available at the scene.
- **Call for law enforcement if the danger is serious or persistent,** especially if the patient makes threats or if a weapon is present.

Most emotional crises present little or no danger to responding personnel, but a degree of caution is essential to reduce the chance that anyone could get hurt. A proper assessment is the very first step when dealing with a distressed patient. The assessment of a patient in a crisis should vary only a little from the assessment conducted by prehospital providers for practically any medical call. Start by sizing up the situation. Listen carefully to the dispatch and obtain as much information about the situation and the patient or patients involved. Think safety, safety, and more safety. If things sound or appear very strange or out of the ordinary, call for police support (**Figure 3-2**).

Keep It Simple

Safety is the first consideration, and simplicity is the second major concern. Field situations are often chaotic, confusing, and noisy. There are competing issues, all of which demand attention. Emergency service personnel do not have the luxury of time. Assessments must be easy to perform, quick, accurate at identifying risks, and efficient.

In the emergency services, we learn many mnemonics to help us remember a wide range of tasks to assist people with a medical crisis. Some of them still apply in crisis intervention and the management of behavioral emergencies. Do not be afraid to use familiar devices to help you do your job. For instance, most of you are familiar with the SAMPLE assessment tool, in which each letter has a specific meaning:

- **S**igns/symptoms
- **A**llergies
- **M**edications
- **P**ast medical history
- **L**ast oral intake
- **E**vent that led to the current situation

Use the SEA-3 assessment tool described later in this chapter to help you determine the signs and symptoms. Listen to what the patient tells you and observe his or her behaviors. Ask about allergies and medications, because toxicity and other changes in blood chemistry may produce some behavioral emergencies. The past medical and psychological

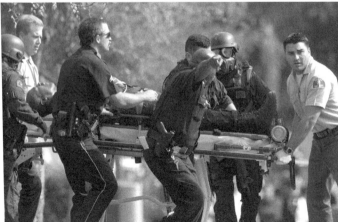

Figure 3-2 Make sure you have sufficient help on hand to manage a crisis situation safely.

history can provide insights into the current and future psychological reactions. The old adage that history—what someone has done or experienced—is the best predictor of future behavior is true for behavioral emergencies as well. The last oral intake is important in crisis intervention, especially if that oral intake was alcohol or other substances of abuse. We also know that if patients have not eaten recently, their blood sugar and hydration levels may be low. That, in itself, may reduce thinking capacity and alter human behavior, especially if the patient is diabetic. Finally, the events that preceded the arrival of the emergency responder may exert a huge influence on current behaviors.

As you gather information about a patient in crisis, keep in mind the conditions in the patient's environment. Human behavior can change dramatically if the circumstances surrounding that patient change or if conditions become severe. Human behavior can change if the brain is:

- Chilled
- Overheated
- Dehydrated
- Starved of nutrients
- Toxified
- Traumatized
- Starved of oxygen
- Exposed to an altitude in excess of 10,000 feet
- Exposed to sudden and excessive alterations in atmospheric pressure
- Severely stressed

Consideration of this list is typically more useful than complicated assessments. A simple, commonsense approach generally works best. The OPQRST mnemonic serves as an additional reminder of simple questions the provider can ask the patient. It is presented here with some slight modifications to make it more applicable to crisis situations.

- **Onset.** When did this feeling or situation first begin?
- **Provocation.** What happened to trigger your reaction?
- **Quality.** How pervasive, repetitive, or persistent are your feelings?
- **Radiation.** Is this distress radiating out to other areas of your life?
- **Severity.** On an ascending 0–10 scale, how intense is your distress?
- **Time.** How long do you think this distress will continue? Do you have any sense of what has to happen to alleviate your pain?

Your main objective in assessment is to learn enough about the patient and the patient's condition to be able to treat and transport the patient safely while reducing risks to yourself and others nearby.

Get the Assessment Done

Time is one of your biggest enemies in a crisis. Complete assessments early and quickly. Once you have completed the critical assessment, you have completed much of the path. The knowledge you gain about the patient gives you power to make decisions and manage the patient appropriately.

Keep in mind that, even though you are able to proceed to the next stage, assessments are never comprehensive or complete, in part because situations, moods, and behaviors are constantly changing. New information may arise, and that should trigger further assessment efforts on our part. Assessment should be an ongoing process as long as you are working with a patient in crisis. In other words, do not

In the Field

The SAMPLE assessment tool provides a standardized method of gathering information about the patient.

In the Field

The OPQRST assessment tool can be modified to provide valuable information about the current status of the patient.

become complacent and remember that you must continue to assess the situation. Be prepared for almost anything. Do not let your guard down: Doing so can make you vulnerable to uncomfortable surprises and a potential failure in patient care management.

The Multi-Axial Approach to Crisis Assessment

If you had a clinical assignment in a psychiatric center during your training, you might remember observing a skilled mental health professional use a multi-axial assessment tool to perform a thorough assessment. The multi-axial assessment evaluates information on several different behavioral axes. In essence, it is a way of breaking complex human behaviors down into more manageable categories that provide a relatively clear picture of a specific human being at a particular point in time. An axis is a domain of behaviors or a set of signs and symptoms aligned in such a manner that they lead to certain conclusions about the person. The signs and symptoms usually form a single category. That is, each axis assesses a distinct area or realm of information about a person. Together, several axes help mental health professionals decide upon the seriousness of a person's condition and the treatments that might be necessary.

The *Diagnostic and Statistical Manual of Mental Disorders, Fourth Edition, Text Revision (DSM-IV-TR)* of the American Psychiatric Association, the guidebook that mental health professionals use to determine a specific diagnosis, presents five separate axes for assessment. The five axes allow the professional to determine a patient's psychological profile. The following are the components of the multi-axial assessment:

- **Axis I** identifies *clinical disorders* that need psychiatric attention (eg, mood disorders, anxiety disorders, and disorders usually identified in childhood or adolescence).
- **Axis II** identifies *personality disorders* (eg, antisocial disorder, obsessive-compulsive disorder, and paranoid personality disorder) and *mental retardation*.
- **Axis III** identifies *general medical conditions,* in particular, medical conditions made worse by the psychological conditions or vice versa.
- **Axis IV** assesses *psychosocial and environmental problems* (eg, relationships, social environment, education, legal issues, housing situation, occupation, and economic conditions).
- **Axis V** provides a *global assessment of functioning* in the form of a scale of human behavior that ranges from superior performance down to persistent danger of harming oneself.

Comprehensive evaluations like the multi-axial assessment help mental heath professionals select appropriate and effective treatments for their patients. However, as this brief overview suggests, the multi-axial approach to assessment is complex, and it is challenging to learn and apply. The multi-axial assessment plan is impractical and beyond the level of training of most emergency personnel working under field conditions.

Mental Status Examination

The mental status examination (MSE) is a relatively standard and systematic examination of a person's state of mind. It is similar to the history and physical examination physicians routinely perform when examining a patient. The mental status examination is somewhat less complex than the multi-axial assessment procedure described above, but it still requires a fair amount of knowledge and expertise in the area of mental disorders. Despite its relative simplicity, the MSE can contribute useful information to the multi-axial assessment that a mental health professional performs.

The main categories of a mental status examination are:

1. **Appearance:** physical characteristics, weight, physical appearance, wounds, scars, grooming, cleanliness, odors, dress, jewelry, glasses
2. **Behavior:** gait, combativeness, gestures, twitches, excessive activity, excitability, reduced activity, hostility, playfulness, cooperation, friendliness, interestedness, attentiveness, defensiveness
3. **Speech:** speed, slurred, mumbled, stuttering, volume, quality, quantity
4. <u>Mood</u> and <u>affect</u>: <u>euphoria</u>, sad, grieving, depressed, panicked, fearful, anxious, tense, agitated, <u>apathetic</u>, irritable, angry, mood swings, ambivalent feelings, appropriateness of mood, flat emotions, labile
5. **Thought process:** the way a person thinks; mental disorder, psychosis, illogical, magical thinking, concrete thinking, abstract thinking, flight of ideas, incoherent, repetitious
6. **Thought content:** what the person thinks; poverty of thought, <u>egomania</u>, <u>hypochondria</u>, obsessive, compulsive, bizarre content, delusional, paranoia, grandiosity
7. **Perceptions:** hallucinations (auditory, visual, olfactory, tactile), <u>disassociation</u>, <u>depersonalization</u>, <u>derealization</u>, multiple personality, <u>agnosia</u>
8. **Cognition:** general level of intelligence, education, degree of concentration, attention
9. **Consciousness:** disoriented, clouded, stupor, delirium, coma, dreamlike state
10. **Orientation:** to person, place, and time
11. **Memory:** remote memory deficit, recent past deficit, immediate recall deficit
12. **Judgment:** critical judgment, automatic, impaired
13. **Insight:** understanding of one's own psychological functioning, impaired insight, denial, externally focused, true insight

The MSE focuses on an assessment of noticeable signs and symptoms. Its main drawbacks are its length and complexity, because it takes more time to complete than most prehospital personnel have available for assessment purposes. Training and skill development are important for the proper use of the MSE, and most emergency personnel lack such training. Nevertheless, awareness of the key components of the mental status examination may offer some insight into assessing people in a crisis. It is presented here with that thought in mind.

Field Assessment of Crises and Behavioral Emergencies

Emergency service personnel must keep the big picture in mind. Look for broad or obvious indicators of problems. The more symptoms and the more obviously disturbed the behaviors, the greater the level of impairment. The danger to a person increases as the level of impairment or dysfunction becomes more severe. Every multi-axial assessment and each mental status examination should include a <u>global assessment of functioning (GAF)</u>. The GAF can be a useful tool for field personnel because it is an outline of broad, general impressions.

The GAF is a 100-point scale that represents the overview or big picture of a person's behavior. It functions as a broad summary or clinical impression of the person's current condition. In one sense, the GAF is an emergency person's best guess about the level of function or lack of function observed in a patient. The lowest score on a global assessment of functioning is 10, indicating imminent harm. People scoring a 10 are a danger to themselves (possibly suicidal) and could be a threat to others (possibly violent or homicidal). A score of 100 indicates superior functioning. The GAF may have some application in prehospital settings. **Table 3-1** outlines key features of the GAF scale.

Sometimes behavior is so obvious that it is easy for personnel to develop a global impression. When emergency personnel have established a GAF for the person in a behavioral emergency or a crisis state, the SEA-3 assessment tool will be useful for responders to develop additional details about the person.

Table 3-1	Global Assessment of Functioning Scale
Score	**Assessment**
10	Imminent harm
20	Possible harm
30	Serious impairment
40	Major impairment
50	Serious symptoms
60	Moderate symptoms
70	Mild symptoms
80	Slight impairment
90	No symptoms
100	Superior function

SEA-3 Assessment Tool

As previously noted, both the multi-axial and mental status examination assessment tools are primarily for use by mental health professionals. At the same time, prehospital providers need simple, practical assessment tools that are applicable under emergency field conditions, and proper field assessment of the patients that they are attempting to assist is urgent. The emergency responder can utilize the SEA-3 assessment tool to perform a brief, five-component evaluation of the person in crisis; the five components are the patient's speech, emotion, appearance, alertness, and activity. It is important to remember that the SEA-3 is based on the mental status examination, but it is a shortened and simplified version of it. This version of the mental status examination was specifically developed for use by prehospital personnel during behavioral emergencies and other crises. The SEA-3 is simple and fast and employs an easily remembered outline. It is a useful guide for rapid evaluation of a person in a crisis state. **Table 3-2** shows the main factors and the primary observations.

The SEA-3 is only a brief screening device that helps the provider determine the stability and general mental functioning of a person in crisis. The SEA-3 is not a full evaluation. Common sense, good judgment, knowledge of behavioral emergencies, and experience will compensate for the shortcomings of the SEA-3. **Table 3-3** summarizes various assessment tools according to the criteria of safety, simplicity, speediness, and appropriateness for use in the field.

Table 3-2	The SEA-3 Assessment Tool
SEA-3 Factor	**Questions to Ask or Observations to Make**
Speech	Quantity and quality of speech, as well as the flow and the organization of the content of the speech
Emotion	Dominant mood, appropriateness of mood, absence of emotion, euphoria, depression, anger, hostility, fear, anxiety, apprehension
Appearance	Unkempt, unclean, clothing disheveled, dirty, atypical, unusual or bizarre, unusual physical characteristics
Alertness	Oriented to person, place, and time, has insight into internal psychological reactions, can judge personal behavior as appropriate or not, memory and intellectual functions appear intact, stream and content of thought appears appropriate, hallucinations, delusions, thought disorders
Activity	Appropriateness of facial expressions, posture, movement, and interactions with helper

The Assessment Process

The assessment tools described are useful, but we have to use them with specific goals in mind. Ultimately, we are trying to develop an action plan to resolve the crisis or move the person to the right resources to help that person manage the problem. There are several important steps in the development of a specific action plan for a person in a state of crisis.

First, establish a positive contact with the person in crisis. Begin by approaching the individual in distress. Introduce yourself and ask the person how you might be of assistance. Ask yourself whether what you observe of the person's behavior matches what you have been told by the dispatcher. Introduce your partner and any others on your crew. Treat people with kindness and respect, and establish rapport with the person.

Second, interview the person involved in the situation and gather information from

Table 3-3 Assessment Tool Summary

Assessment Tool	Focus on Safety	Simple	Speedy	For Field Use
Multi-Axial	Yes	No	No	No
MSE	Yes	No	No	Partially
GAF	Yes	Yes	Yes	Yes
SAMPLE	Yes	Yes	Yes	Yes
OPQRST	Yes	Yes	Yes	Yes
SEA-3	Yes	Yes	Yes	Yes

that person first. Going to others first can be interpreted negatively by a distressed person. Gather personal identification information such as the person's name, age, occupation, marital status, and address. Question others present about their relationship to the primary person. Find out who is involved in the current situation. Ask if those involved are related to each other. Find out if there are any children involved. Ask those involved who they view as a possible help or as someone who may be harmful in the situation.

Third, determine the nature of the current problem. Ask about what is occurring now. Find out what has happened just prior to the arrival of help. Determine if there is any recent history of the situation, then ask if there is a past history of the situation. It is important that all possible sources of information be considered. The sources of information include, but are not limited to, family members, friends, and witnesses.

Fourth, use assessment tools to gain additional insight into the situation and the reactions of those involved; the results of such assessments will also guide the subsequent steps. Utilize the components of SAMPLE and OPQRST, as well as the SEA-3 evaluation tool, to gather information about the person. Ask yourself what your instinct tells you about the situation. Attempt to rule out medical conditions (as opposed to those of psychiatric nature). Consider these decision points: Is the situation new or chronic? Does the situation appear to be stable, escalating, or receding in intensity? Is the current level of intensity mild, moderate, or severe? Is there a life threat (suicide or violence)? Is the person in or out of control of himself or herself? Is the situation strictly within the person (depression or psychosis) or between the person and others (family conflict)? Is the person distressed predominantly because of a situation (fire, flood, disaster, or terrorist event)? Is the person adequately coping with the problem? Does the person need additional support or resources? What would help most right now? Who can help now? Are resources available, willing, and capable of helping?

Fifth, use the information from the assessments to make an action plan. Aim at simple, brief, and practical action plans that can be put into effect immediately. Crisis action plans may need to be innovative and organized for application in close proximity of the person's usual activity area or comfort zone. Crisis action plans should help to establish expectations of positive outcomes or resolution. Emergency personnel should encourage the person to maintain hope that the situation is manageable and emphasize that they are making their best efforts to bring about a positive outcome. A crisis action plan should be thoughtful, organized, and focused on getting something done to resolve the crisis. All crisis action plans should be developed in cooperation with the person or people involved in the situation. Crisis action plans must include provisions for referral to hospitals, social service agencies, law enforcement, or other resources if those services are necessary

> ### In the Field
>
> The assessment process consists of six components:
>
> 1. Establish a positive contact and gather information.
> 2. Interview those involved.
> 3. Determine the nature of the problem.
> 4. Use assessment tools.
> 5. Make a crisis action plan.
> 6. Implement the crisis action plan immediately.

Finally, implement the crisis action plan immediately. Check on the success of the plan. Alter the plan if necessary. Maintain the plan if it is working. Dispense with the plan if it achieves its goals and it is no longer necessary.

Final Thoughts

Assessment is a vital aspect of every patient contact for prehospital personnel. Logical and systematic assessments help responders manage their patients efficiently and effectively. Assessment consistency helps avoid mistakes. A good assessment is a starting point for outstanding patient care. The assessment tools discussed in this chapter will have importance for all of the chapters that follow.

Selected References

American Psychiatric Association: *Diagnostic and Statistical Manual of Mental Disorders, Fourth Edition, Text Revision (DSM-IV-TR)*. Washington, DC, American Psychiatric Association, 2000.

Caroline NL: *Nancy Caroline's Emergency Care in the Streets*, ed 6. Boston, MA, Jones & Bartlett Publishers, 2008.

Everly GS Jr: *Assisting Individuals in Crisis*, ed 4. Ellicott City, MD, International Critical Incident Stress Foundation, 2006.

Mitchell JT, Resnik HLP: *Emergency Response to Crisis*, Ellicott City, MD, Chevron Publishing Corporation, 1986. Reprinted from original.

Scheiber SS: The psychiatric interview, psychiatric history, and mental status examination, in Hales RE, Yudofsky SC (eds): *Essentials of Clinical Psychiatry*, ed 3. Washington, DC, American Psychiatric Press, 1999.

Stedman's Medical Dictionary for the Health Professions and Nursing, ed 5. Baltimore, MD, Lippincott, Williams, & Wilkins, 2005.

Wise MG, Strub RL: Mental status examination and diagnosis, in Rundelland J, Wise MG (eds): *Textbook of Consultation Liaison Psychiatry*. Washington, DC, American Psychiatric Press, 1996, pp 66–87.

Zimmerman M: *Interview Guide for Evaluating DSM-IV Psychiatric Disorders and the Mental Status Examination*. Washington, DC, American Psychiatric Press, 1994, pp 3–6.

Prep Kit

Ready for Review

There are many assessment tools that can be used for evaluating patients with behavioral emergencies. When choosing one for the prehospital environment, make sure that it is safe, simple, and speedy.

Assessment tools such as SAMPLE, OPQRST, and SEA-3 provide the evaluator with a consistent format that, when used properly, ensures that all necessary information is gathered.

Mental health professionals use the *DSM-IV-TR* of the American Psychiatric Association to diagnose mental disorders. A complete psychological evaluation is called a multi-axial assessment.

Complex and lengthy mental status examinations exist for use by mental health professionals. However, in the prehospital environment, the SEA-3 assessment tool is a simple and helpful tool. It allows the emergency responder to evaluate a patient's speech, emotion, appearance, alertness, and activity.

A thorough prehospital assessment consists of six components: (1) establishing a positive contact and gathering information, (2) interviewing those involved, (3) determining the nature of the problem, (4) using the proper assessment tools, (5) making a crisis action plan, and (6) implementing the crisis action plan immediately.

Vital Vocabulary

affect The observable emotion or feeling, tone, and mood attached to a thought; one's emotional presentation to the evaluator.

agnosia The inability to identify or recognize common people or objects that would normally be familiar.

apathetic Condition in which a patient exhibits a lack of emotion; indifferent.

axis A domain of behaviors or a set of signs and symptoms aligned in such a manner that they lead to certain conclusions about the person. Axes include: clinical disorders, personality disorders, mental retardation, general medical conditions, psychosocial and environmental problems, and the GAF.

depersonalization A state in which someone loses the feeling of his or her own identity in relation to others in the family or peer group or loses the feeling of his or her own reality.

derealization An internal perception that an individual is living through a dream or in a movie, or that one is outside of oneself and looking on as a spectator to their own experience.

Diagnostic and Statistical Manual of Mental Disorders, Fourth Edition, *Text Revision* (DSM-IV-TR) A guidebook published by the American Psychiatric Association that sets forth diagnostic criteria, descriptions, and other information regarding the classification and diagnosis of mental disorders.

disassociation An unconscious separation of a group of mental processes from the rest, resulting in an independent functioning of these processes and a loss of the usual associations.

egomania Extreme self-centeredness, self-appreciation, or self-content.

euphoria An exaggerated or abnormal sense of physical and emotional well-being that is usually not based on reality or truth and is inappropriate for the situation and disproportionate to its cause.

global assessment of functioning (GAF) scale A tool outlined in the *DSM-IV-TR* that is used to give a numeric value to a person's overall daily function.

hypochondria A morbid concern about one's own health and exaggerated attention to any unusual bodily or mental sensation.

mental status examination (MSE) A tool used by mental health professionals to evaluate the state of a person's mind. MSEs vary in length and look at various characteristics of one's behavior, mood, affect, thought process, judgment, and memory.

Prep Kit | continued

mood The pervasive feeling, tone, and internal emotional state of a person; how one feels.

multi-axial assessment An approach used in assessing the overall status of a patient.

SEA-3 assessment tool A brief, five-component tool used for a quick evaluation of the person in crisis. It is used to evaluate a patient's speech, emotion, appearance, alertness, and activity.

Assessment in Action

Answer key is located in the back of the book.

1. When assessing the patient, it is important to recognize that many medical situations can mimic psychological conditions.

   A. True
   B. False

2. One of the best predictors of a patient's current psychological condition is his or her history.

   A. True
   B. False

3. From the following list, select the one that is NOT a component of the multi-axial assessment tool.

   A. Psychosocial and environmental problems
   B. Global assessment of functioning
   C. SAMPLE history
   D. Clinical psychological disorders

4. A patient's mood is best evaluated by:

   A. looking at how the person is sitting during the interview.
   B. asking the person how he or she is feeling.
   C. evaluating the person's motor responses by having the person close his or her eyes and touch the nose with the index finger.
   D. noting the person's inability to focus on your questions during the interview.

5. From the following list, select the one that is NOT a component of the SEA-3 assessment tool.

   A. Activity
   B. Alertness
   C. Affect
   D. Appearance

Responding to the Emotional Crisis

EMS personnel need common sense, compassion, confidence, and courage as they respond to a crisis, but arrogance will not serve anyone's best interests. P. J. Plauger, a technical writer, observed, "My definition of an expert in any field is a person who knows enough about what's really going on to be scared." As EMS personnel, you frequently serve as the most readily available medical "experts" during an emergency. You are in an enormously responsible position and you should be a little scared. Decisions you make may seriously affect, positively or negatively, both the people you are trying to help and you.

You would be wise to keep a little wariness in mind as you respond to any emotional crisis. Being a little scared on a call helps you to stay alert and nimble enough to respond to subtle and significant changes, both in the situation and in the person's reactions. Some appropriate anxiety during a call can help a responder make the best decisions for patient care. Circumstances can change rapidly, and what is safe at one moment may not be safe the next.

From the very moment an ambulance response begins, the crew must use its assessment skills as well as its people skills to gather information, make plans, and initiate the right care, at the right time and under the best circumstances that can be arranged. A combination of the seven primary principles of crisis intervention with good prehospital medical skills and the assessment tools discussed in Chapter 3 helps EMS providers maximize the chances of achieving a successful outcome.

Expertise is not something that is issued automatically with graduation from an EMS program, the police academy, or a mental health educational program. Presuming that one is an expert in a behavioral emergency can be dangerous for everyone involved. The key to success in managing emotional crises is incorporating the specialized skills such crises require into the established routines for excellent everyday prehospital care. True expertise will follow with hard work and a considerable amount of field experience over the course of one's career.

Clarify Big Issues First

While you are on the way to a call, ask yourself if you and your partner have sufficient information to manage the call. Typically, there is insufficient information, and most EMS crews begin the call somewhat blinded. Rarely can dispatch personnel provide all of the information that the EMS crew needs. Therefore, as Chapter 3 outlines, the crew must adopt a flexible strategy to gather the facts as quickly as possible once on the scene and complete an assessment that is thorough enough to make a plan of action.

Once you are on the scene, it is vital that you determine whether you or any of the first responders are in immediate danger. If you are in danger, call for backup support and for law enforcement authorities. Do not proceed until reasonable resources are present to maintain control over the situation.

Next, determine whether the victims are in danger. If they are, get help and get it fast. If the victims need protection, call law enforcement (**Figure 4-1**). Add whatever other resources might be necessary under the circumstances. Proceed only when safety and security issues have been addressed.

Behavioral Emergencies

There are innumerable crises that can befall people, but only about a dozen types turn into life-threatening emergencies (**Table 4-1**). The twelve most common and potentially life-threatening behavioral emergencies that require immediate assessment and intervention are:

- Suicidal thinking and actions
- Irrational rage reactions (caused by both personality disorders and psychosis)
- Uncontrollable panic attacks
- Adverse reactions to alcohol and other dangerous substances
- Adverse reactions to medication causing behavioral changes
- Severe withdrawal symptoms
- Delirium or confused states and excited delirium
- Eating disorders
- Severe mental illness causing disturbance in mood, thought, and behavior

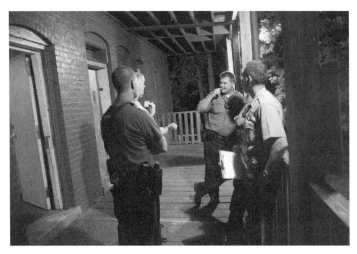

Figure 4-1 If you are in danger, call for backup support and for law enforcement authorities.

Table 4-1 Common Life-Threatening Behavioral Emergencies

Behavioral Emergency	Signs and Symptoms	Response
Suicidal thinking and actions	Depression, hopelessness, helplessness, worthless feelings	Assess, contain, disarm, transport to hospital
Irrational rage	Clenched fists, reddened face, threats, forced speech, spitting, violent actions	Keep your distance, call for police, attempt verbal calming, restraint, transport to hospital
Uncontrolled panic attack	Feeling one cannot breathe, erratic quick movements, feeling overwhelmed, fearful, terrified, shaking, wide-eyed	Calm; reassure; assess medically; administer oxygen; quiet the frantic environment; reassure with a calm, quiet voice; transport to hospital for further evaluation and possibly treatment
Alcohol and drug reactions	Drunkenness; incoherent, slurred speech; uncontrolled actions; unconsciousness	Complete assessment, treat according to priority of symptoms, follow protocols for intoxicated or overdosed person
Adverse medication reactions	Strange, unusual behaviors; shock; rash; mental confusion or disorientation, including hallucinations, delusions, illusions; thought disorder; anaphylactic reactions	Assess for medical complications; treat symptomatically by protocols; contain, protect the person; transport to hospital for further evaluation and treatment
Severe withdrawal symptoms	Always a potential with drugs and medications; wide range of physical and mental symptoms possible; may be life threatening, especially if respiratory or cardiac symptoms are present	Assess, stabilize, treat symptoms; try "talk down" procedures; call police if violence erupts; transport to hospital for further evaluation and treatment
Delirium, confusion; excited delirium	Mentally confused, disoriented, agitated, may appear angry, frustrated, excited, pacing, paranoia, panic feelings, inattentive	Assess, calm, reassure; assess for drug use; contain, do not antagonize or joke; gently encourage cooperation; quiet the environment; transport to hospital for further evaluation and treatment
Eating disorders	Significant threat to health, especially if prolonged; signs of starvation; obsessive behaviors	Assess, discuss eating behaviors; encourage person to go to the hospital immediately; most cases require medical treatment and psychological care
Severe mental illness	May become dangerous; self-destructive behaviors or threats of violence toward others; hallucinations, delusion, illusions, serious thought disorder, and significant behavioral change	Rule out conditions;, do not joke, tease, ridicule; encourage cooperation, be respectful; obtain history, treat symptomatically, call police if danger to self or others is present; most patients need further evaluation and treatment; sometimes medication must be administered by a physician

(Continued)

Table 4-1 (Continued)

Behavioral Emergency	Signs and Symptoms	Response
Threats or acts of aggression	Look for overt signs such as puffing of cheeks, pounding fists, spitting, verbal assaults, cursing, clenched fists, direct threats	Assess fully and cautiously; calm and quiet the environment; contain the person; call the police and do not endanger yourself, have police restrain if necessary; transport to a hospital for further evaluation and treatment
Abuse of children, elders, or handicapped persons	Look for evidence of abuse, perpetrator behaviors, physical injuries, burns, bite marks, tie marks, missing teeth, hair pulled out, broken long bones, stories that make little sense, threats to the victim, signs of neglect in the environment	First, protect and care for the victim, call the police, try to encourage those present to allow you to transport the person to a hospital so that treatment can begin; do not leave the victim until the police arrive; police may be necessary to protect rescuers or to arrest the perpetrator
Severe emotional shock	Classic signs and symptoms of shock, including weak pulse, labored breathing, dry mouth, mental confusion, fainting, sudden, prolonged, intense headaches, cascading into catastrophic physical collapse	Assess medically; treat symptoms, especially unconsciousness, inattentiveness, respiratory distress or poor decision making, unresponsive cardiac; quiet environment, reassure, provide guidance to family and friends, transport to hospital for further evaluation and treatment

- Acts of aggression, acts of violence, and homicidal aggression
- Abuse of children, elders, and handicapped persons
- Severe emotional shock cascading into catastrophic physical collapse

Any one of the dozen conditions on the list can pose a significant threat to life and safety. The individual, or the people around the individual, including rescuers, may be in danger. Sometimes a person in one of these behavioral emergencies is an imminent threat to himself or herself and to others simultaneously.

Most behavioral emergencies with a significant life threat are covered thoroughly in other chapters in this book. There are a few, however, that may demand rapid evaluation and intervention to keep them from escalating into even more serious conditions. EMS personnel may have a significant influence in bringing these conditions under control while the patient is still in the field.

Panic Attacks

Panic attacks are bursts of intense fear that produce powerful physical reactions such as difficulty breathing, racing heart, nausea, dizziness, profuse sweating, and muscle tenseness. In essence, a panic attack is a powerful physical and emotional flight-or-fight stress response when such a high-intensity response is clearly unnecessary. Panic attacks may have a specific trigger based in an exposure to some stressful circumstance or a reminder of a stressful circumstance, or they may be spontaneous and unexpected with no specific cause. Some panic attacks are triggered by excessive nicotine, caffeine, alcohol abuse, thyroid problems, and certain medications. Sometimes they can occur while a person is asleep.

About a third of the general population experiences a panic attack in the course of their lives. However, only about 2% of people who experience panic attacks develop a more serious problem, panic disorder, which is a persistent and repetitive condition with frequent panic attacks over time. More women than men suffer from panic attacks and panic disorder, but men are not free of the problem. Additional research on the causes of panic attacks is currently under way.

Sometimes a person may have only one or two panic attacks and then the condition disappears. Some people have panic attacks periodically throughout their lives. If panic attacks occur frequently, or if a person's behavior changes substantially after the panic attacks, the person may have a panic disorder and should be evaluated for psychological treatment. Treatments for panic attacks and panic disorder are very successful and most people usually reduce the number and intensity of their panic attacks and resume normal life functions.

Panic attacks alone have little power to cause someone bodily harm or death. From a physiological point of view, they are fairly harmless. The behaviors that accompany or result from panic attacks, rather than the attacks themselves, are more likely to be the threats that could endanger people. As panicky feelings increase, clear thinking and controlled behaviors decrease. A person experiencing a panic attack may run into traffic or be frightened into behaving in a dangerous manner, such as unnecessarily jumping from a ship into the ocean when rescue is on the scene but not yet ready to rescue the passengers.

The symptoms of a panic attack can be quite alarming. Often a person feels overwhelming fear or terror. Most people feel like running away or hiding. Many people have difficulty breathing or find themselves breathing rapidly. Some feel as though they are choking and may experience nausea and gastrointestinal distress. Some even experience chest pain, dizziness, profuse sweating, chills, and body and extremity shakes. People who have experienced a panic attack often describe a racing heart and fear that they will die from a "runaway" heart. Some others say they can hear their heart beating loudly in their ears.

If it is the person's first panic attack, he or she should be seen by a physician to rule out heart attack, asthma, metabolic problems, or other serious medical conditions. If you reassure the person, provide oxygen or breathing space, and quiet the environment; the person typically begins to recover within about 15 minutes. Such recovery is a good sign that you are dealing with a panic attack. Nevertheless, make sure to ask the person if this is the first time he or she has ever experienced anything like this. If it is the first time for such an experience, then you need to encourage the person or a family member to let you take the person to the hospital. At the very least the person and the family should be advised that the individual should be evaluated by a physician.

Because they tend to have less impulse control, adolescents with panic attacks are more at risk for suicide attempts or completions. Therefore, it is extremely important that they be seen by medical personnel in a hospital or in a physician's office. It is not uncommon for panic attacks to result from some traumatic event in the young person's life. Examples would include sexual assault, child abuse, molestation, or witnessing some highly traumatizing event such as the death or maiming of a loved one. A friend's suicide may also contribute to self-destructive thoughts. Panic attacks in teenagers should be taken quite seriously and almost always require further evaluation and possibly medical or psychological treatment.

Although prehospital medical personnel and other emergency workers might recognize key signals that a person is having a panic attack, a medical professional should be the person who ultimately makes that diagnosis. In most cases the condition can be relieved by a short course of counseling, but sometimes medical treatment may be required. This is especially true if the panic attacks occur repeatedly. It is better to be conservative and bring the person to a physician or emergency department than to ignore a panic attack.

In the Field

Even if you do not see any reason why the person is experiencing a panic attack, the condition is very real to the person and it should be treated as a medical condition until a physician determines otherwise.

It is important to inquire about medication use or other substances that might have contributed to the onset of the attack. Inquire about nicotine, caffeine, and alcohol use, as high doses of any of those substances can trigger or intensify a panic attack. Finally, inquire about recent illnesses and psychological traumas or shocks; the most frequent cause of a panic attack is a history of exposure to some significant traumatic experience. Information about whether the patient has a history of panic attacks and the current physical condition of the victim will be crucial for hospital personnel.

To help a person having a panic attack regain a sense of control, pay close attention to what the person tells you; although it will not resolve the problem completely, just being listened to can help reduce the tension and distress behind a panic attack. Encourage the person to relax and breathe slowly. Decrease stimuli in the environment. Speak slowly, calmly, and softly, but make sure you are loud enough to be heard. Reassure the person that you are there to assist. Let the person know that he or she is safe and that the sensations of panic will subside soon. Reassure the person that he or she is not going crazy and is not in immediate danger of dying, and remind the patient that if he or she can talk, then he or she can breathe.

Be gentle, patient, and confident, and be ready to repeat yourself. Take your time and do not rush the person. Encourage the person to take in a few deep breaths and let them out slowly and evenly; you can try counting slowly as the person breathes or encourage the patient to do so. Have the person progressively tense and relax muscle groups from the feet and then up the legs and body, ending with the arms, neck, and face. Keep instructions brief, clear, and to the point.

When assisting a person who is experiencing a panic attack, it is important to calm the environment, calm the person, and help the victim regain self-control. Because most panic attacks last between 5 and 20 minutes, time is on your side and a little supportive intervention can go a long way. When you complete your intervention with a panicked person, encourage the person to undergo a thorough medical evaluation.

Severe Emotional Shock

Severe **emotional shocks** can produce immediate physiological reactions such as a dangerous drop in blood pressure, a weak, racing pulse, and profuse sweating that can jeopardize a person's physical well-being (**Figure 4-2**). It is common for people to go into psychogenic shock and faint, collapse, and even sustain physical injury. The person may be glassy-eyed, feel weak and dizzy, and appear to be stumbling and uncoordinated. People may also blanch white in the skin or appear ashen gray. Sudden cardiac arrest has occurred after some people became aware of the death of a loved one, especially if the death was sudden or if it was the result of traumatic circumstances. If you see signs of psychogenic shock, get the person seated or lying on the floor immediately. If the person faints, assist him or her to the floor or ground. Typically the patient will recover consciousness in just a few minutes. Do not allow the person to get right back up when he or she awakens. A few more minutes of rest will help to restore normal heart rate and blood pressure. The suggestions below will be helpful for emergency personnel who are dealing with people in severe emotional shock.

First, bring the person to a safe and secure location immediately and decrease the amount of stimuli. Quiet the environment by lowering the noise level. Get unnecessary people out of the immediate area.

When you have created a safe, secure, and quiet environment, turn immediately to the patient's physical needs. Provide treatment according to the symptoms and as the circumstances require. Make sure the person is breathing and has a heartbeat. Treat for shock if necessary. Put a blanket between the person and the floor to cut down on

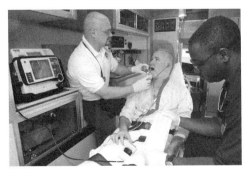

Figure 4-2 Emotional shock can produce dangerous physiological reactions.

heat loss. Keep the person warm, but do not overheat. Medical care may include oxygen. Raising the level of the legs may help. Provide cool water to drink. Avoid administering medications, especially any with depressant effects. Check vital signs frequently.

Throughout, be calm and speak softly, but loud enough to be heard by the person. Be kind and gentle. Try to anticipate a person's needs. Fulfill the person's requests if possible. Distressed people will appreciate the expression of sympathy and concern. Remember that people in a state of emotional crisis tend to be literal thinkers. If you say everything will be alright, they hear you quite literally and then become upset when everything is not really alright. Be cautious not to use wording that might reverberate in a very negative way later, such as "You'll be fine." It is better to say something such as, "I know you are very distressed right now and things are not going well. I will try to do whatever I can to help you through this difficult and painful situation."

If the distressed person jokes a little, that is fine. It is a very bad idea, however, for the person providing support to try to be funny. Under tense circumstances, the distressed person usually interprets attempts to be humorous as insensitive and unkind. These persons often cannot get the joke, because distress makes them concrete or literal in their thinking processes, or the persons may be offended that you are not taking the situation seriously. Humor from a support person has a much greater chance of being harmful than it does of being helpful. This is especially so in the early stages of contact with a distressed person, family, or group.

Remember, in a stress reaction, the brain is bathed in a flood of stress-related chemicals that focus the brain on cues to safety or danger. The chemicals of distress help people review their memories for anything that might be useful in the immediate acute crisis state. The chemicals seriously interfere with the brain's capacity to process abstract thinking such as jokes, psychological theory, or theological discussions. After the acute stages of a crisis reaction, when people calm down and are with people they know and trust, humor may be more appropriate. Proceed cautiously and do not try to lighten up a person's mood.

Throughout the experience, remember to protect a person's right to privacy. Do not discuss a person's situation with people who have no need or right to know. Confidentiality is an important factor in crisis communications. A distressed person should be able to trust that what he or she tells you will not be shared with others, and written medical records are protected by federal law. To maintain privacy and reduce the confusion that results from the involvement of too many people, restrict the number of people that discusses a patient's medical condition with the patient. In prolonged situations in which a change of shifts may occur, the rule of thumb ought to be only one primary communicator per shift.

Finally, as the circumstances unfold, regroup people into natural groupings such as family, friends, work groups, and neighborhoods. If there are no natural group members available, do not leave the distressed person alone.

Throughout the experience, keep in mind that the greatest concern with a person in severe emotional shock is for the person's immediate physical well-being. Psychogenic shock can be deadly if it continues without alleviation.

Excited Delirium

When a person is experiencing a severe disturbance in his or her level of consciousness and mental status, he or she is experiencing delirium. The condition usually occurs within a brief time frame, typically within 1 to 3 hours. The characteristics of delirium are disorientation to time, place, and other aspects of environment. It becomes increasingly difficult for the delirious person to focus or sustain attention. The person is easily distracted. Perceptions may be disturbed, and hallucinations are possible. A state of delirium can be caused by a number of potentially life-threatening conditions, including infection, head trauma, high fever, and adverse reactions to medications or illegal drugs. Anyone in a delirious state requires rapid medical evaluation and treatment.

When a person is delirious, he or she may exhibit behavioral changes that may serve as warning signals for EMS crews. A delirious person may be oppositional, defiant, irritated, angry, paranoid, and quite aggressive (**Figure 4-3**). If EMS crews get angry and demanding or if they try to exert force or make threats, a delirious person will usually escalate his or her aggression and may resort to violence. Restraining a delirious person is difficult and often dangerous, because the person may have unusual strength. Sometimes a delirious person has a remarkably high tolerance for pain and intense resistance to force. It is not unusual for as many as eight people to be required to restrain a delirious person. The disproportionate force required to subdue and control some delirious people leads to the discussion of excited delirium.

Excited delirium is not a recognized medical or psychiatric condition; it should be used only as a descriptive term, and it is often used in describing extreme drug reactions. In the 1980s, the term typically was used to describe behaviors associated with stimulant drugs like cocaine or methamphetamine, for example, as part of a longer phrase such as "cocaine-induced excited delirium." More recently, the term was shortened to excited delirium and is used to explain a sudden death that occurred after a person was restrained in a forceful or violent manner. The term has already been used, in a few cases, as a defense of law enforcement personnel against charges of excessive force or police brutality.

In almost every case of sudden death that occurred while the victim was restrained or in custody, the death occurred during or shortly after a period of intense physical activity such as running away from police, strenuous fighting, being restrained by multiple police officers, being shocked by Taser™ devices, or being placed in restraining devices such as straitjackets or full-body restraints. In some cases, the intense physical activity ends and everything appears to be returning to normal when the person suddenly stops breathing or goes into cardiac arrest.

Autopsies confirm that the majority of victims of excited delirium had ingested cocaine or amphetamines. Thus, some argue that the abuse of cocaine and amphetamines is what actually causes the sudden death of a restrained person; proponents of this explanation suggest that a burst of adrenalin may supercharge the heart and cause cardiac arrest. Some suggest that chronic use of cocaine and amphetamines may weaken or damage the heart and sensitize the brain to overreact to stimuli, thus triggering erratic behaviors, paranoia, delirium, high body temperature, and, ultimately, an overload on the cardiac muscle, resulting in cardiac arrest. Other experts contend that it is the severe psychological stress associated with being chased, captured, and restrained that produces the overload on the system and causes the death. Researchers are continuing to study the matter, but are far from drawing any definite conclusions.

First when managing a delirious person, secure the environment. Reduce stimuli and ensure privacy. Remove anyone who is antagonizing the situation. It is not advised that you work alone. You should have a partner with you whenever you are working with a delirious person. There are many physical and mental reactions that the person might have, and you will certainly need help in managing the case. It is also unsafe for you to work alone, because the patient may become agitated or even violent.

Second, obtain an adequate history about the person and his or her behaviors. It is extremely hard to do the right things to help someone if you have no idea what is going on. It is important to ask the person or family member about any new medications that the person may be taking. Be aware of any other medications that the person may

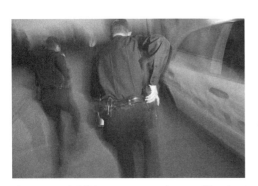

Figure 4-3 A delirious person may be oppositional, defiant, and aggressive.

be using, especially any that have behavioral side effects or adverse reactions when combined with other drugs. Some medications as well as some illegal drugs may cause delirium, impaired mental status, emotional instability, psychomotor retardation or acceleration, and psychotic symptoms.

Third, be alert to the mental confusion and heightened agitation that is often present in people who are delirious. Pay close attention to declining level of consciousness and mental status (the SEA-3 mental status examination is a useful tool in these cases). Note any increase in irritability as you question the person and be aware that some people will react quickly and negatively when they are questioned, challenged, directed, or ordered.

Fourth, do not provoke or continue to use psychological pressure if the person's condition appears to worsen. Do not excite, confront, or agitate people who are already in a delirious state. Calm verbal communications will usually help more than confrontation. Often, if EMS personnel avoid threats and force, the situation may settle down and the person might regain some appropriate orientation.

Along the same line, attempt to contain behavior and avoid restraints, especially if the individual is not an immediate threat to self or others. Avoid rushing the person. Such pressure usually heightens distress and intensifies the delirium.

Should force become necessary, use the lowest level of force required to control the person. Learn and practice proper restraining techniques before attempting them under field conditions. Be familiar with and adhere to the state laws, local directives, and general guidelines for the use of restraints that apply in your jurisdiction.

Anyone in a delirious state increases the potential for physical injury of EMS personnel, and there is an elevated risk that actions taken by EMS and law enforcement personnel will injure the delirious person. Utmost caution is highly recommended in every case.

Restraints

"As a matter of law, any individual who chooses to restrain someone may be charged and found responsible for the intended and unintended impact."—Dr. Michael G. Conner, 2006

EMS personnel should always pause before engaging in actions to restrain a person. Ask yourself, "Is restraining this person truly a last resort? Have we tried every other alternative before deciding to restrain? Is the person a threat to either himself or herself or to another nearby person? Do we have enough help and the proper equipment to properly restrain a delirious person without causing harm?" The following guidelines will help you determine the need for restraints and offer suggestions for accomplishing a safe patient containment.

Restraining a person is always a last resort. You should exhaust every possible alternate means to control a delirious person before deciding to use restraints. Try calming, talk-down procedures first, but stop using such procedures if the person becomes more agitated. Increased agitation is a common reaction in certain substance abuse cases, such as phencyclidine (PCP). Immediately cease the effort to talk a person down if there is a strong negative reaction to verbal efforts.

When utilizing such techniques, appeal to a person's reason. Ask for cooperation so that you can protect the person from harm. Reassure the person that you have his or her best interest in mind. Sometimes letting a person know that the police are standing by can be helpful, but do not use this information too early in the negotiations with the person, as it typically will only need to be offered if the circumstances are deteriorating. On occasion, the choice between going calmly with a medic crew or having to be forced to go to the hospital by the police will cause the angry, upset, or delirious person to calm down and cooperate. If the circumstances do not improve, law enforcement personnel may be required. They have training to manage such cases and medics usually do not.

In the Field

Restraining a Patient

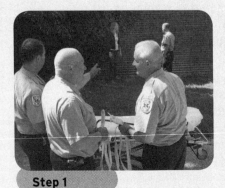

Step 1

Assemble 4 or 5 rescuers and have the stretcher or carrying device and soft restraints nearby. Designate a leader.

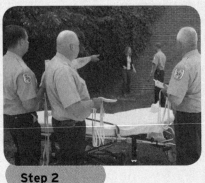

Step 2

Assign positions to each team member: four extremities and the head.

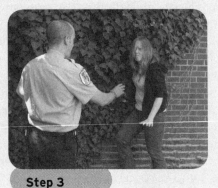

Step 3

If possible, corner the patient in a safe area.

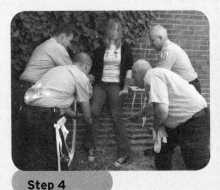

Step 4

On the direction of the team leader, move together toward the patient.

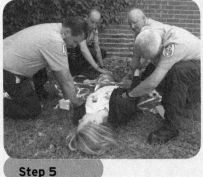

Step 5

Each team member should grasp the assigned body part and carefully, with the least amount of force, bring the patient to the ground.

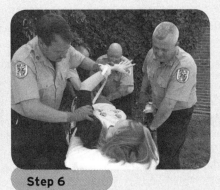

Step 6

Carefully place the patient on the stretcher or carrying device in a face-up position.

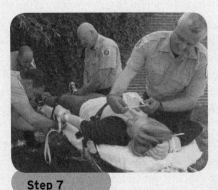

Step 7

Tie the patient with soft restraints at each wrist and ankle as well as the chest and pelvis with sheets. If the patient is spitting, place an oxygen mask or surgical mask on his or her face.

Treat the person as a person with a problem, not a problem person. Your own attitude toward the person may calm or exacerbate the behaviors you are encountering. Work slowly and do not rush the person while you are trying to negotiate better behavior on his or her part.

If the person you are trying to help displays a weapon, back out and wait for law enforcement personnel. It is foolish to risk being injured by an angry or upset person. Sometimes backing out of the immediate area and not presenting any type of a threat can allow the person to gain control of himself or herself. A little time may be all that is lost, and you may gain a more cooperative patient. Remember, your interactions with an upset and distraught person do not need to be instantaneous unless the person is in a life-threatening situation.

Do not display restraining equipment when you are still attempting to talk with and calm the person. The distressed person is likely to interpret that as an imminent threat, and the person will react as if under attack.

If restraining someone is necessary, use restraints that are humane and have the least potential to cause physical injury. Never use belts, wires, or electric cords. Never leave the person in a face-down position. Once a person is restrained, a member of the EMS crew must monitor the person's mental status and breathing continuously. Once applied, restraints should be left in place until hospital personnel evaluate the person and determine that it is safe to remove the restraints. If the patient's medical condition worsens, you may have to remove the restraints.

The decision to use restraints is a serious one that almost always has negative consequences. Weigh all the options and consider all the potential outcomes before moving toward restraints. It is wise to call in law enforcement personnel and fully brief them on the mental and physical condition of the person before engaging in any efforts to restrain the person. Ask yourself, "Are we doing what is necessary for the well-being of the patient and are we avoiding violations of a person's rights?" If the questions cannot be answered with a "yes," then you should slow down your actions and rethink the situation. If circumstances require you to move ahead with restraints, then do so with all due caution and concern. Aim at helping to restore order and control, not hurting or punishing.

> ## In the Field
>
> Never restrain a patient as punishment for his or her actions. Restraints should only be used as a last resort to help maintain the patient's safety.

Legal Issues

Every patient, no matter how physically sick, emotionally distressed, or mentally disordered, has rights. The first right is to be treated with dignity and respect. The second right is to be properly medically treated by appropriately trained personnel who adhere to common standards of practice. Disregard for those elementary rights sets up the conditions for legal actions against prehospital personnel.

Local, state, and federal laws cover virtually every aspect of prehospital care. It would be foolish to function in a prehospital environment without being very familiar with the laws that apply to EMS providers. Make yourself aware of these laws, and always remember that it is your responsibility to know your legal responsibilities and rights. Numerous books and professional articles thoroughly cover the legal responsibilities of EMS personnel. Anyone encountering legal action as a result of his or her prehospital work would be wise to consult with an attorney who is familiar with the laws that apply to prehospital care.

Sample Patient Bill of Rights

A patient has the right to:

- Respectful care given by competent workers.
- Know the names and the qualifications of his or her caregivers.
- Privacy and access of medical information as outlined by local, state, and federal laws.
- Privacy with regard to his or her medical condition. A patient's care and treatment will be discussed only with those who need to know.
- Have his or her medical records treated as confidential and read only by people with a need to know. Information about a patient will only be released with permission from the patient or if permitted by law.
- Good quality care and high professional standards that are continually maintained and reviewed.
- Make decisions regarding his or her care and has the right to include family members in those decisions.
- Information from the EMS provider in order to make informed decisions about his or her care. This means that patients will be given information about their diagnosis, prognosis, and different treatment choices. This information will be given in terms that the patient can understand. This may not be possible in an emergency.
- Full information about any research studies in which he or she has been given the option to participate. A patient may refuse to participate in any research study. A patient who chooses to participate has the right to stop at any time. Any refusal to participate in a research program will not affect the patient's access to care.
- Refuse any drugs, treatments, or procedures, to the extent permitted by law, after hearing the medical consequences of refusing the drug, treatment, or procedure.
- Care without regard to race, color, religion, disability, sex, sexual orientation, age, or national origin.
- Be given information in a manner that he or she can understand. A patient who does not speak English or is hearing or speech impaired has the right to an interpreter, when possible, at no cost to the patient.
- Upon request, access all information contained in the patient's medical records within a reasonable time frame. This right may be restricted as allowed by law.
- Have information in the medical record explained to him or her.
- Treatment that avoids unnecessary discomfort.
- A copy of his or her bills. A patient also has the right to have the bill explained.
- Request help in finding ways to pay his or her medical bills.
- Access people or agencies to act on the patient's behalf or to protect the patient's rights under law. A patient has the right to have law enforcement or social services contacted when he or she or the patient's family members are concerned about safety.
- Be informed of his or her rights at the earliest possible time in the course of his or her treatment.
- Make advance directives (such as a living will, health care power of attorney, and advance instruction for mental health treatment) and to have those directives followed to the extent permitted by law.
- Personal privacy and to receive care in a safe and secure setting.
- Be free from all forms of abuse or harassment.
- Appropriate assessment and management of pain.
- Be involved in resolving dilemmas about care decisions.
- Have his or her complaints about care resolved.
- The family/guardian of a child or adolescent patient generally has the right and responsibility to be involved in decisions about the care of the child. A child or adolescent has the right to have his or her wishes considered in the decision making as limited by law.

Patient Responsibilities

Patients are responsible for:

- Providing correct and complete information about their health and past medical history.
- Reporting changes in their general health condition, symptoms, or allergies to the EMS providers.
- Reporting if they do not understand the planned treatment or their part in the plan.
- Following the recommended treatment plan they have agreed.
- Treating others with respect.
- What happens if they refuse the planned treatment.
- Paying for their care when applicable.
- Respecting the property and rights of others.

Our EMS providers are committed to protecting your health information, which is a right you have and one detailed in the federal Health Insurance Portability and Accountability Act (HIPAA) of 1996. If you have any questions or requests, please contact our administrative offices at _____.

Adapted from: Cotswold Medical Clinic, 200 Greenwich Road, Charlotte, NC 28211. Retrieved from: *http://practices. novanthealth.org/cotswoldmedical/about_us/patient_rights.jsp, June 20, 2007.*

Emergency Vehicle Operations

The most common legal problems encountered by prehospital personnel are associated with emergency vehicle operations. On an ascending scale from least to most problematic would be violations of motor vehicle laws, property damage, injuring a person not under your care, accidents with a patient on board, further injuring a patient in an accident, and, worst of all, contributing to the death of a patient. Excessive speed, stress, and distractions are significant factors in emergency vehicle accidents. Proper emergency vehicle operator training, cautious driving, and adherence to motor vehicle laws help to protect EMS personnel (**Figure 4-4**).

Patient Consent

People have a right not to be touched. They also have a right to refuse emergency medical care. It is always best to obtain a person's permission before touching or treating the person. <u>Actual consent</u> is direct verbal or written permission to provide emergency medical care. <u>Implied consent</u> is an assumption that a person who is unconscious or otherwise unable to communicate actual permission for treatment would, in all probability, agree to treatment if he or she were capable of communicating such permission. For children 17 years and younger, parents or legal guardians take on the responsibility of authorizing emergency medical care. In the absence of parents or guardians, life-saving medical

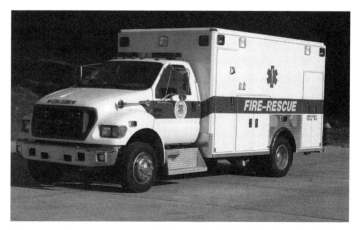

Figure 4-4 Proper emergency vehicle operator training helps to protect EMS personnel.

care may be provided in an emergency. Again, the assumption is that a parent or guardian would want the child to be treated.

Patient Refusal

Unless patients are mentally incompetent or otherwise unable to make decisions in their own best interest, they may refuse medical care. Sometimes there are good reasons for refusing care; a patient may not trust the skills of the medical provider or might simply not like the medical provider assigned to the case. In some circumstances, a person might remember an extremely painful experience with a medical treatment.

If you suspect that a person is not capable of making a sound judgment about medical care, it is best to call law enforcement and explain the situation to them. Police can aid in the decision to treat or not to treat and can serve as witnesses in the case of legal actions against you. Additionally, police departments and mobile crisis teams usually have the authority to write an emergency petition (see below), which legally mandates that the individual must go to the emergency department for a psychological evaluation.

Crime Scene Preservation

Many emergency medical scenes are also crime scenes. EMS personnel have an obligation to preserve the crime scene as near to its original condition as possible. EMS personnel should move and touch as little as they can when they are working a medical emergency in the midst of a crime scene (**Figure 4-5**). They should make every effort to remember as much detail as possible about the scene and the position of the injured people when working within the internal perimeter of the crime scene. Be cautious in handling items that may serve as evidence. Clothing with body fluids, for example, should be placed in paper bags, not plastic. Make sure any materials that may serve as evidence are turned over to law enforcement as quickly as possible. Write notes or draw diagrams about the circumstances of patient care on the report forms. Those records often become part of the evidence presented in courtrooms.

Reporting Requirements

Every state has mandatory reporting requirements for prehospital EMS personnel. The most common is that child abuse cases must be reported to child protection agencies or to the police. Requirements to report elder abuse, felony crimes (including sexual assault), injuries sustained as a result of violence, animal bites, and some infectious diseases are also common. Be familiar with the reporting requirements that apply in your jurisdiction and follow them precisely.

Scope and Standards of Practice

The scope of practice includes the limits of one's authorization to provide care. Surgery, dental work, psychiatry, and the practice of law, for example, are well beyond the scope of practice for prehospital personnel. Emergency medical personnel should not do anything that falls outside of their scope of practice. When they do function within the scope of their authorized services, they should always be aware of and adhere to the standards of practice. The standards of practice are the commonly accepted methods of performing procedures that are within the scope of prehospital care. If an EMT used a leg traction splint on an elbow injury, he or she is acting

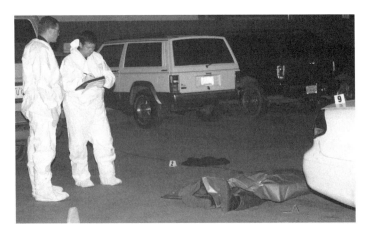

Figure 4-5 Always be cautious when handling items that may be evidence in a crime.

in a manner that violates a standard of practice and would be liable for the damages the patient would most likely sustain. Likewise, an attempt to perform psychotherapy with a distressed individual is also a violation.

Duty to Act

It is presumed that if you are functioning in an official capacity, such as serving as a crew person on an ambulance, you are obligated to provide emergency medical care to the patients who are assigned to your unit. There is also an obligation for an emergency unit to stop to render assistance at an accident scene or to call for another unit if already carrying a patient to the hospital. In some states, physicians and nurses are required to render assistance at an accident scene if there are no other emergency services already functioning at that scene.

Good Samaritan Laws

These laws provide some protection from legal liability for people who assist others in emergencies. They will not protect people who do not follow standards of care or who act in dangerous and irresponsible ways. Reasonable and prudent behavior is always required when rendering aid to others. For example, if a person is behaving in a manner that indicates a threat to self or others, emergency personnel cannot leave the person alone and leave the scene simply because the person refuses help.

Negligence

If a person with a duty to act does things that he or she should not do, the person may be <u>negligent</u> by acts of <u>commission</u>. Administering a psychoactive drug that the paramedic has not been approved to give without direct authorization of a physician is an act of negligence by commission. On the other hand, if a person with a duty to act does not do something that he or she should do, then the person may be negligent by acts of <u>omission</u>. Not conducting a full head-to-toe assessment on an intoxicated subject simply because the subject smells bad would be considered negligence by omission. Charges of negligent behaviors are typically filed only when injury or damages occur as a direct result of a blatant disregard for proper procedures. Errors in judgment are usually not considered negligence.

Abandonment is a form of negligence; it occurs when prehospital personnel begin to assist someone and then leave the person without providing for alternate forms of assistance. Prehospital personnel can be held responsible for abandonment, especially if damages or further injuries occur. Prehospital providers must be cautious to not abandon patients who may be experiencing mental or cognitive disorders that would make them incompetent and hence unable to make the reasonable decision to refuse service.

Impaired patients may require additional care. A good rule of thumb to follow whenever you are dealing with an impaired patient, regardless of the cause of that impairment, is to provide more than the ordinary care. If a person is impaired, he or she is less capable of self-care. The EMS crew must do more to take care of that patient than would be necessary for a person who is able to provide at least some care for himself or herself.

Mentally disturbed or mentally incompetent patients may not always be normal, nice, or easy to deal with, but they still require emergency medical care. Not caring for the mentally disturbed and incompetent person is an invitation for legal complications if the patient sustains further injury or death because of your refusal to help the person.

Patients Expressing Threat to Self or Others

Emergency medical personnel must take actions that are in the best interests of saving human lives when they encounter individuals expressing threats to themselves or others. EMS providers must do everything they can to contain the crisis, remove the person from danger, and transport the person to a medical facility for further evaluation and care. In some cases, restraints may be necessary and law enforcement personnel may be required.

If threats of harm are made against specific people, those people have a right to know that they are the target of someone's rage. You have an obligation to notify police about the threats and the person who is the target must be warned of the possible danger by the police or a representative social service agency.

Emergency Petitions

All states have mechanisms in place to take a person who is a danger to self or others into custody for purposes of psychiatric evaluation and treatment. The specific procedures vary from state to state, so EMS personnel are encouraged to be thoroughly familiar with the procedures in their state. In some states, mobile crisis teams and law enforcement can write and serve the petition. In other states, courtroom procedures are required before the individual can be evaluated. In these situations, testimony is heard and the judge issues or denies the request for emergency petition. Law enforcement then takes the person into custody and transports the person to the emergency department. In special situations, the police will ask EMS providers to provide the transport.

Do Not Resuscitate Orders

Do not resuscitate (DNR) orders that have been signed by the patient's physician should be followed. Resuscitation efforts in opposition to properly developed and signed DNR orders may place EMS crews in legal liability. Additionally, the resuscitation procedures produce enormous distress for the sick person's family. Family members had accepted the inevitability of a loved one's death and now emergency personnel are attempting to resuscitate the person. The family often sees this as a violation of the patient's right to die with dignity. The family is also insulted that the patient's wishes are being ignored. On the other hand, it is a particularly bad idea to comply with DNR orders that are made up on the spot by the sick person's relatives or friends. DNR orders are written in advance of the cessation of breathing and heartbeat. They are signed by a physician, and they are not something that family and friends can make up in the heat of the moment.

Failure to Adequately Communicate With the Patient

Failure to communicate with a patient, a parent, a guardian, or appropriate family members causes unnecessary anxiety and frustration for those in need of information. With enough provocation, frustration eventually gives way to expressions of irritability, intense anger, and rage. In a considerable number of cases, anger is a major contributing factor to medical lawsuits. Every effort should be made by all parties involved to be professional and to provide adequate information whenever possible.

When communicating with a patient, ask the person if he or she understood what was just stated. Ask the person if he or she has any questions. Take a few minutes to answer the questions and to go over any details that the patient needs to know more about. Be careful with your wording, and make sure that specific aspects of medical care are presented in a manner that helps the person understand what is being done and why. Be prepared to repeat anything that is unclear, and make sure you simplify the words to match the needs of the patient.

When communicating with parents, guardians, or the relatives of impaired patients, be precise and concise in your presentation. Stop periodically and ask if there are any questions so far. Then proceed to provide enough information to guide them in patient care.

If you are having difficulty communicating with someone for any reason, allow another person to try to communicate for you. A partner, a nurse, a physician, or another family member may be able to help when communications become difficult. Sometimes you may need to write things down to assist in the communication. Avoid giving information to strangers. That is a serious violation of patient confidentiality.

Generally you can avoid having to use a translator. But, on occasion, a language barrier makes it impossible for you to communicate with a sick or injured person by any other means. Please ask the translator to be cautious and use words that match the meaning of your words as exactly as possible. The translator should be careful to express the patient's meaning as clearly as possible to you.

Situations involving potential organ donations should be given special attention. Know the organ donation guidelines for your jurisdiction and communicate quickly and effectively with the authorities who manage the donor program (**Figure 4-6**). Failure to do so jeopardizes precious organs that might be vital to survival for other people. Recognize that even in a time of crisis or traumatic death, family members may want to discuss donating the organs of a loved one to help others.

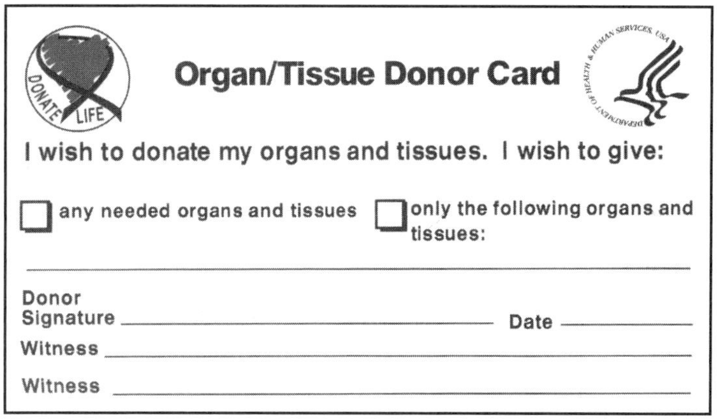
Organ/Tissue Donor Card

I wish to donate my organs and tissues. I wish to give:

☐ any needed organs and tissues ☐ only the following organs and tissues:

Donor Signature ____________ Date ____________

Witness ____________

Witness ____________

Figure 4-6 Organ donation card.

EMTs and paramedics take on an important responsibility with regard to patient confidentiality, and they must ensure that patient confidentiality is protected. Federal, state, and local laws have been strengthened over the last several decades, and violations of patient confidentiality put EMS personnel in a vulnerable position for legal actions. Specifically, the Health Insurance Portability and Accountability Act (HIPAA) of 1996 provides strict guidelines on managing a patient's confidentiality and the penalties for failing to meet the guidelines set forth by the law. HIPAA specifically relates to the transmission of patient records, especially by electronic means. Emergency personnel should be aware of the laws that apply to them regarding patient confidentiality.

Final Thoughts

The list of legal concerns seems long and complicated. Thankfully, the actual number of legal actions taken against prehospital personnel is quite small in comparison to the huge number of emergency medical cases handled by EMS personnel each day. The best protection against a negative legal situation is thorough knowledge of the laws that apply to emergency medical care, training, common sense, adequate supervision, and adherence to commonly accepted standards of care.

Behavioral emergencies can be high-risk situations, and they should not be taken lightly. Emergency medical personnel should approach them with more than the ordinary care that they display on routine medical calls. There may be risks of injury or death for the victims and the rescuers, and careless handling elevates the risk of legal complications. That being said, do a good job and do not let fear of legal action inhibit your ability to make a difference in the lives of others.

Selected References

Aguilera DC: *Crisis Intervention: Theory and Methodology*. ed 8. St Louis, MO, Mosby; 1998.

American Psychiatric Association: *Diagnostic and Statistical Manual of Mental Disorders, Fourth Edition, Text Revision (DSM-IV-TR)*. Washington, DC, American Psychiatric Association, 2000.

American Psychiatric Association: Practice guideline for the assessment and treatment of patients with suicidal behaviors. *Am J Psychiatry*, 2003;160(suppl).

American Psychological Association: Answers to your questions about panic disorder. Available at: http://www.printthis.clickability.com/pt/cpt?action=cpt&title=Answere+to+Questions+Abo. Accessed May 1, 2007.

Antai-Otong D: *Psychiatric Emergencies,* ed 2. Eau Claire, WI, PESI Healthcare, 2004.

Anxiety Disorder Association of America: Statistics and facts about anxiety disorders. Available at: http://www.adaa.org/mediaroom/index.cfm; 2003. Accessed December 6, 2006.

Beck AT, Rush AJ:Cognitive therapy, in Kaplan HI, Sadock BJ (eds): *Comprehensive Textbook of Psychiatry,* ed 6. Baltimore, MD: Williams & Wilkins, 1995.

Beers MH, Berkow R (eds): *Merck Manual of Diagnosis and Therapy.* ed 17. Whitehouse Station, NJ, Merck, 1999.

Benner AW, Isaacs SM: "Excited delirium": a two-fold problem. *Police Chief,* 1996;(6).

Carkhoff RR: *The Art of Helping.* ed 2. Amherst, MA, Human Resource Development, 1977.

Cohn BM, Azzara AJ: *Legal Aspects of Emergency Medical Services.* St Louis, MO, Saunders Publishing, 1998.

Compton WM: The role of psychiatric disorders in predicting drug dependence treatment outcomes. *Am J Psychiatry,* 2003;160:890–895.

Conner MG: Excited delirium, restraint asphyxia, positional asphyxia and "in-custody death" syndrome: controversial theories that may explain why some children in treatment programs die when restrained; 2006. Available at: http://www.educationoptions.org/programs/articles/Sudden Death.htm. Accessed January 23, 2007.

Dhossche DM: Suicidal behavior in psychiatric emergency room patients. *South Med J:* 2000;93(3).

Dubovsky SL, Davies R, Dubovsky AN: Mood disorders, in Hales RE, Yudofsky SC (eds): *Essentials of Clinical Psychiatry,* ed 2. Washington, DC, American Psychiatric Association, 2004.

Gutman DA, Musselman DL, Nemeroff CB: Neuropeptide alterations in depression and anxiety disorders, in Den Boer JA, Ad Sitsen JM (eds): *Handbook of Depression and Anxiety: A Biological Approach.* New York, NY, Psychiatric Research, 2003.

Hamilton PM: *Psychiatric Emergencies: Caring for People in Crisis.* Comptche, CA, Wild Iris Medical Education, 2007.

Health Insurance Portability and Accountability Act of 2003 (HIPAA). U.S.C.45C.F.R. 164.501.

Healthwise Inc: Panic attacks and panic disorder–topic overview; 2005. Available at: http://www.webmd.com/anxiety-panic/tc/Panic-Attacks-and-Panic-Disorder-Topic-Overview. Accessed May 1, 2007.

Jamison KR: *An Unquiet Mind.* New York, NY, Knopf, 1995.

Mason T, Chandley M: *Management of Violence and Aggression.* Philadelphia, PA, Churchill Livingstone, NY, 1999.

Mitchell JT, Resnik HLP: *Emergency Response to Crisis.* Ellicott City, MD, Chevron Publishing Corporation, 1986.

Mitchell JT: Stress management, in Jones SA, Weigle A, White RD et al, (eds). *Advanced Emergency Care for Paramedic Practice.* Philadelphia, PA, JB Lippincott Company, 1993.

NANDA International: *Nursing Diagnoses: Definitions and Classification, 2005–2006.* Philadelphia: Author; 2005.

National Institutes of Mental Health. NIH News: gene more than doubles risk of depression following life stresses; 2003. Available at: http://www.nih.gov/news/pr/jul2003/nimh-17.htm. Accessed August 12, 2008.

Negrete J: Clinical aspects of substance abuse in persons with schizophrenia. *Can J Psychiatry,* 2003;48:14–21.

Plauger PJ: Computer language (March, 1983). Available at: http://quotationsbook.com/author/5744. Accessed August 12, 2008.

Caroline N: *Nancy Caroline's Emergency Care in the Streets.* Sudbury, MA: Jones & Bartlett; 2008.

Schneid TD: *Legal Liabilities in Emergency Medical Services.* London, England, Taylor & Francis, 2001.

Shields J: Panic attacks (eMedicineHealth). Available at http://www.emedicinehealth.com/script/main/art.asp?articlekey=58904&pf=3&page=1: Accessed May 1, 2007.

Stewart J: Excited delirium (CBS News; 2003). Available at: http://www.calpoliceimage.org/excited_delirium_dec.htm. Accessed January 23, 2007.

Sullivan L: Tasers implicated in excited delirium deaths. National Public Radio. Available at: http://www.npr.org/templates/story/story.php?storyId=7622314. Accessed June 21, 2007.

Varcarolis EM, Carson VB: Shoemaker NC: *Foundations of Psychiatric Mental Health Nursing.* ed 5. St Louis, MO, Saunders-Elsevier, 2006.

Webb JM, Carlton EF Geehan DM: Delirium in the intensive care unit: are we helping the patient? *Crit Care Nurs Q,* 2000;22(4).

Prep Kit

Ready for Review

- Remember that the key to any successful crisis intervention is based on seven principles: simplicity, brevity, innovation, practicality, proximity, immediacy, and expectancy.

- Panic attacks are bursts of intense fear that produce powerful physical reactions such as difficulty breathing, racing heart, nausea, dizziness, profuse sweating, and muscle tenseness. These symptoms are often quite alarming for the patient and can even scare some emergency responders.

- While most panic attacks are psychological in nature, the symptoms can often mimic serious medical problems. When in doubt, patients should be transported to an emergency department for evaluation.

- In some overwhelming situations, emotional shock can occur. Emotional shock is also known as psychogenic shock and can present with fainting, weakness, glassy eyes, dizziness, and lack of coordination. In most cases, positioning the person supine will allow the body to begin the compensation process.

- Calm, compassionate, psychological support should be provided to the person in emotional shock. Remember to take care of physical needs first, such as proper positioning, oxygen administration, or cool water to drink.

- Excited delirium is not a recognized medical or psychiatric condition. It is a descriptive term that should be used only to describe the extreme manifestations of drug use, usually cocaine or amphetamine. The term is commonly used to describe a sudden death that occurs after a person has been restrained in a forceful or violent manner.

- Restraining a patient in crisis is always a last resort. Every effort to calm the patient verbally should be used. Realize that the successful intervention might take an extended amount of time.

- All patients have rights. Everyone should be treated with dignity and respect. Trained providers should always adhere to the standards of practice for their profession. Remember that patients do have the right to refuse emergency care unless they have been placed under an emergency petition by a mental health professional or law enforcement officer.

- As an emergency responder, you have a duty to act and provide proper and ethical care for the patient in crisis. However, failure to act within the law is known as negligence and can occur by two means. Negligence by commission is the act of doing something outside of the scope of practice or in error. Negligence by omission is failing to treat the individual as another competent provider would, given the same situation.

Vital Vocabulary

actual consent Direct verbal or written agreement by the patient to accept a medical intervention.

commission A form of negligence that occurs when the EMS provider with a duty to act performs assessments or procedures that in turn harm or create injury to the patient.

emotional shock An acute and severe emotional condition that can produce immediate physiological reactions that can jeopardize a person's physical well-being.

excited delirium A term used by medical examiners to explain why people—often high on drugs or alcohol—die suddenly while in police custody. Symptoms are said to include extreme agitation, aggressive, violent behavior, and incoherence.

implied consent An assumption that a person who is unconscious or otherwise unable to communicate actual permission for treatment would agree to treatment if he or she were capable of communicating such permission.

negligence Professional action or inaction on the part of the EMS provider that does not meet the standard of care expected of similarly trained and prudent health care professionals and that results in injury to the patient.

omission A form of negligence that occurs when the EMS provider with a duty to act fails to

Prep Kit | continued

perform assessments or procedures and this failure in turn harms or creates injury to the patient.

panic attack Periods of time marked by intense fear, opposition, and physical discomfort in which an individual feels helpless or as if he or she is about to lose control or even die.

panic disorder An anxiety disorder in which an individual has recurrent panic attacks or has apprehension about the possibility of future attacks.

Assessment in Action

Answer key is located in the back of the book.

1. From the following list, select the one that is NOT true of excited delirium.

   A. The phrase excited delirium is commonly used to explain when a patient dies of sudden death while being restrained in a forceful or violent manner.
   B. Excited delirium is seen in patients who are not only in respiratory or cardiac arrest, but also under the influence of illicit drugs such as cocaine or methamphetamines.
   C. Excited delirium is considered by the American Medical Association to be both a medical and psychological condition.
   D. Death in individuals with excited delirium usually is accompanied by a burst of adrenalin from the patient's own body.

2. The decision to physically restrain a patient is a serious one. Pick the statement that represents the best philosophy of patient control.

   A. Patients should always be secured and transported in a prone or face-down position.
   B. Once applied, restraints should remain in place until the patient can be evaluated by hospital personal and determined to be in a safe environment.

   C. EMS providers do not have time to wait for the arrival of the police in some cases where the patient has a weapon.
   D. A direct aggressive approach is the best manner for gaining control of the scene where the patient is experiencing a psychological crisis.

3. Knowledge is paramount for you and your partner prior to arriving at the scene of a behavioral emergency. Which of the following is NOT necessary to know before arriving on location?

   A. Are you going to be in immediate danger upon arrival at the scene?
   B. Do you have adequate knowledge about what is going on (for example, why are you being called there)?
   C. Is the victim in danger of self-harm?
   D. Is the patient abusing alcohol or any illicit substances?

4. True or false? Behavioral emergencies and patients with psychiatric histories rarely experience the disease process alone. These conditions usually involve and often stress many friends and family members of the patient.

   A. True
   B. False

5. Patients who have a history of panic attacks will commonly:

   A. report symptoms similar to that of a heart attack, such as chest pain or shortness of breath.
   B. acknowledge that their attacks can be triggered by excessive use of alcohol, caffeine, or nicotine.
   C. experience overwhelming fear or terror.
   D. all of the above.

Chapter 5

Assisting Large Groups

Under certain conditions, a crowd of curious onlookers can turn into a cooperative group that helps you or an uncontrolled mob that threatens you. Much depends on how you treat the crowd. Furthermore, much depends on your power of persuasion.

It is difficult to understand crowd behavior or to predict it accurately. Crowd behavior and the combination of many different personalities in the same location and at the same time is inherently unstable (**Figure 5-1**). There are, however, several psychological theories that contribute to our understanding of human behavior in crowds.

Theories of Crowd Behavior

The first is the <u>contagion theory</u>. Crowds may exert tremendous influence on individuals, causing those individuals to act quite differently in the crowd than they would as individuals. We sometimes refer to this as mob rule. The crowd atmosphere or mood can strongly influence the crowd members to participate in activities that people would normally avoid if they were functioning only as individuals. The members of the crowd may be more submissive to leadership exerted by some dominant leaders.

A good example of contagion for emergency personnel is when a person in a crowd starts shouting to a potential suicide victim on a ledge, encouraging the person to jump. Before long, many others in the crowd take up the chant and the person contemplating suicide falls under enormous pressure. Individual members of the crowd would most likely never engage in such behavior without a crowd.

Emergency personnel should take a position that is very visible to the crowd and should raise their hands with flat palms showing toward the crowd. Fists will normally be interpreted as a sign of threat; flat

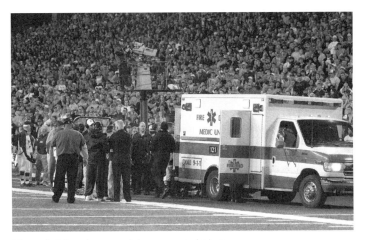

Figure 5-1 Crowds can work for you or against you.

palms are a sign of calming or restraint. Using a megaphone or having the emergency person with the loudest voice yell, ask the crowd to be quiet. Let the crowd know that their behavior might cause the death of a distressed human being. Ask the crowd to allow you to do what you can to help the person without further interference. Then proceed to do what you can to save a life.

The second theory of crowd behavior is the <u>convergence theory</u>. Like-minded people may come together and form a crowd that ultimately acts on goals held by the individuals who make up the crowd. It is not the crowd, therefore, that makes them act in certain ways; people join the crowd so they can act on goals they already hold. The members of the crowd came to the crowd with a set of wishes, ideas, or beliefs. They find leaders within the crowd who are willing to help them achieve their objectives. The individuals within a crowd are active, willing participants in the activities of the crowd and choose to take part in the crowd's actions for personal motivations.

Emergency personnel see convergence when a crowd gathers and many of the members already believe that EMS personnel do not pay much attention to members of their particular ethnic group. If EMS personnel are taking a little too long to transfer a person to the hospital, crowd members see the delay as a sign of bad treatment. This is so even when medics are working very hard to stabilize a patient. The crowd begins to exert a growing, hostile pressure on the EMS crew.

The safest procedure for the emergency personnel is to speed up their actions and do only what is absolutely necessary. Get the patient into the ambulance immediately and drive away from the crowd. If necessary, the ambulance can be pulled to the side of the road or into a parking lot in a safe zone where additional stabilizing measures can be taken before proceeding to the hospital.

The third key theory regarding crowd behavior is the <u>emergent-norm theory</u>. In many ways, this theory is a combination of both the contagion and convergence theories previously described. Crowd behavior may not be predictable, but it does have some rational elements. Similar interests draw people together and then certain behaviors emerge from the crowd. One person does something, and others in the crowd follow that person's example.

Rules in the crowd develop as time passes and as the situation evolves. Someone suggests something and the crowd members decide to do it. As if in a theater production, every person in the crowd eventually takes on a role. They may be leaders, followers, silent bystanders, or even opponents. The pressure mounts in the crowd for everyone to play their roles. If people fail to play within the crowd's structure, the remainder of the crowd may ignore them, reject them, or even attack them. A crowd may split into factions that conflict with one another or may turn its frustration onto the authorities or even against innocent people. Smaller groups within a crowd may be more organized and able to flock together at crucial moments and do things that influence the behaviors of the larger crowd. This is often how a riot begins.

The emergent-norm theory is at work when emergency personnel are called to treat a person who was injured by an angry crowd. The person may have started off as a member of the crowd, but did not appear enthusiastic enough and the crowd members turned on the person and beat and kicked the person until he or she dropped.

The safest action for the emergency personnel is to have the police respond to protect the emergency medical crew. If the police are not there and the situation is deteriorating, get the patient out immediately. If the crowd blocks your exit, use your best powers of persuasion to convince the crowd members that they really do not want to be responsible for a person's death. Sometimes convincing one person in the crowd who appears to be a leader is far easier than trying to convince the entire crowd. A leader in the crowd might influence the crowd to let you pass with your patient.

Crowd Management

Emergency personnel face many challenges in controlling a crowd. Numerous factors add to the complexity of a crowd situation. Emergency management planners spend a huge amount of time working over the details of planned events to ensure a safe, efficient crowd control program for all of the participants in a community activity. Some of the factors they have to consider are:

1. **The type of crowd.** Is the crowd a stationary crowd, as in a theater or stadium, or is the crowd mobile or fluid, such as a crowd gathered on a county fair ground where there are many activities going on simultaneously in different areas of the campus? Knowing the type of crowd helps emergency personnel to plan the deployment of emergency equipment, access and egress routes, and the placement of barriers to assist in crowd control.

2. **The reason the crowd has gathered.** Is the crowd a political rally gathered in protest over some controversial issue? Or is the crowd gathered together at a fun festival? Is the crowd mostly made up of children or teenagers or is it mostly adults? Fun festivals usually do not turn hostile. Injured or ill people are generally brought to a first aid station or emergency personnel go to the location of the injured on foot or by bicycle or golf cart. Protests, on the other hand, are more volatile, and people react to what leaders say and do. Emergency teams usually take up positions outside of the perimeter of the crowd and are ready to move to trouble spots as the needs arise. The key to successful response is excellent communications not only within one agency but among the various emergency organizations.

3. **The size of the crowd.** The bigger the crowd, the greater the challenge in managing it. A crowd of 12 people is obviously much easier to direct and control than a crowd of 12,000 people. Bigger crowds demand more resources, including security personnel, more rest room facilities, more access and egress points, more food and water, and greater numbers of staff.

4. **The space that contains the crowd.** Enclosed spaces must have a much higher level of life-protection policies, procedures, and equipment, including, for example, sprinkler systems, fire extinguishers, cardiac defibrillators, first aid kits, emergency lighting, and signs indicating routes of evacuation. A fenced-in open field must have enough exits to evacuate the area in the shortest possible period of time. Emergency equipment is usually maintained on mobile units under these conditions. Units or elements of those units are moved to trouble spots as required.

5. **The mood or attitude of the crowd members.** Is the crowd happy or angry? Is alcohol being served? Are crowd members using substances in addition to or other than alcohol? Is there anything going on that might excite or upset the crowd? What can potentially destabilize the crowd? An unhappy crowd in which alcohol and other substances are being consumed becomes more potentially threatening to emergency personnel, and crews will need to be more cautious.

6. **The needs of the crowd.** What does the crowd want? Is it entertainment or information or instructions? Is there some political agenda? Are they seeking religious inspiration? Has the weather turned bad and the crowd is seeking shelter? Consider the factors that are driving the crowd's behavior.

7. **Movements within the crowd.** Is everyone in a mobile or fluid crowd moving in the same direction? Are there small sub-groups gathering and moving through the crowd as units? This behavior may be similar to gang behavior or pack behavior, and it may turn dangerous, especially if the pack is beginning to disrupt the crowd's movement and cohesiveness.

8. **Physical issues.** Environmental concerns include such features as walkways, access and egress routes, choke points or bottlenecks, and physical barriers. Weather conditions can contribute to a deterioration in the mood of the crowd. Crowd control demands that event organizers consider, plan around, and develop operational procedures to compensate for obstructions and other physical features of a facility.

9. **Presence or absence of law enforcement personnel.** Is the gathering covered by an adequate number of law enforcement personnel? Is the event employing private security personnel? What is the level of training and experience of the security personnel? How soon can police be on the scene if they are required? Does the nonsecurity staff know what to do in an emergency?

10. **Procedures for the distribution of important information.** Are there public address systems? Are there battery-powered megaphones available in the event of a power failure? How is information about dangerous conditions distributed to the crowd? How is the staff notified of emergencies? How are new instructions communicated to staff and to the crowd itself?

Organizing a crowd control program is a complex and time-consuming process. Field personnel, however, are more likely to be involved in crowd situations with little or no preparation. EMS providers must think their way through a potentially dangerous situation and use their powers of persuasion.

The Use of Bike Teams

The use of bike teams is a relatively new concept in the EMS arena. Historically, police agencies have used bike teams for access in crowded conditions that make vehicle access difficult. Given the success of law enforcement bike teams, EMS providers across the United States have implemented bike teams as well.

Bikes teams are particularly useful when crowds are gathered in fairly large areas of territory and there is an insufficient number of emergency personnel to cover all of the potential threats (**Figure 5-2**). Bikes are used where larger vehicles could not operate easily. Bikes are often used during marathons. The runners are moving constantly and it would be dangerous to have large ambulances moving from site to site. Bike teams can maneuver through alleys, along narrow sidewalks, and on parallel side streets to keep up with the runners.

These specialized teams require many hours of training on everything from bicycle maintenance and shifting gears to how to fall correctly and how to use the bike properly for crowd control. Bicycles help to move the emergency personnel quickly to hot spots in a crowd or to the scene of an injury. Police can calm a disruptive situation and medical personnel can treat the injured. Typically the bikes are used to go around the perimeter of the crowd or to get ahead of a moving crowd and to reach the points where problems have occurred.

The International Police Mountain Bike Association (IPMBA) is the primary supporting organization for bike medic teams, and certified instructors have modified the police courses for EMS providers. EMS

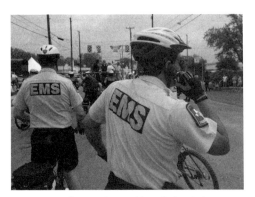

Figure 5-2 Bikes can be used to get ahead of a moving crowd and reach the scene of an emergency.

providers should not think that they can start a bike team simply by buying a few mountain bikes and saddle bags. Bike teams are expensive and team members must be in good health and dedicated to many hours of rigorous training. (For more information, go to www.ipmba.org.)

Informing and Directing Crowds During the Emergency Response

The majority of situations involving emergency personnel will involve spontaneous crowds rather than planned gatherings. Spontaneous crowds are those that gather in the immediate aftermath of an accident or an injury. Sometimes the people who make up the crowd are attracted to the scene by the sirens of responding units.

Emergency responders must be ready to use their people skills and their ability to communicate with the crowd (**Figure 5-3**). Ignoring a crowd when it is experiencing a rising level of tension generally backfires on field personnel and may trigger negative reactions and unexpected dangers. Crowds need information and direction to maintain good behavior. Without instructions, crowds tend more toward chaos.

Information and guidance are among the most pressing needs within a crowd. Leaders who share information usually fill the <u>information gap</u>, which is the discomfort that arises when some people have information others do not. Emergency personnel who are willing to share information can reduce crowd tension levels significantly. People with information are typically viewed as leaders by the crowd and have a greater chance of positively influencing crowd behavior. A failure to provide vital information to a crowd leaves the crowd without a positive influence, making the situation more likely to spiral out of control. Information is among the best tools available for crowd control during crises.

Supplying information to crowds can be difficult, but following the ten essential principles maximizes your ability to maintain control of a situation and effectively reduce a crowd's tension level.

1. All information presented to a crowd must be *accurate*. Accuracy refers to the truthfulness of the information. Every effort should be made to ensure that the information is factual. On some occasions, the information that is available will not be accurate. You may end up presenting it as if it were accurate, because it is the best information available and you believe it is correct. More accurate information then appears and you will have to correct the false information. It is best to apologize, explain how the discrepancy occurred, and then present the most accurate information available. Without doubt, such a circumstance will cause a disturbance in the group, but the disturbance caused by an accidental presentation of faulty information is nothing in comparison to what occurs in a crowd when someone has provided deliberate lies, coverups, and misinformation. Such negative behaviors generate anger and hostility in a crowd and the outcomes are unpredictable and can become violent.

2. All information should be *current*. Current means that the information is up-to-date or the most recent. When information comes into a command post or to an emergency operations center, it should be dated, and the time of arrival of the information should be noted. The person delivering the information should be questioned about the source of the information, when it was obtained, and how the information came about. If in doubt about how current the information is, supervisors should have the information confirmed by a second source, preferably one who is at the scene of the emergency or near the source of the information.

3. Information given to a crowd must be *timely*. Information should be presented as quickly as possible and when it is suitable to provide it. It would not be suitable, for example, to give information if that information would jeopardize the safety of the emergency services

personnel or if it would be a disclosure of private, personal information about an injured person. In law enforcement cases, some information may be withheld to preserve the integrity of the case or to avoid threatening the investigation.

It is certainly suitable to give information that might prevent injuries. For instance, you are at the scene of a building fire and you notice a wall appears to be leaning toward a group of fire fighters. Timely information can help the fire fighters to evacuate from the area. Delayed information might threaten their lives. Two courses of action are appropriate. Warnings need to be communicated by radio or shouted to the unit supervisor, and the overall command must be interrupted and informed of the danger.

Imagine that a large crowd gathered near the wall. If it collapses, bricks and other debris might be thrown in the direction of the crowd. The crowd needs this information so that the people might back away from the wall before any potential dangers can be turned into realities.

4. Information needs to be *concise.* People need short bursts of information during a crisis. Lengthy discourses are hard for people in a crowd to hear and absorb. Long paragraphs may raise, instead of lower, the level of tension in a crowd. Here is an example of a concise message. "Ladies and gentlemen, please listen carefully. We are investigating a potential danger and we need your cooperation. You are in no immediate danger. Emergency personnel are arriving to assist us. As a precaution, we need to evacuate the building in an orderly manner. Please walk to the exit closest to your location. Follow the instructions of the staff. Once outside, please move away from the building and gather on the parking lots as far from the building as possible. There we will give you additional information as it becomes available. Please go now to the exits without delay." The message addresses the intended recipients, makes a statement about what is going on, and provides precise instructions.

5. Information should be *simple.* Remember, people cannot deal with complex concepts during a crisis. Choose straightforward, uncomplicated words. Hit the main issues: what is happening, what the danger is, what needs to be done, and the specific steps the crowd needs to take to avoid the danger. Do not make the message long. Keep it short and to the point. Typically a message to a crowd should contain no more than three or four points.

6. Authorities should deliver information with *confidence.* Crowds are more likely to listen to people who are certain in their knowledge and able to express themselves convincingly. Select a person to deliver the information who can speak well in public, is loud enough to be heard, and is perceived by most people to be knowledgeable and experienced. A person within the organization who has good leadership skills is usually the best person to provide information to a crowd. It is important to avoid an air of arrogance because that will usually anger a crowd and make a tense situation worse.

7. A crowd needs *practical* information. Useful information and practical guidelines help the crowd take actions that help the emergency personnel complete their tasks. People feel more in control of a disturbing circumstance if they have a set of specific steps they can take to manage the problem and keep themselves and their family members safe. As much as possible, people should be given a step-by-step approach to handle the situation. Avoid too many steps, because the instruction will then appear complex and unachievable. Make sure you are telling people to do things that they can actually accomplish. When

Mayor Rudolph Giuliani addressed the people of New York after the attacks on the World Trade Center on September 11, 2001, he issued concise, precise, and practical instructions. He told the crowds not to wait for public transportation, but to walk north and exit Manhattan by means of the bridges to the other boroughs or to New Jersey. He was seen by many as the leader not only because he was mayor, but because his suggestions were simple, concise, and easily followed.

8. The most important information should be *repeated*. Many people do not hear something the first time it is said. A good summary that is repeated several times after an important announcement is helpful. A good example for a crowd gathered at a county fair might be "Please, may I have everyone's attention for an important safety announcement. The weather service is reporting a line of violent thunderstorms approaching our location from the west. There is a strong possibility of extremely strong winds, hail, and heavy rains with as much as two inches of rain per hour. The storm is expected to reach our location within a half hour. Please be alert for signs that a storm is approaching and be prepared to take cover immediately. The main exhibit hall and the two large picnic pavilions near the information booth are now available as severe weather shelters. Vendors please secure loose materials in your exhibit area." The main elements of the message may then be repeated as a summary. "This is a safety advisory. A severe thunderstorm is expected within 30 minutes. Be prepared to take shelter immediately. The main exhibit hall and the two large picnic pavilions near the information booth are now available for shelter."

9. It is generally best to make announcements using *positive terms*. For example, if you are trying to evacuate an area it is better to say, "First Street and Third Street are the best routes out of town," rather than, "Do not use Second Street." Many people during a crisis do not hear the "not" and respond to the rest of the message as if it were the most important information.

10. When it is possible, respectfully *enlist the assistance* of a person in the crowd who appears to be in a positive leadership position. It might go like this, "Sir (or Ma'am), you seem to be a leader in this group. I was wondering if you could help us out here by asking these people to clear a pathway so we can move the injured person to the ambulance." If people feel valued and important, they are more than likely to use their influence with the crowd to stimulate the crowd to take certain positive actions.

Information Push

When dealing with a spontaneous crowd, emergency personnel need to get important information out to the crowd members. It is not appropriate to engage the crowd members in long discussions and negotiations. Emergency personnel have a certain amount of information that may influence and guide a crowd and keep tensions under control. They also have a limited amount of time in which the information is to be delivered. An **information push** provides direction to a crowd and avoids stimulating additional unwanted emotional responses in the crowd members. An information push should aim at providing answers to five questions: *who, what, when, where,* and *why.*

Identify who you are and who is involved in the situation. Next, tell people what has happened and what measures are being taken to manage the problem. Provide specific, precise, and concise directions to the crowd and encourage the crowd members to assist each other. Let people know when things are likely to happen and where they are going to occur.

In the Field

When providing information to a crowd, remember the 5 Ws: who, what, when, where, and why.

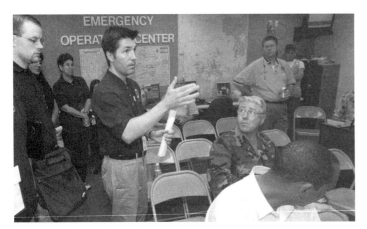

Figure 5-3 Emergency responders must be prepared to communicate with crowds during an emergency.

If possible, try to tell people why authorities have made certain decisions.

Most large group interventions will be relatively spontaneous. A crowd is doing something that needs to be altered or is not doing something that needs to be done. An emergency person using a bullhorn, a public address system, or at least with a loud voice must address the crowd and provide them with information and directions. Always be respectful of people and do nothing to antagonize a crowd. You are an agent of crowd control, but only if you remain in control of yourself. To stay calm, take a few deep breaths, gather as much information as you can, determine what the crowd needs, and provide the crowd with appropriate information and direction. Address the crowd with confidence and respect and express yourself as a leader.

Common Crowd Emergencies
Mass Transit Situations

In a mass transit situation you have what amounts to a crowd in a confined space. It is a more complicated situation because you will be dealing with injuries, possibly deaths, and a fairly large number of upset people who have just experienced a frightening event. The uninjured may be in the way of emergency personnel and will need to be removed from the area to allow emergency personnel to work properly. Sometimes the space available is so small that the uninjured cannot move out of the way. The people may need to be removed one at a time as the rescuers locate them. Under those circumstances people should be directed to stay where they are and wait for the emergency personnel to reach them. They should also be encouraged to assist people who are wounded until the emergency personnel can reach them. There are a few essential elements of dealing with the psychological needs of a crowd involved in a mass transit incident, including:

1. A rapid response of sufficient emergency services resources to assure the crowd that the authorities are involved and are handling the situation (**Figure 5-4**).

2. The presence of a calm, organized, and decisive leader who directs the emergency services crews and who makes frequent announcements to the passengers about what is going on and why things might be taking longer than people like.

3. Providing the crowd with specific instructions, such as, "If you are not injured, we need you to go out the exit nearest to you and our personnel will meet you and guide you once you are outside. Please do not take your belongings with you right now. It is most important that you get out as quickly and as safely as you can. If you need assistance we will be with you as quickly as we can. Please be patient and try to help each other."

4. Gather the nonwounded people together and let them know what is being done to provide alternative transportation, lodging, food, and other important information. Reassure them that the wounded are being cared for as quickly as possible.

5. Reunite people with their families and friends as soon as possible. Some will want to go to the hospital where their loved ones are being treated. Arrangements should be made as soon as possible to accommodate them.

Mass Hysteria

Hysteria is a condition of intense anxiety that causes individuals to behave in irrational, disorganized, and sometimes dangerous ways. The more intense the level of anxiety, the greater will be the level of erratic behavior. Hysteria can be transferred from individuals to groups. When that occurs it is given the label mass hysteria.

Among the most famous cases in United States history is the Salem witch trials during the 1600s. The individual hysterical reactions of a few colonial teenaged girls to their personal anxieties became the source of unwarranted accusations against adults in their town. Soon the townspeople joined in the growing frenzy and people faced trials, convictions, and actual deaths on the basis of invented charges. Almost 30 people were executed before the hysterical reactions calmed and rational thinking was restored to the population of Salem, Massachusetts.

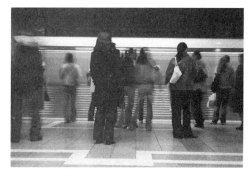

Figure 5-4 Mass transit emergencies require rapid response of sufficient emergency services resources to assure the crowd that the authorities are involved and are handling the situation.

In its extreme, mass hysteria can cause a crowd to panic, bolt, and run wildly. Like a stampede of animals, the crowd will run over anything and anyone in its path. Once hysteria generates panic, there is virtually no chance that talking to the crowd is going to have any effect. Emergency personnel need to protect themselves and take evasive actions to avoid the crowd. People can be crushed to death if they get in the way of a hysterical and panicked crowd. The only recourse for emergency medical personnel is to avoid being in front of the crowd. Get behind the crowd and care for the wounded. Police will have to employ riot control tactics to break the crowd into smaller components and then contain them. Until that occurs, considerable damage may be caused by the unruly crowd.

Obviously, every effort must be made to prevent hysteria from gripping a crowd. Announcements, information, guidance, and direction are the key elements in maintaining calm and control in a crowd. Anyone who is agitating the crowd should be quickly removed by the police before things escalate into the dangerous, uncontrolled behavior of mass hysteria.

Parade

Always think "perimeter" when working a parade (**Figure 5-5**). Stay on the perimeter, move around the perimeter, respond from the perimeter, and return to the perimeter. Only law enforcement personnel should be within the perimeter. Prearrange access and egress points and work with law enforcement to maintain those corridors during the parade. If, out of necessity, you need to cross a parade route to handle an emergency, move with the flow of the parade, not against the flow. Progress diagonally across the parade as you move with the flow of the parade.

As our parents told us, mind your manners. Even in an emergency it is helpful to show respect to the crowd. Saying please, excuse me, I'm sorry, and thank you can help to keep the crowd's resentment of your intrusion at a low level. Extract your patient from the parade route by the shortest, least disruptive route possible and then have your medic unit meet you and your patient at the exit point.

Protests

Protests, by their very nature, have a potential to turn nasty. If a crowd senses that it is not being listened to, it may escalate its volume and its activities to gain attention. Additional frustration may lead to negative actions. Depending on the responses of event organizers and law enforcement's skill in managing the crowd, things will either get better or worse. Emergency personnel should never take sides in a protest. You are the professionals and the issues may not be your issues. It is best to stay out of the issues while you are functioning in an official capacity.

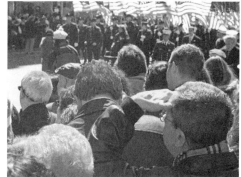

Figure 5-5 Always think "perimeter" when working a parade.

Most of the time, the emergency personnel stay with their units and avoid direct contact with a protest crowd. An ambulance makes a wonderful target of opportunity for an angry crowd to show the authorities just how upset they are. It is better to have uniformed teams of medics strategically placed with aid kits around the perimeter of the crowd. Keep the ambulance away from the main body of a protest. Coordinate your functions and locations with law enforcement personnel. Keep communication links intact and inform command of your movements and the conditions that exist in your area. If you have to respond to an emergency, extract your patient by the easiest and safest means of egress and get to a safe area where an ambulance unit can rendezvous and remove the patient to the hospital.

Riot

A riot is the most dangerous form of work with a crowd. In some ways it is similar to a mass hysteria situation, because it is a rapidly moving crowd. In other ways, a riot is far more dangerous. In mass hysteria people are usually running away from some perceived threat. In a riot, there is mob rule and a general state of lawlessness. A mob in riot mode often selects targets and then proceeds to attack them. People hurt others or destroy or steal things simply because the opportunity is present and there are insufficient law enforcement personnel to maintain order. Rioters may turn their rage on innocent people who just happen to be in the wrong place at the wrong time. Serious injuries and deaths can occur. In a riot, the mob takes delight in expressing its frustration on people, buildings, and property.

Move away from the angry mob and stay out of range of thrown rocks, bottles, and other missiles. Never work alone. Do not enter the danger zone without law enforcement protection. Orders and instructions to an angry mob are usually made by means of a megaphone. That does not necessarily mean that the rioters will listen to the information or the instructions, but it is worth a try.

Medical care and evacuation of the wounded can take place only when law enforcement can gain a more or less secure route of access to the wounded. Move the patient out of danger and then treat. No one can guarantee that a safety zone can be maintained in the middle of a riot or that thrown objects will not strike the emergency personnel. Removal of the patient, therefore, is essential for the safety of both the patient and the emergency personnel. The other option is to wait until the rioters move to a different location and then assist the wounded. That is a difficult choice to make, but the safety of the emergency personnel is among the highest priorities.

Disasters

Disasters are often defined as powerful destructive and disruptive events that overwhelm the resources of the local community (**Figure 5-6**). Disasters can also attract large crowds of spectators. Emergency personnel must consider many things during a disaster response. They must gain access to the scene; establish a perimeter; develop a command structure; communicate with the dispatch center; call for a comprehensive response; pinpoint a staging area; assess, triage, and treat the wounded; stabilize the situation; and prepare for a complicated and extended operation. In other words, they are busy.

In addition, emergency personnel must provide information and direction to crowds that might include survivors, relatives, and friends of the dead and injured, well-meaning but unhelpful do-gooders, onlookers, souvenir hunters, opportunists, and media personnel. Separation of these people into different categories can be helpful. For instance, gathering all of the survivors in one area can help with triage functions. Moving the media personnel to another area will allow the Public Information Officer to more easily provide accurate information, instructions, and specific directions to vantage points for camera work.

The Crisis Management Briefing (CMB) provided by trained Critical Incident Stress Management (CISM) teams is a very useful tool for crowd control. The CMB process is briefly described in the next section of this chapter.

Terrorist Attack

Terrorism can be the worst form of a disaster. It causes enormous disruption to daily life. Terrorism is deliberate and purposeful violence against people to further political, philosophical, or religious objectives. It is essentially psychological warfare.

Among the many problems presented by terrorism, emergency personnel will be faced with the iceberg effect: Just as three quarters of an iceberg is hidden below the surface of the water, the number of psychologically wounded people in a terrorist event will far exceed the actual number of wounded or dead. From the earliest possible point, emergency personnel must bring calm and organization to a terrorist event. They must show that there is sufficient help to manage the scene and that the authorities are making every effort to deal with the effects of the attack.

People who gather in crowds near the site of a terrorist attack should not be ignored. Instead they should be cautioned about dangers, directed to safe areas, and given information about managing the psychological impact of the situation. The CMB described below can be very helpful in providing people with reassurance, information, and guidance.

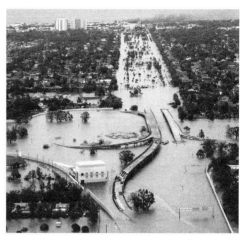

Figure 5-6 Disasters are powerful, destructive events that overwhelm the resources of the local community.

Crisis Management Briefing

Crisis Management Briefing is a tool used to provide an organized and structured information session to a large group of people. The CMB is often used when people with a common interest in a traumatic event have come together. For example, if a town has been flooded, community members may assemble in a town meeting format to gain information from the authorities. On occasion, emergency personnel may be involved in presenting a portion of this large group crisis intervention process.

The CMB is a short informational meeting with the specific purpose of providing practical information to a large group of people who have already experienced, or who are about to experience, a distressing event, with the intention of reducing the stress of that event. The group process remains in the cognitive (thinking) domain and avoids or limits discussions in the affective domain (emotions). The CMB is organized and provided by a trained CISM team. The emphasis in a CMB is on information, instructions, guidelines, directions, and cautions for people dealing with an upsetting or traumatic event.

When participating in a crisis management briefing, it is important to maintain a sense of confidence and follow the organizational structures in place. If you show that you know what you are doing, the crowd will feel safe and more at ease. The effort should be coordinated and conducted jointly with personnel from a local CISM team. The CISM personnel and the emergency personnel should meet in advance to determine the most important information and the best way to deliver that information. Usually the representative of the CISM team introduces the process and the participants.

Once introduced by the CISM team member, an emergency services person may tell the group what has occurred and what is currently happening to resolve the crisis. The meeting that the CISM team conducts with the emergency personnel before the CMB should guide the emergency personnel participating in the CMB to provide the most helpful information (**Table 5-1**). The presenter provides facts about the situation as well as directions and guidance related to the incident. It is especially important that the operations personnel use this opportunity to instruct people about safety issues. For example, "Please do not turn on any lights or electrical appliances in your home until emergency teams check your homes for the presence of natural gas. The leak

In the Field

Focus of the Crisis Management Briefing

- Information
- Instructions
- Guidelines
- Directions
- Cautions

in the area was extensive, and although it has been stopped, gas may have settled in closets and in basements and may explode with the spark from a light switch or other electric appliance. We are checking each home as quickly as we can. It is best not to enter your home until we have cleared it of danger." Emergency personnel should also answer questions to clarify the information.

Provide information about the stress reactions the group may be experiencing. Place emphasis on explaining and normalizing the stress reactions of the group's members (**Table 5-2**). When you let people know, for instance, that having disturbed sleep is normal after a traumatic event, they feel more in control, and they feel normal and healthy. Provide practical suggestions on stress management and specific methods to deal with an emotional crisis. Advise people about proper nutrition, rest, physical exercise, and discussing the traumatic stress with someone they trust. A final question-and-answer period is allowed before summarizing the meeting.

A trained CISM team will handle most of the work in a CMB. Before the CMB, the CISM team will advise the emergency personnel about the role they would play in the CMB as well as the type and amount of information they are expected to present. The CISM team takes on the most challenging aspects of the presentation, and members are trained to handle the most difficult questions.

Final Thoughts

Quick thinking and the ability to deliver a clear, concise, and accurate message is crucial to managing crowds and maintaining your safety under field conditions. Handling a large group of distressed people is just another aspect of crisis intervention. The primary principles and practices of crisis intervention are as applicable with a crowd as they are with individuals.

Table 5-1 Suggested Issues for Presentation in a CMB

- Facts
- Estimated time to resolve the problem
- Existing dangers
- Damage estimates
- Emergency procedures under way
- Casualty reports
- Available resources
- Information about safety, security, shelter, food, and water
- Information to dispel rumors and lower anxiety
- Brief descriptions of the typical signs and symptoms of distress
- Information to mitigate the emotional reactions
- Any information that guides people to appropriate behaviors, such as checking in on elderly people in the neighborhood until the situation is resolved
- Information to assist children, the elderly, and any other special populations
- Suggestions on diet, exercise, rest, sleep, decision making, and problem solving
- Any other important information

Selected References

Berk RA: *Collective Behavior.* Dubuque, IA, Wm C Brown, 1974.

Buford W: *Among the Thugs: The Experience, and the Seduction, of Crowd Violence.* New York, NY, WW Norton & Co Inc, 1990.

Everly GS Jr, Mitchell JT: *Critical Incident Stress Management (CISM): A New Era and Standard of Care in Crisis Intervention.* Ellicott City, MD, Chevron Publishing Corporation, 1999.

Everly GS Jr: Crisis management briefings (CMB): large group crisis intervention in response to terrorism, disasters, and violence. *Int J Emerg Ment Health,* 2000;2:53–57.

Johnson NR: Panic at the Who concert stampede: an empirical assessment. *Soc Probl,* 1987;34:362–373.

Lee GS: *Crowds: A Moving Picture of Democracy.* New York, NY, Doubleday Page & Company, 1913.

McPhail C: *The Myth of the Madding Crowd.* New York, NY, Aldine de Gruyter, 1991.

Mitchell JT: *Group Crisis Support: Why It Works, When and How to Provide It.* Ellicott City, MD, Chevron Publishing Corporation, 2007.

Table 5-2 Methods for Coping With Stress

- Deal with urgent issues immediately.
- Non-urgent issues may have to wait a bit.
- Re-establish routines and schedules as soon as possible.
- Get rest when you can.
- Eat nutritious foods.
- Be cautious of fatty foods, sugar, and excessive salt.
- Limit (or eliminate) caffeine intake.
- Avoid substance abuse. (Alcohol is not your friend when it comes to stress.)
- Avoid smoking or use of tobacco products. Nicotine has a direct, negative effect on the nervous system.
- Get some physical exercise. It helps to reduce stress chemicals in the body. At the very least, take a walk.
- Keep a journal if you can. Some days are better than other days. The journal helps you to see a big picture of progress or setbacks.
- Remember, almost everyone around you is suffering from distress. At various times, most people will get a bit irritable. Try not to take it personally.
- Avoid big life changes in the midst of a crisis.
- Think things through and avoid impulsive decisions.
- Talk to people who care about you.
- Keep your mind occupied, but do not overdo it.
- Try to maintain a positive mental attitude.
- Flexibility helps in the midst of chaos.
- Avoid self-blame and guilt feelings. They almost never help.
- Disturbing thoughts, dreams, and nightmares are common in the early stages of a major situation, but usually recede over time.
- Prayer and meditation may be helpful to some.
- Reach out to help others. It often helps you.
- It is not a good idea to be alone all the time.
- Listen to others.
- Spend time with people who are worse off than you appear to be. Help them when you can.
- Let people have private time when they need it.
- Do not tell people that they are lucky. They do not feel that way. Instead, just let them know that you are sorry they are going through a bad experience.
- Serious sleep disturbances, feelings of intense sadness, uncontrollable emotions, suicidal or homicidal thoughts, and any self-destructive actions are all indications that a person needs immediate intervention. Get help, without delay.
- If things are not getting better for you, especially more than three weeks after the event, call for help from professionals. There are many things that can be done to help you.

Mitchell JT, Everly GS Jr: *Critical Incident Stress Debriefing: An Operations Manual for CISD, Defusing and Other Group Crisis Intervention Services*, ed 3. Ellicott City, MD, Chevron Publishing Corporation, 2001.

Moscovici S: *Social Influence and Social Change.* New York, NY, Academic Press, 1976.

Turner R, Killian LM: *Collective Behavior*, ed 4. Englewood Cliffs, NJ, Prentice Hall, 1993.

Prep Kit

Ready for Review

- Assessing and managing large groups of people can be challenging and unpredictable. However, by understanding the theory of how crowds react, the emergency responder can begin to prepare for the crisis at hand.

- Contagion theory is also referred to as mob rule. Basically this means that the mood or atmosphere of those involved in the event can strongly influence people to respond differently than they would as individuals.

- Convergence theory implies that like-minded people come together and form a crowd that ultimately acts on similar goals. Crowd members will then find individual leaders with the same wishes, ideas, or beliefs to help them achieve their objectives.

- Emergent-norm theory is based upon the theory that people with similar interests are drawn together and then certain behaviors emerge from the crowd itself. As a result, the rules that guide the crowd are very fluid and change as the situation evolves. At some point, everyone takes a role in the crowd, be it leader, follower, silent bystander, or opponent.

- The management of crowd scenes requires advance preparation. Emergency personnel can only be effective if organizations have spent time planning for a variety of large group scenarios. Many factors should be considered during the planning process, such as the types of crowds that may gather in your community, why they gathered and their needs, what resources are available, and how you will share information.

- Law enforcement and EMS agencies have effectively used bike teams for quick response at large gatherings. Bicycles allow for a rapid response and an ability to navigate areas where cars and ambulances cannot enter.

- During any large group event, it is important for crowds to receive information so the scene remains under control. For the optimal outcome—a safe scene—the emergency responder should follow ten basic principles to reduce tensions; information should be accurate, current, timely, concise, simple, practical, repeated, positive, given with confidence, and shared by leaders in the group.

- The Crisis Management Briefing (CMB) is a short informational meeting with the specific purpose of providing practical, stress-diminishing information to a large group of people who have already experienced, or who are about to experience, a distressing event. The emphasis of the CMB is on information, instructions, guidelines, directions, and cautions for people dealing with an upsetting or traumatic event.

Vital Vocabulary

contagion theory Crowds exert tremendous influence on individuals, causing those individuals to act quite differently in the crowd than they would as individuals; also known as mob rule.

convergence theory Like-minded people come together and form a crowd that ultimately acts on similar goals held by the individuals who make up the crowd.

Crisis Management Briefing (CMB) A meeting to present stress management information, typically to a large, mixed group of people who experienced a traumatic event. The CMB emphasizes practical, immediately useful information to manage the crisis situation. The CMB focuses on a cognitive discussion instead of an exploration of emotions. It is useful in reducing anxiety and distress in the group members.

emergent-norm theory Theory that combines factors from both the contagion and convergence theories; similar interests draw people together, and then certain behaviors emerge from the crowd itself.

information gap An uncomfortable feeling that arises when some people have information and others do not.

information push The process of providing information and direction to a crowd aiming to answer questions such as who, what, when, where, and sometimes why. This information is given in an effort to avoid stimulating addition-al unwanted emotional responses in the crowd members.

Assessment in Action

Answer key is located in the back of the book.

1. A group of individuals gather together to discuss the problems of rising crime in their community. At the meeting, the decision is made to select the local minister as the leader of the group. This is an example of which theory of crowds?

   A. Contagion
   B. Convergence
   C. Emergent-norm

2. A 6-year-old girl is hit and killed on her bike in a residential community where the posted speed is 25 mph. The driver appears to be intoxicated and was driving in excess of the speed limit. A group of neighbors and family rally together, go to his home, and assault the driver of the vehicle, rendering him uncon-scious. This is an example of which theory of crowds?

   A. Contagion
   B. Convergence
   C. Emergent-norm

3. From the following list, select the one that EMS personnel might use in the planning phase of an anticipated large gathering, such as a concert or public demonstration.

   A. The reason the crowd has gathered
   B. The type and method for disseminating information

   C. The type of people assembling at the event
   D. The attitude or mood of the crowd mem-bers when they arrive

4. Information is an important need for people involved in a crisis. From the following list, se-lect the one that is NOT an example of some-thing that would be useful for the stressed individual.

   A. An elaborate, detailed discussion of exact-ly how a rescue attempt will be accom-plished
   B. Repeating important information
   C. Practical information or tips on how they can cope or respond during the emergency
   D. Information should be presented with knowledge and confidence

5. The crisis management briefing is a short meeting which provides practical information that will help ease the attendees of some of the stress that they have experienced or will experience in the near future. During the CMB, all of the following are emphasized EXCEPT:

   A. Directions
   B. Cautions
   C. Instructions
   D. Debriefings

Chapter 6

Emergency Response to Violent Events

Muhammad Ali once said, "There are more pleasant things to do than beat up people." A quick view of television news or a reading of the daily newspapers suggests that not everyone agrees. Violence is a part of life in every country in the world. Most people will encounter violence directly or indirectly several times in their lives, and emergency personnel and crisis workers will deal frequently with situations involving violence. Thus, such workers must be aware of the potential for violence and familiar with appropriate procedures to manage violence.

Types of Violence

This chapter discusses five major categories of violence: 1) family violence, 2) school violence, 3) street violence, 4) workplace violence, and 5) violence associated with organized crime, terrorism, or war (**Figure 6-1**). Each has its own set of statistics, and each has particular factors that make crisis intervention work a little more challenging.

Family Violence

Family violence is often called domestic violence. It takes many forms, including physical, sexual, or psychological abuse of a spouse, partner, or child and neglect of family members, and it can involve incest, murder, and suicide. Family violence accounts for approximately 11% of all reported violence.

School Violence

School violence is any form of violence that occurs within an elementary or high school or in a college or university. It ranges from threats to bullying to murder, Internet crimes, vandalism, property damage, sexual harassment, assault, gang violence, attacks on faculty and staff, and suicide. Fraternity or club initiations can sometimes be considered school-based violence. About 12% of high school students reported some form of victimization at school.

Street Violence

As the name implies, street violence is any violence that occurs outside of our homes, workplaces, organizations, or social areas. Street violence includes arson, assaults, threats with a weapon, sexual

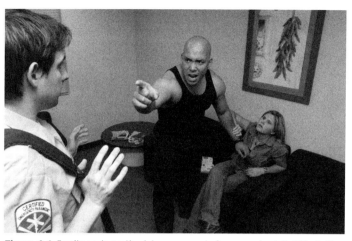

Figure 6-1 Family or domestic violence accounts for approximately 11% of all reported violence.

assault, vandalism, armed robbery, home invasions, drug violence, kidnapping, gang violence, carjacking, and murder. Federal Bureau of Investigation statistics indicate 1.4 million violent crimes occurred in the United States in 2006.

Workplace Violence

Any violence or threat of violence that occurs in the setting of someone's place of employment is classified as workplace violence. Workplace violence may include intimidation and harassment, sexual harassment, assaults, thefts, robbery, stalking, Internet crimes, vandalism, gang violence, suicide, and murder. In the United States, about 18,000 assaults occur at the workplace each week.

Violence Associated With Organized Crime, Terrorism, and War

Identity theft, arson, assault on members of certain ethnic groups, gang violence, murder, genocide, sexual assault as a terror tactic, bombs, hostage taking, torture, attacks against environmental targets, assassinations, trafficking in humans, nuclear, biological, or chemical attacks, slavery, and narco-terrorism are all examples of violence associated with organized crime, terrorism, and war.

Assessment of Violence

Violence is extremely difficult to predict; even experts with years of experience have a difficult time accurately predicting violent acts. At best, most professionals have to take their best guess and are frequently wrong. Always remain alert to the possibility of violence.

Signs of Imminent Threat

Often people mean what they say. If they make clear verbal threats, take them seriously. Violence may not be far off. The more tense a situation becomes,

In the Field

Essential Assessment Questions for Violent Situations

1. What is the category of violence (family, school, street, work, organized crime, terrorism, or war) for this particular event?
2. Is the violent event completed or ongoing?
3. Is the perpetrator still present?
4. Is there a weapon present?
5. Do law enforcement personnel need to be involved?
6. Am I, my partner, or the victims in any immediate danger?
7. Do I have at least one escape route?
8. Is anybody else in danger or at risk of being in danger?
9. Does anyone need emergency medical care?
10. Are there signs of imminent violence?

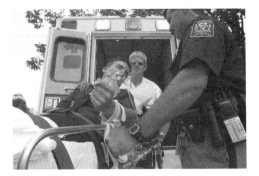

Figure 6-2 When faced with a threatening individual, personal safety must be paramount.

the greater the danger for emergency personnel. Escalating tension (increasing irritability, or hair-trigger reactions to questions or comments) is a sign of increasing danger. Sometimes an enraged person will make provocative statements or insult you in an effort to get you to strike first, so the person will feel justified in responding to the attack.

If you notice aggressive movements toward you or other crisis workers, your position is becoming more vulnerable. Try to put some distance between you and the angry person. Do this immediately and do not wait for further escalation.

Sometimes you will notice that the enraged person is spitting when he or she speaks. Other signs, including puffing one's cheeks, pounding a fist against the other hand or an object, or stomping one's feet, also represent increasing danger for the field provider. Be alert for some of the other signs of increasing rage. They include:

- Bulging neck veins
- Reddened face
- Gritted teeth
- Muscle tension around the jaw
- Threatening gestures
- Threatening posture
- Display of a weapon
- Clenched fists
- Wild or staring eyes

A person who is dangerously aroused is filled with emotional tension and more energy than he or she can control. She may pace constantly or demonstrate physical agitation. He may push an emergency services person who gets too close, slam a fist into a wall, throw something, or slam a door. The best predictor of future behavior is past history. If family members and friends report that this person has been violent in the past, especially if the violence has been frequent, then the current situation is even more threatening.

SEA-3 Evaluation for Violence

- **Speech:** Is it forced, loud, abusive, threatening, disordered, or psychotic?
- **Emotion:** Is anger, rage, fear, or phobia present?
- **Appearance:** Is anything about the appearance perceived as threatening? Is the subject disordered or disheveled? Does the person have glaring eyes or puffing cheeks? Is the person making threatening gestures or handling a weapon?
- **Awareness:** What is the person's level of consciousness and orientation to person, place, and time? Is the person aware of surroundings? Does the person give appropriate responses to questions and engage in appropriate interactions with crisis intervention personnel?
- **Activity:** Is there pacing, acting aggressive, clenching fists, or threatening gestures? Is there anything else causing you concern?

Not everyone who is violent or on the verge of violence is mentally unstable. Some people who are under extraordinary stress can become violent. Others with a metabolic imbalance or who are taking certain medications or abusing substances might also become violent. Evidence of alcohol and other substances of abuse, including anabolic steroids, especially when combined with the other signs presented in this chapter, is a particularly worrisome situation. Alcohol and many other abused substances reduce inhibitions and thus eliminate the main control system for human behavior.

General Guidelines for Managing Violence and Threats of Violence

When faced with a threatening individual, personal safety should always be paramount (**Figure 6-2**). Avoid entering a danger zone unless absolutely necessary. If you are engaged in an unexpectedly dangerous circumstance, some of the general guidelines presented in this section may help you to avoid injury and even death. Situations change rapidly, and one must be extremely alert and ready to react to escape or to protect oneself and one's colleagues.

> ## In the Field
>
> Slow down! A potentially violent situation is no time for you to rush. Move slowly, deliberately, and cautiously.

Use every available source of information before entering into a potentially dangerous situation. Listen to the dispatch and gather information from family, friends, police, and witnesses. See if there is any known history regarding the individual. Is the person saying anything or are there any noises? Can you see, hear, smell, taste, or feel anything that indicates danger for you or your crew?

Think before you do or say anything. Are there consequences or benefits to what you are about to do or say? Avoid working alone. Even if you are a police officer, it is very dangerous to be working in isolation, away from fellow emergency personnel. Stay in a safe place if you sense danger to yourself or others. Never take unnecessary risks. Do not close in, corner, threaten, challenge, or otherwise appear to be a risk to the person. Many people with violent feelings will act irrationally and dangerously if they feel pressured or trapped. Never display a weapon and do not make threats to use one; that will almost certainly intensify the situation. Aim at calming things down, not inflaming the person's feelings. Unless it is criminal in nature, most violence is defensive. If you make a verbal or symbolic threat to a person who feels overwhelmed and defensive, you can easily intensify the pressure so much that the person switches from a defensive to an offensive mode.

Decrease stimuli, such as noise, movement, and activity, in the immediate environment. Keeping your emotions under control will help the angry, upset person to calm down and will help you to think more clearly.

Look for at least one or, preferably, two escape routes. Stay close to your exit points in case violence erupts suddenly. Do not stay in a violent situation. Exit the premises immediately if violence erupts. Call for law enforcement assistance once you have moved a safe distance away. If a person becomes violent in the back of an ambulance, immediately stop the unit, turn off the engine, take the keys and portable radio, get out, and move away. Then call for help.

Verbal negotiations are important to lower tension and generate a crisis plan. Only one person at a time should negotiate with the angry, threatening, or potentially violent person. Never argue with a person who is ready and willing to hurt you; the situation is just too volatile. Furthermore, do not provoke the person by laughing, joking, or belittling, or by not taking the person seriously.

Do not lie to an angry, threatening person. The anger or rage may escalate if the person realizes you are lying. Never try to use reverse psychology, in which you say something like, "Go ahead and jump. Nobody will care." The reality is, in a high-stress emergency situation, reverse psychology fails.

Be prepared to offer food and fluids like water or fruit juice to a threatening person. Sometimes hunger may be contributing to feelings of rage. There are several important messages in providing food and nutritious fluids. The person will understand that you care about his or her welfare and is more likely to see you as a friend and not as an enemy.

If a person threatens you with a weapon and you cannot withdraw to a point of safety, let the person know that you are not there to cause harm and that there is no need for a weapon. Ask the person to put the weapon down. Do not make the weapon a focal point by concentrating only on it. Move on to other aspects of the crisis conversation and periodically request that the person put the weapon down on a table, the floor, or the ground. Never try to remove a weapon

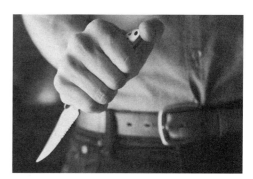

Figure 6-3 Never try to remove a weapon forcefully from a person unless you have been trained to do so.

forcefully from the person unless you have received special training to do so (**Figure 6-3**). Make sure that there is more than enough help to remove the weapon safely. If you are not a trained law enforcement officer, you should wait for law enforcement personnel to arrive to manage the situation. Removal of a weapon is not the role of the prehospital service provider.

If restraints are necessary, follow the protocols that are in effect in your local jurisdiction and use humane restraints. Once in place, it is important to keep the restraints on until the person is evaluated in controlled conditions, such as a hospital, where there is sufficient help to manage the person should the violence return.

SAFER-R Model

Using the SAFER-R model to work your way through the crisis conversation will provide you with time, information, and an opportunity to build trust with the individual in crisis. SAFER-R is a mnemonic for *Stabilize, Acknowledge, Facilitate, Encourage, Recovery,* and *Referral.*

Stabilize the situation. Remove irritating stimuli such as noise, people, and distractions. This can be accomplished by asking people to step back from the scene, turning off televisions, or moving to a different room to talk.

Acknowledge that something distressing has occurred. Recognize and acknowledge the person's anger. Think of alignment in this circumstance. <u>Alignment</u> is a crisis intervention technique in which the person attempting to help expresses understanding of the victim's situation and feelings.

The crisis worker may say something like, "I can see how you would be angry about that circumstance. You know, I would probably be angry about it myself if I were going through it. However, hurting someone is not going to help you or anyone else. Let's see if you and I can come up with some alternatives that might be helpful in resolving the situation without anyone getting hurt." The alignment occurs in two places in this example: 1) when the crisis worker says, "I would be angry about it myself if I were going through it" and 2) when the worker says, "Let's see if you and I can come up with some alternatives." Try to acknowledge your understanding of the person's position without necessarily agreeing with the person, then suggest that you team up together to accomplish the task of resolving the situation peacefully.

Facilitate the person's understanding of the situation. This will also facilitate the person's reaction to the situation. When you are able to discuss the situation calmly and discuss the person's feelings of anger while perhaps lowering the tension, the person's violent threats may subside, because the person feels listened to and understood. Most anger is time limited and, in some cases, the time it takes to listen carefully and voice your understanding may be all that is necessary to remove some of the tension from the situation.

Encourage the person to make an acceptable plan of action. Then implement the plan as quickly as possible. Depending on the circumstances, something like this might help. "Okay, I understand how angry you are and how you want to pay that person back for what he did to you, but hurting someone is only going to get you into deep trouble. Why not walk out with us now rather than have the police involved? You do not want your neighbors to see you struggling with some police officers when you could walk out to the ambulance with us. That way, no one gets hurt and you keep your dignity. Wouldn't you rather handle things that way?"

The rational approach is often helpful, but not always. Sometimes things go badly and the police must be involved to contain the situation. However, rational negotiation and encouragement is worth a try in most cases.

Recovery is evident. The person you are trying to work with is calming down and not as threatening as he or she was when you first arrived. The individual appears to be cooperating with the crisis action plan that you helped to develop with the distressed individual. It is clear that the person is making positive efforts, and progress toward resolution of the state of crisis is evident. As long as no crimes have been committed and the person is cooperating with the crisis plan, law enforcement personnel may not be required.

In a few situations, the crisis reaction may be resolved and the emergency personnel can disengage from the situation and depart from the scene. This is especially so if helpful family members, friends, clergy, or other resources are ready to continue to support the distressed person and help the person to complete the recovery process.

Referral to additional sources of help. It is certainly encouraging that some people may have calmed down with the assistance of crisis intervention personnel. It is a relief when they are calm, cooperating, and pose no immediate threat. If you suspect that the calm is a temporary condition and that the person may still require further evaluation, do not hesitate to refer him or her or transport the person to the hospital. It is quite possible that a few people will be unable to control themselves despite your best efforts. They require further evaluation, medical care, or medications. The closest hospital is usually the best referral for anyone who needs more assistance beyond that delivered by crisis intervention workers. After initial evaluation, the local emergency department can refer the patient to the appropriate facility for additional care.

If a person continues to threaten violence or act in a violent manner, then crisis intervention personnel have no choice but to call in law enforcement personnel to assist in bringing the person under control. This is especially so if there is imminent threat to the person or to someone else.

Assisting the Victims of Violence

The number of violent events each year in the United States is staggering. A woman is battered every nine seconds. There are 4 million cases of battering a year. About 600,000 cases of sexual assault occur each year. Approximately 2 million youths are arrested each year for violent crimes. Firearm-related deaths of youths 15 years of age or less are 12 times higher in the United States than in 25 other industrialized nations. Firearms kill about 12 young people below age 19 years day in the United States. There are 89 suicides in the United States each day, and more than 32,000 each year.

When the violent act has already occurred, you will most likely be dealing with the victims or witnesses to the violence. Many, but not all, perpetrators leave the scene after an act of violence. Do not become complacent and let your guard down. There have been cases in which the perpetrator remained nearby or returned to inflict additional injury on the victim. In such cases, the rescuers may be in grave jeopardy as well. Many perpetrators have opened up the back of the ambulance or entered the emergency department to continue the violence.

Genuine care and concern and a careful, courteous management of the person are the most important aspects of crisis intervention for a victim of violence. There are several important steps to keep in mind when assisting victims of violence.

First, make sure that the victim is either safe or that he or she is removed quickly to a safe location. Do not promise things you cannot control, such as "Don't worry, he won't come back." You cannot say that with absolute certainty. Therefore it is better not to say it at all.

Second, call for law enforcement. Avoid touching or moving items at the location. Remember, you are working within a crime scene. Everything you touch or move creates difficulties for law enforcement personnel. Be careful where you step. If you can remove the person from the crime scene before providing emergency medical care to prevent the destruction of evidence, do so. If the injuries are too severe to move the person, be as careful in the scene as possible. When you place the patient onto your stretcher, recognize that the ambulance sheet may contain important evidence (hair, paint tracings, fibers related to the crime, and body fluids) for the police. There have been cases in which bullets and small weapons have been found under the patient once they were moved over to the hospital stretcher.

Law enforcement personnel need to make vulnerability assessments to determine whether the victim is in danger of a repeat attack. Steps must be taken to protect and assist the victim if the dangers are likely to continue in the future (stalking cases would exemplify this condition).

Third, provide medical assessment and treatment. Assess injuries and provide emergency medical care. First aid must sometimes wait until you ensure the person's safety. Every person has his or her own personal emotional and psychological reactions to a violent episode. Do not expect that everyone will react in the same manner. Be careful not to casually touch the assaulted victim. The victim may feel uncomfortable with touching from a helper unless it is medically necessary. Let the person know what steps will be taken to help him or her and make sure that he or she is willing to be touched.

Informed people appreciate your efforts and become less resistant to treatment. Remove only as much clothing as necessary to provide medical care. Do not strip the clothing off a victim of violence unless it is contaminated with some dangerous substance.

After providing medical care, take care of non-medical physical and social needs. Ask if there is anyone the victim wants notified or called to the victim's location. Be aware of and sensitive to cultural differences. Support religious needs of victims. Call for clergy if the victim requests that service. Do not try to cheer up a victim of violence by lighthearted conversation or jokes. Violence victims do not find much humor in their circumstances. This type of behavior is likely to be interpreted as uncaring and unprofessional.

Allow survivors to tell their stories at their own pace. Show concern, warmth, and caring. If the patient is a victim of a crime, do not encourage the victim to disclose a great deal of detail about the event; the detailed discussions should be reserved for law enforcement personnel. If you allow a victim to say too much about the experience, he or she may be angry when the law enforcement officer has to ask for the same information. Allowing too much discussion before law enforcement is involved causes confusion, mistrust, and anger.

Remember that what a victim tells you is confidential; protect that information. Each person has a right to privacy. However, last-minute statements prior to the death of a patient must be documented and reported to police. They can often provide the name or information about the perpetrator.

In many cases, the first person to assist the victim of violence must gather some important information about the perpetrator. Ask the victim if he or she knows who did this. Try to obtain a brief description of the suspect. The type and color of clothing may be very helpful as is information about gender, race, and use of a weapon. Determine the direction of flight from the crime scene. Give this information to the police as soon as possible. If possible, transmit crucial information via radio communications while the police are responding to the scene; police may notice a suspect fitting the description given by emergency medical person and be able to apprehend the suspect.

Child Victims

According to the US Department of Health and Human Services, child protective services in the United States received over 3.6 million maltreatment referrals in 2006, involving over 6 million children, and 25.2% of these are substantiated as significant threats or actual injuries to children. There were more than 1 million cases of abused and neglected children in 2006, and the numbers vary only slightly each year. Parents and legal guardians were responsible for 82.4% of the emotional and physical neglect of children. In addition, family members are responsible for the deaths of nearly 5% of all murdered youths (about 1,530 in 2006) in the United States.

Violent situations that involve children are always challenging and can result in chaos at the emergency scene. Children and families can be emotionally traumatized simply by the exposure to the scene of violence (**Figure 6-4**). The presence of police, fire, and EMS can scare children and make them afraid of care providers. The response of children can vary, depending upon their age, environment, and home situation. Listed below are some tips for managing children at the scene of violence.

1. *Remove the child from the threatening or violent situation and away from seriously wounded or dead people.* Ensure that the child is safe. Regroup children with trusted adults as quickly as possible. Whenever possible, keep family units together. Try to find someone the child knows and trusts, even if it is not a family member. This arrangement is temporary until responsible, caring family members can be located. Safety, shelter, food, fluids, reconnection to family, and emotional support are a high priority in dealing with child victims or witnesses to violence.

2. *If the child is injured, emergency medical care is essential.* Remember to direct your assessment and care based on the child's developmental age. Be gentle and talk calmly and softly, but loud enough to be heard by the child. Bend down or sit so that you are at or close to eye level with the child. When young children are anxious and upset, they may revert to behaviors more appropriate for younger children. Most children cry or show their distress. Accept this as normal behavior under highly distressing circumstances.

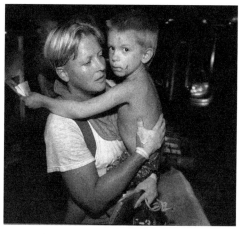

Figure 6-4 Remove the child from the threatening or violent situation whenever possible.

3. *Provide information.* Children need and want information about what happened and about what you or others are doing about it. Be honest with children and attempt to answer their questions, but do not share too much and overload them with detail. If they keep asking for more information, they probably need more information. Address and correct rumors and false alarm issues. Listen to children speak before you try to explain things to them.

4. *Be caring and reassuring.* Children often mirror the reaction of their parents to violent traumatic events. Instruct the parents to try to remain calm and under control. Make sure you remain calm and controlled yourself. This is especially important if the parents are injured and unable to care for the child or if they are absent for some reason. Young children often need holding and hugs when they are distressed. Let children know that it is normal to feel confused, sad, frightened, or anxious and that adults feel those things as well. Be reassuring that those feelings will get better when the situation becomes more controlled and time goes by.

5. *Communicate with children in ways they can understand.* Be kind and reassuring with distressed children. Adults need to hear children speak of their experiences, but children do not need excessive details concerning the experiences of adults.

Do not try to keep everything secret from children. It is an impossible task, and children know that something bad has happened. They may not know the details, but they can tell by the reactions of the adults around them that things are not going well. Let children know that someone will take care of them during and after the situation. The challenge in working with children is to acknowledge that a bad thing has happened and then to be reassuring and encouraging in a manner that avoids stirring greater distress in the children.

Let children know that even though their parents are upset, scared, or sad, their parents can still take good care of them. Children need to be included in any family recovery process. They have genuine anxieties, fears, and reactions to violence and need plenty of support to manage their crisis reactions.

When a child witnesses violence against a family member, he or she is likely to be extremely distressed. The serious injury or the death of a parent is particularly upsetting. Children should be removed from traumatic scenes as quickly as possible. Someone should be assigned to stay with and care for the child until the other parent or an appropriate family member is located and brought to the child.

If the child has been abused by his or her parents, the child should remain in the care of medical or social service agencies until appropriate caretakers can be identified. Obviously children are not returned to the care of the abuser(s) until the environment is rendered harmless. Field personnel should remove abused children to the care of a hospital emergency department. There are legal reporting requirements in every U.S. state and within the legal codes of many other nations. Report all child abuse cases to the law enforcement authorities. In turn, those agencies typically bring the cases to the attention of the social service agencies, which then take on the responsibility of finding safe shelter and appropriate care for the children.

If emergency personnel are treating a child and they begin to suspect child abuse, they should report it to the hospital authorities or to law enforcement personnel immediately. In most cases social service agencies review the cases and determine if the children are under actual threat.

Final Thoughts

Emergency personnel cannot prevent all acts of violence or cure all of the ills that violence causes. However, crisis workers can provide help to people who have experienced violence. These efforts may help some people avoid violence. Skilled, sensitive care may mitigate some of the effects of violence on family members, bystanders, and others.

Selected References

Carll EK: *Trauma Psychology: Issues in Violence, Disaster, Health, and Illness, Vol 1, Violence and Disaster.* Westport, CT, Praeger Publishers, 2007.

Carll EK: *Trauma Psychology: Issues in Violence, Disaster, Health, and Illness, Vol 2, Health and Illness.* Westport, CT, Praeger Publishers, 2007.

Davies J: *Confidentiality and Information Sharing Issues for Domestic Violence Advocates Working With Child Protection and Juvenile Court Systems.* Washington, DC, National Council of Juvenile and Family Court Judges, 2000.

Forster EM: *Howard's End.* London, England, Edward Arnold Publishers, 1910.

Gibson M: *Order From Chaos: Responding to Traumatic Events.* ed 3 rev. Bristol, England, The Policy Press, 2006.

Hogan LJ (ed): *Terrorism: Defensive Strategies for Individuals, Companies and Governments.* Frederick, MD, Amlex Inc, 2001.

Krebs DR: *When Violence Erupts: A Survival Guide for Emergency Responders.* Sudbury, MA, Jones & Bartlett Publishers, 2003.

Mitchell JT: *The Quick Series Guide to Suicide Prevention.* Fort Lauderdale, FL, Luxart Communications, 2004–2006.

Mitchell JT, Resnik HLP: *Emergency Response to Crisis.* Bowie, MD, Robert J Brady Company, 1981.

Patterson WM, Dohn HH, Bird J, Patterson GA: Evaluation of suicidal patients: the SAD PERSON Scale. *Psychosomatics,* 1983;24:343–349.

Roberts AR: *Crisis Intervention Handbook: Assessment, Treatment, and Research,* ed 3. New York, NY, Oxford University Press, 2005.

Rosenburg MB: *Nonviolent Communication: A Language of Life,* ed 2. Encinitas, CA, PuddleDancer Press, 2005.

Tunnecliffe M: *A Life in Crisis: 27 Lessons From Acute Trauma Counseling Work.* Palmyra, Australia, Bayside Books, 2007.

US Department of Health and Human Services, Administration for Children and Families, Administration on Children Youth and Families Children's Bureau: Child Maltreatment 2006. Available at: http://www.acf.hhs.gov/programs/cb/pubs/cm06/index.htm. Accessed April 15, 2008.

US Department of Health and Human Services: *Identifying and Responding to Domestic Violence: Consensus Recommendations for Child and Adolescent Health.* Washington, DC, DHHS, Office for Victims of Crime, 2004.

US Department of Health and Human Services: *Recovering Your Mental Health, Dealing With the Effects of Trauma: A Self-Help Guide.* Washington, DC, DHHS, Substance Abuse and Mental Health Services Administration, 2005.

US Department of Health and Human Services: *Communicating in a Crisis: Risk Communication Guidelines for Public Officials.* Washington, DC, DHHS, 2002, 2006.

US Department of Justice: *Juvenile Offenders and Victims: 2006 National Report.* Washington, DC, US Department of Justice, Office of Justice Programs, National Center for Juvenile Justice, 2006.

US Department of Justice Programs: *Extent, Nature, and Consequences of Rape Victimization: Findings From the National Violence Against Women Survey.* Washington, DC, National Institute of Justice, 2006.

Prep Kit

Ready for Review

- There are five categories of violence discussed in this chapter: family or domestic, school, street, workplace, and those acts associated with organized crime, terrorism, or war.

- Each year, an astounding number of individuals in the United States are affected by some type of violent event. Emergency responders are often the first on the scene and can be instrumental in beginning the recovery process for the victim, both medically and psychologically.

- The safety of the emergency responder is paramount. Care cannot be provided if you also become a victim. Always wait until police have secured the scene before responding to the location. In some cases, you should wait a substantial distance away until law enforcement officers on location give permission to enter the scene.

- In threatening or volatile environments, it may be necessary to load the patient into the ambulance immediately and move to a new location to begin care.

- The concept of alignment is often successful in working with violent individuals as you try to express your understanding of their situation and feelings.

- Working with children at the scene of violence is often very challenging and stressful for all parties involved. Because children follow the cues of their parents and other persons of authority, it is important to make every effort to remain calm and professional at all times. Your composure will reassure children that they are safe and that you are someone to be trusted.

Vital Vocabulary

alignment A crisis intervention technique in which the person attempting to help expresses understanding of the person's situation and feelings.

domestic violence See family violence.

family violence Includes physical, sexual, or psychological abuse of a spouse, partner, or child and neglect of family members. It can involve incest, murder, and suicide.

school violence Any form of violence that occurs within the school system, including elementary, middle, or high schools and colleges or universities. The violent acts can include threats to murder, bullying, Internet crimes, vandalism, property damage, sexual harassment, assault, gang violence, attacks on faculty and staff, and suicide.

street violence Any form of violence that occurs outside of homes, workplaces, organizations, or social areas. The violent acts can include arson, assaults, threats with a weapon, sexual assault, vandalism, armed robbery, home invasions, drug violence, kidnapping, gang violence, carjacking, and murder.

violence associated with organized crime, terrorism, or war Any form of violence involving organized crime groups, acts of terrorism, or war. The acts of violence can include identity theft, arson, assault on members of certain ethnic groups, gang violence, murder, genocide, sexual assault as a terror tactic, bombs, hostage takings, torture, attacks against environmental targets, assassinations, trafficking in humans, nuclear, biological, or chemical attacks, slavery, or narco-terrorism.

workplace violence Any form of violence or threat of violence that occurs in the setting of someone's place of employment is classified as workplace violence, such as intimidation, harassment, assaults, thefts, robbery, stalking, Internet crimes, vandalism, suicide, or murder.

Assessment in Action

Answer key is located in the back of the book.

1. A 4-year-old girl witnessed the brutal death of a neighbor in front of her home during a drug deal. From the following list, select the one that best describes the little girl's response.

   A. She will be scared and cling to her mother.
   B. She is not going to want to know what happened.

Prep Kit | continued

C. She is not going to understand what occurred.

D. She will grow up always living in fear of her neighborhood.

2. You respond to a domestic scene where a husband has stabbed his wife with a kitchen knife. Upon arrival you find that the husband has fled the scene and that the wife has minor defensive wounds to her hands and arms. She states that her husband said he was "going to get a gun and come back and kill her." What is the MOST appropriate action for you at this time?

A. Notify the police that the perpetrator has left and that the scene is secure.

B. Dress her wounds with sterile gauze and wait for the police to arrive.

C. Lock the apartment doors and wait for the police to arrive, during which you can conduct a detailed survey and provide treatment.

D. Quickly dress her wounds and move promptly to the ambulance. Then lock the patient compartment door and drive to the hospital, notifying police of your destination.

3. All of the following are indicators of potential violent patients EXCEPT:

A. Aggressive actions such as stomping of the feet or puffing out of the cheeks.

B. Spitting at the provider.

C. Cursing or degrading comments toward the EMT or police.

D. All of the above are indicators.

4. Aggressive actions such as hitting a wall, threatening EMS providers, repeated gestures, and pacing represent which component of the SEA-3 evaluation for potentially violent patients?

A. Activity

B. Emotion

C. Appearance

D. Awareness

5. The removal of irritating stimuli, such as noise, loud music, or family members, best represents which component of the SAFER-R model for potentially violent patients?

A. Acknowledgment

B. Stabilization

C. Encouragement

D. Facilitation

Chapter 7

Suicide: An Extraordinary Case of Violence

In the novel, *Howard's End,* E. M. Forster wrote, "The crime of suicide lies in its disregard for the feelings of those whom we leave behind." <u>Suicide</u> is likely to leave loved ones, professionals, and crisis intervention personnel with many disturbed feelings and a long list of unanswerable questions. Around the world, about a million people a year take their own lives. Teenagers and young adults, ages 15 to 24 years, are the most vulnerable (**Figure 7-1**). All suicides are difficult for family members as well as for people who work in crisis intervention and emergency services. The self-inflicted deaths of young people can be particularly distressing for everyone.

Why Do People Commit Suicide?

There is rarely one single reason why individuals choose to end their lives. The reports from most people who have attempted to commit suicide but survived to share their experiences generally confirm that a combination of forces drive people toward this drastic, final, and permanent solution to what is typically a temporary problem. There are many factors that contribute to suicide. <u>Hopelessness</u> coupled with feelings of <u>helplessness</u>, <u>haplessness</u>, and <u>worthlessness</u> are the most common recurring themes in first-hand reports from survivors of suicide attempts.

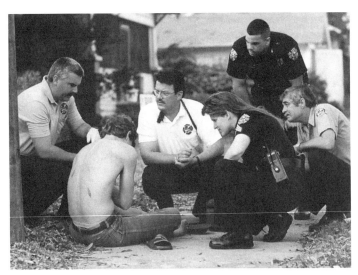

Figure 7-1 Teenagers and young adults are the most vulnerable to suicide.

Isolation, social problems, and loneliness are very closely associated with psychological depression, and depression is a key underlying factor in the majority of suicides. Add alcohol or substance abuse to the feelings of hopelessness, isolation, guilt, loneliness, and depression, and the potential for suicide increases dramatically. Alcohol and other abused drugs diminish a person's capacity for rational thought as well as mental and emotional inhibiting mechanisms. In addition, some prescription medications can increase the risks of suicide, even when the medications are taken properly.

Suicide is often triggered by intense personal loss, like the death of a loved one. Other triggers include the end of a relationship or struggles with sexual identity. Some teenagers, and even adults, react so strongly to public humiliation or embarrassment that they contemplate suicide. For example, if a person is arrested and therefore humiliated before family and friends, that person might conclude that suicide is the only way out of the emotional pain caused by the public humiliation.

Financial problems, legal issues, significant illness, divorce, retirement, and being fired from one's job are all factors that generate an enormous amount of stress. People have less-clear thinking processes and may feel emotionally overwhelmed when they are stressed or frustrated. As a result, they may think that suicide would make all of their frustrations and stresses go away. They are unable to consider the devastating impact of their actions on their loved ones or may even believe that their loved ones would be better off without them.

Chronic mental problems such as depression, schizophrenia, bipolar disorder, or post-traumatic stress disorder (PTSD) can all contribute to suicide. All of these disorders can be characterized by disordered thinking. Some disorders, particularly schizophrenic conditions, can cause hallucinations, including hallucinations that someone is telling the person to kill himself or herself. PTSD can include vividly reliving traumatic events, including events when the person was in danger, which can cause the person to believe the surrounding environment is posing threats; this is particularly problematic for people who have experienced war and for people who have been assaulted.

When combinations of the above factors are present, people may move from general and unfocused <u>suicidal thoughts</u>, or <u>suicidal ideation</u> of suicide, to <u>suicidal gestures</u>. Suicidal gestures are actions that indicate that one is considering suicide. Examples include taking a tiny amount of a prescription drug or writing a suicide note to show to friends and family to get their attention. Another gesture is making non-lethal hand signals that indicate that one is thinking of suicide, such as pointing to one's head with an imaginary gun.

Early assessment of potential suicides is important. It should be done before the progression from thoughts about suicide to suicidal gestures can move into the suicidal actions that are classified as <u>suicide attempts</u>. Emergency personnel should listen carefully and try to determine if the person is suicidal (**Figure 7-2**). Do not ignore hints that indicate a suicide attempt is being planned. The objective when one suspects that suicide is being considered is to get the person to a professional who can further evaluate the person and decide if the person

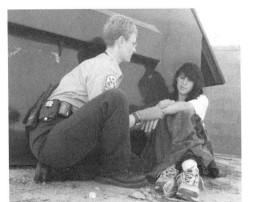

Figure 7-2 Listen carefully to patients who may be suicidal.

needs to be in a treatment program. The person typically needs professional support, but that is always
determined by mental health professionals, not by
field personnel.

> **Four Steps Toward Suicide**
> - Ideation or thoughts about suicide
> - Suicidal gestures
> - Suicide attempts
> - Completion of the suicide

Some people skip the suicidal gestures and
move directly into suicide attempts. The person who
is contemplating suicide may take one or more deliberate actions that are dangerous and possibly lethal.
If we took every suicidal gesture or attempt seri-
ously and referred people for professional help, many people might decide not to take the final step
toward suicide. Transfer the person to the hospital. Alert hospital personnel about your suspicions
and suggest that a psychiatric consult might be helpful. What you do not say in a case of suspected
suicide potential can be harmful or can possibly result in a loss of life.

The final step in the progression that ends in a self-inflicted death is the <u>suicide completion</u>.
Crisis intervention efforts prior to the completion of a suicide aim at prevention. Once a suicide is
completed, crisis intervention efforts must then focus on the support of family, friends, and colleagues who will suffer the long-term effects of the loss.

Suicide Assessment: When Suicide Is Possible or Threatened

The process of assessing the patient for suicidal thoughts is a complex one that can be made more
complicated by the presence of underlying medical or psychological conditions. The emergency
provider's goal is to perform a quick, yet thorough, assessment (see Chapter 3 and the section
below) and transport the patient to the most appropriate facility. In most cases, the best place to
transport the person is to the hospital.

Take every suicidal threat or gesture seriously. Never disregard a direct or overt suicidal
statement such as "I want to die." Usually a person's discussion of suicidal thinking will be less
obvious. These less-than-obvious suicidal indicators are called covert indicators of suicidal threat.
They can include actions as well as words. Giving away cherished possessions, buying a handgun,
and saying things like "No one would miss me if I went away" all fall under covert indicators.

After introducing yourself, begin your assessment. Talk to the person and ask questions
about the person. Be respectful, kind, caring, and empathetic. Keep your voice calm; do not rush
the discussion. Accept and validate any emotions the person may express. Do not think that you
will cause a person to make a suicide attempt just because you are talking to him or her. In fact,
an open discussion about suicide may be a relief to the person who is contemplating it. The person is in emotional pain and the more comfortable and confident you seem, the greater the chance
is that the person will talk to you and work with you to resolve his or her crisis. Find out about
recent and past history and anything that was particularly distressing that led the person to think
that suicide was his or her best option.

Being confident is important, but never allow yourself to become too self-assured. It is foolish
to think everything is fine and under control just because you are present. Do not take unnecessary
risks. For example, lock yourself onto a ladder when working with a person at a height above the
ground; a suicidal person can easily turn homicidal if the person makes up his or her mind to commit suicide and can easily take you with him or her if you just happen to be in the way.

The usual order of questions to a potentially suicidal person is as follows:

1. **Recent history**. "Why did you call the ambulance today? Can you tell me about what has
   happened today to make you feel this way? Can you describe your feelings right now?"

2. **Past history.** "It would help me to understand what you are going through if you can tell me when you started feeling this way. What is the history of this situation?"

3. **Direct questions about suicide.** "It sounds to me that you are under enormous stress right now. Sometimes when people are under stress they think of harming or killing themselves. Are you having any thoughts like that? Do you know anyone who has taken his or her own life?"

4. **Suicide plan.** "You just mentioned that you sometimes think of killing yourself. Do you have a plan in mind for killing yourself?"

5. **Availability and lethality of method.** "You said that you would probably just take some pills or use a gun. Do you have a gun in the house or a supply of medications?"

6. **Alternatives that might keep you safe.** "What would have to change to prevent you from taking your own life? How about if we considered together some alternatives that might work for you? Let's work together on this." You can also ask the person to promise not to commit suicide without first calling for help.

You can ask many questions in each segment of the interview. You do not have to stick with the examples shown above. Every case will be a little different. What works one time may not work the next. You may have to adjust as the person provides information about his or her feelings and intentions. Direct questions about one's suicide potential are the best route. Avoiding the issue altogether gives the impression that you are uncomfortable with the topic. If that is the case, the person will not want to talk to you and will suppress his or her true feelings. It is important that you acknowledge and validate the person's feelings.

If you determine that the person has an event or a situation that is causing hopeless, helpless, hapless, and worthless feelings and that the person is contemplating suicide, then you must consider the *plan, method,* and *lethality.* The more detailed the plan, the more lethal the method, and the more available the means of suicide, the greater is the threat.

If you are having a hard time remaining objective in the case of a suicide threat, let someone else take over the negotiations. Hints that you are having trouble in the communications include getting emotional, getting distracted, losing focus in the discussion, and having distressing thoughts of someone you knew personally who committed suicide.

People are not permanently suicidal. In most cases, the suicidal threat declines over time. The immediate impulse can diminish in as little as 45 minutes. The first 24 to 72 hours tend to be the most dangerous time because the person is in a heightened state of agitation and thinking processes are impaired.

There are a few factors that can help you in your efforts to save the person's life. One is time. The longer you can keep the person from taking any self-destructive actions, the greater is the chance that he or she will not commit suicide. Also working in your favor is a condition called *ambivalence.* Ambivalence in a suicide situation means that a person is unsure if he or she really wants to die. Many people do not want to die as much as they want the pain of their situation to end; they believe that suicide is the only way to end the pain. Such confusion may allow the person to calm down and think more clearly. People may then find options that they were having trouble seeing when they were most upset. The mobilization of various resources to help the person is also useful. When family and friends gather around and support the person, he or she may lose the desire to kill himself or herself. Therefore, never remain the only one helping. Do not promise not to tell anyone else. You need resources to complete the assessment and to move the person toward professional therapy. Work toward getting appropriate resources lined up. Promising not to tell anyone defeats the main objective of preventing the suicide.

Cues to Suicide

While not all suicides can be predicted, the majority will have some similar characteristics or cues that might be recognized by friends and family. Be sure to ask those who know the person best if they have witnessed any of the following cues.

Overt Clues to Suicide

Overt clues to suicide suggest more immediate threat and require immediate action. Overt clues include:

- Making funeral arrangements for oneself and letting people know about the details of those arrangements
- Buying a weapon
- Telling someone that he or she wants to die and having a plan to commit suicide; the greater the detail of the plan, the more imminent the suicide
- "Practicing" a suicide
- Feelings of extreme frustration with everyday issues
- Feeling extremely sad, confused, despairing (loss of meaning for life), or upset

Crisis intervention is necessary when there are overt clues. "Practicing" includes behaviors like loading a gun and pointing at oneself or climbing to a height and standing on the edge to see what it might feel like to begin the final act. People expressing feelings of extreme frustration with everyday issues are usually agitated, are obviously upset, and may appear driven or on a mission; any attempt to discuss things with them is usually rejected, and they are unusually angry and react vigorously to slight stimuli such as questions from a friend or relative.

The intensity of the emotions suggests that the person is in immediate threat, and crisis intervention personnel must work to quickly reduce the tension and bring the person to a hospital where assessment and professional care can be started. Be aware that some people may be much less agitated or obviously upset; many people experience a deadening of emotions and a feeling of being outside themselves or disconnected from family and friends.

Covert Clues to Suicide

Covert clues to suicide are more difficult to interpret, but may eventually lead to suicide, especially if combined with many clues over time. Covert clues include:

- Drinking excessively or using other substances of abuse
- Increase in risk-taking activities
- Expressing feelings of loneliness, isolation, hopelessness, helplessness, haplessness, and worthlessness
- Spending excessively, beyond what one can afford
- Loss of clear, logical thinking; very rigid thinking; loss of positive thinking and a sense of no future
- Heightened anxiety and expressions of worry and concern or difficulties making every-day decisions
- Feelings of rejection
- Changes in personality, including lowered job performance, loss of interest in things that used to be fun or exciting, and giving away prized possessions
- Sleep disturbance
- Deteriorating personal hygiene, such as cessation of bathing or shaving or dirty hands and face

SAD PERSONS

Sex: Males are more likely to commit suicide than females.

Age: The age group with the highest risk is 15- to 24-year-olds.

Depression: Depression is present in the majority of cases.

Previous exposure: Knowing someone who committed suicide or previous attempts increase the risk.

Ethanol (alcohol) or drug abuse: Drug use lowers inhibitions and may increase depression.

Rational thinking: The person's ability to think rationally is impaired.

Social support: A person with few social supports has higher risks.

Organized plan: A person who has put together a plan is at higher risk.

No spouse or significant other: People who are single are a higher risk.

Sickness: Illness or injury, especially if chronic, increases the risk.

Covert clues may include saying things like, "I can't take any more. Nothing works for me. Everything keeps going wrong. I don't see any way out of this mess."

The SAD PERSONS Checklist

Suicide assessment can be very complex and detailed. The mnemonic SAD PERSONS helps crisis personnel determine if someone is a significant threat to himself or herself.

Crisis Intervention in Cases of Suicide

Your immediate goal is to reduce the risk of suicide and to move the person who is contemplating suicide toward professional help. Do not be afraid to bring up the issue of suicide and to discuss it openly. A suicidal person feels supported if the issue is addressed as part of a normal conversation; the person feels that the crisis worker has heard the cry for help. Be calm and do not sound shocked that the person is thinking about suicide. Take your time when speaking with a suicidal person. Rushing will not help the individual, it will only intensify the pressure. Remember that you cannot solve all the problems; your goal is crisis intervention. Trying to solve all of the issues that led the person to this point is an unrealistic goal.

It is helpful to emphasize the temporary nature of the problem and that it would be a tragic mistake to take such a drastic final action for a problem that can be solved by other means. Try to get the person to explore other possible options, including going to the emergency department for evaluation and help.

Do not argue with the person. It is an argument that you will not win. Instead, accept the feelings expressed. Acceptance is not the same as agreement. Acceptance means that you can understand the person's point of view, not that you agree with the person's choice of suicide. If you agreed, you would not be making efforts to save the person's life.

A suicidal person may ask that you promise not to tell anyone else about his or her desire to commit suicide. Never agree to keep the person's suicidal threat to yourself. Simply state the fact that you must get appropriate help for the person and that can only be done by letting some key people know that their assistance is required. You do not want to be the only person helping in a suicidal crisis. That burden must be shared with others; it is too much for one person to bear. Remember, your primary aim is to negotiate the suicidal person into accepting professional medical and psychological assistance.

Once you begin to work with a suicidal person, you cannot leave him or her alone, even for a moment. You and other emergency workers can only disengage from the person when you have delivered the person into the care of medical or mental health professionals. If, while you are working with a suicidal person in a state of crisis, the suicidal threat escalates and appears imminent, you should make every reasonable effort to prevent the suicide. That includes calling in the police and having the person taken to a hospital even against his or her will (**Figure 7-3**).

At the same time, always be aware of the intensified dangers to rescuers who attempt to stop a suicide in progress; do not take unnecessary risks.

   If a suicide attempt has occurred before you arrived, treat the person medically and notify the police. The person should be brought to a hospital for further medical and psychiatric evaluation. The person will require psychiatric intervention to resolve the issues that led to the suicide attempt.

Steps to Safety for People Threatening Suicide

Helping a suicidal person is not an easy task. It takes time, emotional energy, excellent listening skills, and a genuine concern for a troubled person. The outline below presents ten steps required to bring a suicidal person to safety.

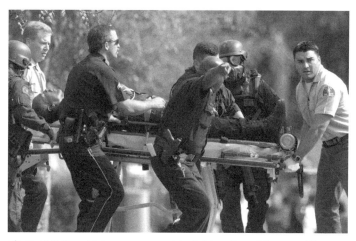

Figure 7-3 Do not take unnecessary risks. Call in police reinforcement if you feel that the person is a danger to self, others, or emergency personnel.

   1. *Secure the environment.* Eliminate or reduce stimuli or distractions. Remove unhelpful people or anyone who provokes the person from the area. Confine the person to a single room if possible. Turn off radios, televisions, and stereos. Keep your own communications radio at a low volume, but keep it available in case you need to call for assistance. Except for your partner or one or two appropriate emergency personnel, do not permit people to enter and leave the room in which you are talking with the suicidal person.

   2. *Develop trust and rapport.* Treat the person as a human being who needs understanding and assistance. Address the person by name. Avoid sarcastic remarks, and do not joke with the person. Take the information about the person's problems, fears, and anxieties seriously.

   3. *Engage in a thorough risk assessment.* Ask if the person is suicidal. Ask about plan, methods, and means. Ask about previous attempts. The SAD PERSONS guide will be helpful in remembering which questions to ask.

   4. *Develop a greater understanding of the person and the issues that led up to the current situation.* Once you have a grasp of the current situation, ask some questions about the recent past and what might have contributed to the current problem.

   5. *Keep the focus on the main problem.* The idea is to expand your understanding of the person but not to probe for unnecessary details. You only need those details that relate to the current crisis.

   6. *Explore alternatives to suicide.* A suicidal person often develops tunnel vision and may have trouble thinking about different approaches to his or her problems. Start expanding the list of alternative actions by asking the person if he or she has any idea what will be helpful right now. If the person cannot come up with any possible alternatives, you can suggest several things that might be helpful. They will probably be rejected, but do not give up. Talk to the person a little more. Ask a few more questions and then bring up another suggestion or two. With gentle persistence you may be able to get the person to cooperate with a plan to step back a little from rigid thinking.

   7. *Select the best option from the available alternatives.* Sometimes you may have to negotiate partial arrangements because you cannot obtain complete cooperation with a set of alternatives. For example, you may first work on getting a suicidal person to sit down so that the immediate danger of falling from a high place is reduced. Next you may get the person to accept some food. When you can convince the person to trust you and accept food, you further reduce the danger of an impulsive action. As blood sugar goes up a little, thinking usually improves.

8. *Develop a practical action plan.* The plan should include going to the hospital with EMS or family members. As the suicidal person develops a few alternatives, such as going with you to the hospital and agreeing to counseling, you will need to build in some details. For instance, you will need the person to put down a weapon or step away from a danger zone and walk toward a safety zone. Then you will need to talk with the person about the steps necessary to get to a place where the person can receive help. The steps the person must take may entail lying on the ambulance cot and being moved to the ambulance, or the police may need to speak with the person. Some jurisdictions require a police officer to accompany the suicidal person to a hospital. In some cases the person may insist upon walking out of the area. Everything can be negotiated, and hard and fast rules may need to be altered. The key objective always remains getting the person to safety and to professional care.

9. *Implement the crisis action plan immediately.* Tell the patient what you are doing as you do it. "John, it is now time to put that action plan we were just discussing into play. The first thing we are going to do is go downstairs. A police officer will speak with you for a few minutes. Remember, they have to do that, and they are not there to hurt you. I will stay with you, as I promised, until you are safely in the hospital. When the officer finishes speaking with you, you will go to an ambulance. The police officer may come with us to the hospital. When we get to the hospital I will introduce you to the nurse and let the person know a little about what you have been going through. The people at the hospital will then check on your physical condition and find the right kind of help for you. Okay? Alright, let's move toward the stairs now."

10. *Refer the patient to the emergency department.* The person will need evaluation and professional treatment.

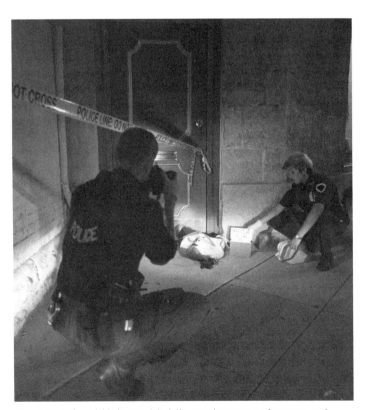

Figure 7-4 If a suicide is completed, the area becomes a crime scene and should be treated as such.

Managing the Completed Suicide

When suicide occurs in a community, family members and friends are thrust into profound shock, confusion, and grief. The emergency worker may find himself or herself dealing with the survivors rather than with someone who is contemplating suicide. The following suggestions may guide crisis personnel in their efforts to alleviate the distressed loved ones.

First Contact With the Situation

If a suicide is completed in your presence, call the police if they are not already on the way and keep the victim's family, friends, and colleagues from entering the area. You now have a crime scene on your hands, and you must treat it as such. Evidence preservation is a high priority in this case (**Figure 7-4**).

The first emergency personnel on the scene should check the body to see if it is still warm and initiate resuscitation procedures if there is any chance of restoring breathing and heartbeat. If the body is cool or rigid, make sure emergency medical personnel evaluate the body to confirm the death. If law enforcement are not yet present, notify them of the situation.

The area around a completed suicide is a crime scene. As such, avoid touching or moving things. Warn family and friends that the police must conduct an investigation and may have to ask some questions that may cause discomfort. Quiet the environment by containing the area, establishing a perimeter, and reducing unnecessary stimuli. That means that no one except law enforcement personnel should be allowed into the crime scene. Some people become loudly emotional when they are dealing with the shock of a suicide of a loved one. It is best to remove them to an area where they can deal with their distress without intensifying the distress of others. Remove antagonistic people, such as neighbors and media representatives, from the area around the family members and friends of the deceased suicide victim.

Supporting the Family and Friends of the Suicide Victim

Some family members and friends are quite aware of the suicide. In all likelihood they called the emergency personnel. Other family members and friends will be coming to the location as emergency teams converge on the area or shortly after their arrival. There is usually a great sense of shock, tension, and distress among the relatives and friends.

- *Gather family and friends in an area away from viewing the body.* Provide them with privacy by posting a police officer at the door. Check on the relationship of new arrivals before allowing them into the area where the family and friends are gathered. When in doubt, ask a family representative if a certain person is to be allowed into the home. Make the family and friends as comfortable as possible under the circumstances. This can be done by moving in extra chairs from another room, seeing if people need water, and assisting anyone with a physical impairment.
- *Ask the family to identify one person* who they would like to have as their representative to communicate with the emergency personnel. This person should be designated by the family as the person emergency personnel could contact first to answer some question or help solve some problems.
- *Be alert to cultural or ethnic concerns.* This is another area in which the designated family representative can be very helpful. Ask about family customs or traditions or issues that would offend the family members. Family representatives can guide you so that you do not inadvertently offend anyone.
- *Express your condolences for their loss* when you begin to communicate with family members. "Mrs. Smith, I am with the police department. I am so sorry to meet you under these painful circumstances. I am sorry, but I must ask you a few questions. These questions may be a bit uncomfortable for you, but I am required to ask them for my report. May I begin?"
- *Do not rush people.* Listen carefully and do not interrupt a person who is speaking to you.

Be aware that in some situations the media, such as television or radio reporters, may arrive at the scene. Your assistance in protecting the family is extremely valuable until someone else can take over this task. Sometimes, especially when a family has difficulty selecting one of their own to be a family representative, a member of the clergy can act as a family spokesperson. Find out what the family needs and provide the family representative with information about what is known about the situation so far.

After you have expressed your condolences to the family and friends and have provided them with general information about the death of their loved one, you may find that nothing else you say seems to be helpful. It is more important then that you attend to the physical needs of the distressed family and friends. Offer practical assistance such as moving furniture out of the way, getting someone a glass of water, or holding a baby for a short time. Silence is an acceptable and appropriate response at times, especially if you are showing support by your presence and if you provide small acts of kindness to the people in need.

Allow people to express their emotions. There may be many simultaneous feelings such as shock, denial, anger, guilt, shame, numbness, depression, and mental confusion. Be patient. Many people in a crisis tend to repeat themselves by asking questions or by expressing disbelief. Shock and mental confusion make it hard for people to understand what you are asking them or telling them. Make sure any questions you ask are clear and simple. The same goes for any statements you make.

After the Initial Shock Subsides

After a period of about 30 minutes, the shock of the announcement of the death begins to subside, and new issues, concerns, and needs begin to arise among the family members and friends. On occasion, family members ask emergency personnel to assist them with solving a problem or making a decision. Listen carefully to the problems they present and, if appropriate, do what you can to help them sort things out and come up with a decision or a solution. There have been situations in which people requested that emergency personnel lead the family in prayer. If emergency personnel are reasonably comfortable in responding positively to such a request, they can be immensely helpful to a distraught family even if they find the request a bit unusual. If the request is uncomfortable for you or if your belief system is very different than that of the grieving family, you would be best to suggest that the prayers ought to be led by a family member or a clergy person. You may then simply bow your head as a sign of respect while a family member leads the prayer. Be careful not to judge people who are distraught. You will most likely intensify feelings of guilt if you do so.

Sometimes the requests the family makes may appear strange. For instance, most emergency personnel would be uncomfortable if asked to sit down and have a cold beer with the family members after the suicidal death of a relative. The invitation does not appear to be an appropriate behavior for the family. The family may not be capable of demonstrating good judgment while in the midst of the turmoil surrounding the suicide of their loved one. It is best to politely decline such invitations by stating that it would violate the policies of the organization.

Under no circumstances should you attempt to interpret a suicide note. You would be making wild guesses, and it is very likely that your interpretation will be wrong. Generally the note should be given to the police for evaluation as evidence. You cannot adequately understand or explain a person's suicide. Do not, therefore, attempt to answer the "why?" question, even though it is likely to be a pressing question for the friends and family. Your mistaken interpretation will anger or frustrate family members, and they will lose their trust in you as a potential helper.

Hearing the distress and pain of the suicide victim's loved ones is not easy, but your presence makes a big difference if you are kind and concerned. As long as the person is not becoming excessively distraught as he or she tells the story of the deceased loved one, let the person tell as much of the story as he or she needs to tell. When a distressed person concludes his or her story, provide reassurance and some feedback. Ask clarifying questions if you do not understand something, but avoid giving advice. You are there to listen to a pained person and to assist the individual through a crisis. Organize whatever resources the family may need, including clergy, friends, and relatives. Do not leave distressed people on their own when they are still in a state of crisis. Your disengagement from the scene follows the arrival and acceptance of support from family, friends, and other resources. You should be involved only enough to facilitate the initial steps of the gathering of this support network.

Supporting Emergency Services Personnel

It is a horrible thing to watch a person take his or her own life. The violence of the suicidal act can leave a permanent psychological scar. Anyone who witnesses a suicide should talk to a member of a crisis response team to obtain guidance on recovering from the tragedy. A single crisis intervention tactic, by itself, is typically not going to be successful in managing the stress of a suicide. A comprehensive, integrated, systematic, and multi-component program of crisis support has a much better chance of achieving positive results. The keys to successful crisis management in a suicide case involve individual and group crisis support as well as large group informational sessions, family support, pastoral crisis intervention, and referrals for additional assistance.

Final Thoughts

Suicide experts tell us that many suicides are preventable if the right kind of help is available early enough. There is no truth to the old belief that if a person is suicidal once, he or she will be suicidal for the remainder of his or her life. In most cases, if adequate help is available, the suicide risk subsides and the person begins to think rationally. What at first may have appeared as a huge and insurmountable problem begins to shrink to a manageable and temporary challenge. People who were once quite suicidal may move on to healthy, happy lives.

Crisis intervention is a crucial start to the helping process. When crisis workers and emergency personnel recognize the suicidal risk, act quickly to intervene, and refer the person for professional assistance, important life-altering changes begin for the suicidal person. Without doubt, crisis intervention makes a life-saving difference.

Selected References

Carll EK: *Trauma Psychology: Issues in Violence, Disaster, Health, and Illness, Vol 1, Violence and Disaster*. Westport, CT, Praeger Publishers, 2007.

Carll EK: *Trauma Psychology: Issues in Violence, Disaster, Health, and Illness, Vol 2, Health and Illness*. Westport, CT, Praeger Publishers, 2007.

Forster EM: *Howard's End*. London, England, Edward Arnold Publishers, 1910.

Gibson M: *Order From Chaos: Responding to Traumatic Events*, ed 3 rev. Bristol, England, The Policy Press, 2006.

Many glossary definitions in this document were adapted from: http://wordnet.princeton.edu (June 2008).

Mitchell JT: *The Quick Series Guide to Suicide Prevention*. Fort Lauderdale, FL, Luxart Communications, 2006.

Mitchell JT, Resnik HLP: *Emergency Response to Crisis*. Bowie, MD, Robert J Brady Company, 1981.

Mitchell JT, Resnik HLP: Emergency Response to Crisis: A Crisis Intervention Guidebook for Emergency Service Personnel. Republished. Ellicott City, MD, Chevron Publishing Corporation, 1989.

Patterson WM, Dohn HH, Bird J, Patterson GA: Evaluation of suicidal patients: the SAD PERSON Scale. *Psychosomatics*, 1983;24:343–349.

Roberts AR: *Crisis Intervention Handbook: Assessment, Treatment, and Research*, ed 3. New York, NY, Oxford University Press, 2005.

Prep Kit

Ready for Review

- As individuals contemplate ending their own lives, it is common for them to move through four steps toward suicide. Those steps are *thought, gesture, attempt,* and *completion.* The process varies, but for most people, the progression toward actual completion develops over time.

- Suicide assessment is a complex technique that requires good information and practice by the provider. During the assessment, it is important to be kind, caring, and empathetic.

- Remember that individuals who are truly suicidal may also be homicidal should you try to interfere. Safety is paramount.

- While there are many reasons that people commit suicide, common threads are feelings of hopelessness, haplessness, and helplessness.

- Using a standardized technique, such as the SAD PERSONS model, will provide the emergency service provider with a way to remember specific questions that are helpful in conducting a thorough suicide assessment.

- Helping the suicidal patient can be stressful and difficult for the emergency responder. It is important to maintain a safe and secure environment for all parties while establishing rapport and trust with the individual. Once life-threatening conditions have been addressed, the process may take an extended amount of time.

- The scene of either an attempted or completed suicide is considered an active crime scene. Be sure to preserve all evidence and do not disrupt the environment.

Vital Vocabulary

haplessness Deserving or inciting pity because bad things just keep happening to the person.

helplessness Powerlessness, as revealed by an inability to act; a feeling of being unable to manage.

hopelessness The despair one feels when he or she has abandoned hope of comfort or success.

suicidal attempts The act of trying to take one's own life through the use of deliberate, potentially lethal actions.

suicidal completion The act of dying as a result of one's suicide attempt.

suicidal gestures Actions that indicate that one is considering suicide.

suicidal ideation The process of having general or unfocused ideas toward harming oneself.

suicidal thoughts See suicidal ideation.

suicide The act of causing one's own death.

worthlessness Feelings that one's life has no value.

Assessment in Action

Answer key is located in the back of the book.

1. The majority of individuals who commit suicide do so primarily because of one cause or event.

   A. True
   B. False

2. You are dispatched to a residence for a patient who is "not feeling well." Upon arriving at the scene, family members tell you that the 17-year-old daughter recently broke up with her boyfriend. Tonight when they returned, they found her in the bathroom, where she had taken a kitchen knife and tried to cut her wrist. In speaking with her, she tells you that she didn't really want to kill herself, she just wanted to see what it would be like. This is an example of a suicidal:

   A. thought.
   B. attempt.
   C. gesture.
   D. completion.

3. While interviewing a 54-year-old female, she tells you that, over the past year, her husband has died and left her without a life insurance policy, she was involved in a crash that totaled her car, and last week she was diagnosed with breast cancer. She says that she simply does not have the will or energy

to go on anymore. This is an example of:

A. hopelessness.
B. helplessness.
C. haplessness.
D. depression.

4. You are very concerned about your EMS partner, because he seems as though he has changed over the past three months. You are aware that he is going through a challenging divorce and was recently reprimanded for being tardy or absent from work on multiple occasions. You also notice that he appears sad and grumpy much of the time now.

Discussing his current situation and asking him about suicide will probably only give him the idea of suicide and may actually lead to him taking his life.

A. True
B. False

5. All suspected suicide scenes must be considered crime scenes and preserved until the scene has been isolated and managed by the police.

A. True
B. False

Chapter 8

Supporting Victims of Death-Related Crises

Epicurus, an ancient Greek philosopher, reminds us how vulnerable we all are to death when he notes, "It is possible to provide security against other ills, but as far as death is concerned, we men live in a city without walls." We witness it in our work, we care for those who are bereaved, and we all will experience death. This chapter aims at helping people who perform crisis interventions and support individuals and families who are suffering through the loss of people they love.

You Do Make a Difference

For many people, death is such a depressing, overwhelming, and disconcerting topic that they find it hard to believe that they can do anything to reduce the suffering of the bereaved. A 2005 study asked family members to evaluate the helpfulness of emergency personnel at the scene of a death of a loved one (**Figure 8-1**). Of 31 families, only one said that more should have been done to try to revive their relative. A large majority of the families (81%) felt that paramedics at the scene had treated the family professionally and in a supportive and gentle manner.

Small mistakes and misstatements, such as mispronouncing the name of the deceased or mistaking a relationship to a particular family member, can be easily magnified and turn an already tense situation into a more painful experience for everyone involved. Before saying or doing anything, always put yourself in the position of the grieving family members and try to determine how your words or actions would sound or appear to them. Always choose the wording or the actions that are simple, appropriate, and most likely to be supportive and help-ful. Wording and actions in the management of the death-related crisis should always minimize the opportunities for misinterpretation. For example, do not say that the person "moved on" or "checked out." Instead, say "died" or "is dead."

The approach you take toward shocked, grieving, and emotion-ally overwhelmed people in the aftermath of a death of a loved one can leave lasting effects on the bereaved. Emergency personnel and other crisis workers enter the lives of distressed people when they are espe-cially vulnerable to further duress. If crisis workers are professional, sensitive, and caring, they do make a significant difference in assisting people through a death-related crisis.

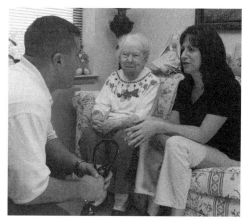

Figure 8-1 Emergency personnel can make a significant difference in the lives of the bereaved in a death-related crisis.

Dealing With Impending Death

For the majority of people, when they first learn that they are dying, their normal world is shat-tered. Their dreams are demolished. The shock of the impending death impairs or otherwise affects their interactions with others. They then engage in the same emotional patterns that are usually associated with the grieving of family and friends after the loss of a loved one (**Table 8-1**).

People facing their own death may initially deny the reality of the threat. They often attempt to bargain their way out of their death and offer some form of change of behavior as a sacrifice to gain the privilege of being spared from death. It is usually not long before the hopelessness of the situation causes anger to set in. People first tend to be angry and frustrated with circumstances; then they may feel angry with other people. Some even turn the anger inward on themselves and persistently blame themselves. Personal responsibility, regrets, and guilt are often the earmarks of anger. Typically, the last psychological stage in the dying process is <u>grief</u>. This stage in the dying process is associated with sadness and a great sense of loss. In grief, people <u>mourn</u> the loss of con-nections to the past as well as an inability to link to a personal future.

Table 8–1	Stages of the Dying Process	
Stage	**Signs**	**Supportive Actions**
Denial	Disbelief in the accuracy of the diagnosis or in the reality or finality of death	Listen; offer kindness, emotional support; do not argue with the denial; offer calm reassurance that the person will not be abandoned.
Bargaining	Would it make a difference if I did this or that?	Gentle acceptance and understanding of how difficult it is for the person to be dealing with the information.
Anger	Frustration and fear lead to anger and irritability	Do not take anger personally, acknowledge anger and validate those feelings, guide anger into useful channels like accomplishing tasks.
Grief	Sadness, sense of loss, and feeling overwhelmed	Offer condolences, respect, kindness; assist in simple tasks.

In some cases people do not go through these stages of dying easily. They may need to repeat several of the phases or may get stuck in one of the stages. Only after having adequate time to work through those stages does a person find the ability to express his or her acceptance of the impending death and say goodbye to those he or she cares about. Some people are unable to accept the reality of the situation even when death is imminent.

There are many things that can assist the dying person. Careful listening is among the most important. It is important that you hear the entire story. Expect the dying person to repeat himself or herself. This is especially true when a person is fearful and confused. Be patient and do not be annoyed by the repetition of the same information. It is part of the process of coming to terms with what might be, for some, a very lonely and frightening circumstance.

Acknowledge, accept or **validate** the feelings expressed by those who are dying. Never attempt to argue with a person's emotions. It is an impossible argument, and it causes a person to feel misunderstood and isolated. Instead, provide as much information as is necessary, but at a pace and at the level that the dying person requests. Ask if the person wants to discuss the situation. Many emergency personnel are surprised by a dying person's willingness to discuss impending death. At the same time, never attempt to pressure a person into talking about the circumstances. Death, after all, is a very private experience. Be sensitive and kind, and do not rush a person who is talking about anxieties and fears. Express understanding and concern. Avoid giving false hopes. Make sure that communications to a dying person are consistent; discrepancies can be devastating to the morale of a dying person.

Try to fulfill reasonable requests of a dying person. Do what you can to make the person as comfortable as possible. Never promise things over which you have no control. For example, do not make statements such as "I am sure the insurance company will pay for all this medical care." If you have to move a person in pain, do so gently. Do not hesitate to engage in a prayer if the person asks you to pray with him or her and you are comfortable praying. If you are very uncomfortable with the request, you may gently decline. You may ask the individual who wishes to pray to lead the prayer. Even if you are not praying, assume a respectful position and remain silent while the person prays. If you do engage in prayer at the request of the dying person, avoid preaching. Never attempt to convert the dying person to your belief system.

You may be surprised by a person's request for a prayer, especially if you know that the individual was not very religious. Just because a person may not have been very religiously observant when he or she was healthy, it does not mean that he or she will not engage in religious observations as death approaches. Ask if the person would like to speak with a spiritual advisor.

Dying is a highly stressful process. Many emotions will arise, including fear, regret, guilt, sadness, dependency, frustration, and anger. It is not unusual for dying people to express strong emotions toward people who are present, but who do not have responsibility for the person's unhappiness. Try not to take angry outbursts personally. They are rarely meant to hurt and are more a sign of fear and frustration.

As long as a person is capable of doing things for himself or herself, encourage the person to do so. If you do too much for a dying but still capable person, you will cause the person to feel inadequate and most likely elevate the sense of loss of function and control. Help people continue to care for themselves. When they are no longer able to care for themselves, it is important to engage other people, such as family members or close friends, in the helping process. You do not want to take on the responsibility of caring for the dying person. It is more appropriate to attempt to keep family members and friends engaged in supporting and caring for the dying person.

Helping a person prepare for death is not among the easiest of tasks, but it is among the most noble. It is both a great burden and a great privilege. Once a dying person has accepted the certainty of death, he or she often feels enormous appreciation and gratitude for whatever a concerned person does to assist them, no matter how insignificant that contribution might seem.

Making the Death Announcement

A death announcement is one facet of managing a death-related crisis in which emergency and crisis intervention personnel are likely to have a profound effect. A death announcement may have significant negative impact on the mental and physical health of the people receiving the news. There are cases in which heart attacks, cardiac arrests, and impulsive suicides were the direct result of abrupt, insensitive, or callous death announcements. Caution is, therefore, required. The Emergency Health Services Department's death and dying course at the University of Maryland Baltimore County teaches students that nearly everyone who was older than 7 years at the time remembers in great detail how they were informed of the death of family member or a close friend. The 2 hours immediately surrounding the death announcement were remembered most vividly. People remember what they were doing at the time. They also remember who made the death announcement, the exact words that were used, and whether or not the person was kind and supportive. A death announcement requires a combination of great sensitivity and excellent communication skills. The guidelines in this section will help a person to make a death announcement in a manner that generates the least disturbance, given the circumstances, on the people receiving bad news (**Figure 8-2**).

It was once common practice that medical personnel in hospitals or the military or emergency services chaplains working in field conditions carried the primary responsibility for making death announcements. In some cases, a single police officer was assigned the grim task of informing a family that a family member had died or been killed. Although that practice continues, it is becoming more common for teams of people trained in crisis intervention to deliver news of a death. The team approach reduces the pressure formerly placed on one person to bear the entire responsibility for informing the family of the death of a loved one. The team approach also helps should the people being notified have a medical problem as a result of the shock associated with the announcement. In addition, a team provides multiple important viewpoints and can contribute those views to the understanding of the family and friends of the deceased.

Depending on the circumstances, a death notification team may include a CISM team member, a physician, a nurse, a paramedic, or a police officer who work in concert with a chaplain or a mental health professional. A team consists of a minimum of two people, and a typical team has three or four people. Many times the team is a function of the police or fire department's chaplain's office. One of the team members is assigned a coordinating role and one is usually designated to make the actual announcement. Anyone else on the team will play supportive, advocacy roles. Those assigned to advocacy roles ensure privacy and may make phone calls on behalf of the family. You may be asked to call in relatives, clergy, or other resources as required. You may temporarily deal with media contacts until the family designates a liaison. You also obtain water, food, medications, and other necessities to make those receiving the news as comfortable as possible. In some cases, you may have to monitor blood pressure and other signals of physical distress in people who are already in fragile health conditions. The best approach is to treat symptomatically. If the person shows signs of medical distress, have emergency medical personnel check the person.

Dr. Tracy Cumberland, a death and dying specialist with the Emergency Health Services Department at the University of Maryland Baltimore County, outlines a specific approach to

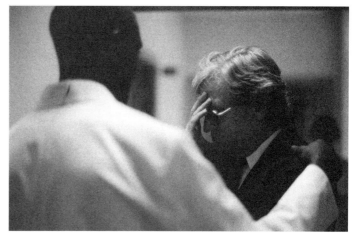

Figure 8-2 Proper handling of the death announcement is an important aspect of the emergency worker's job.

In the Field

Four Steps in Making a Death Notification

1. Pre-death
2. The actual death notification
3. Follow-up
4. Grief

making a death announcement. It includes four phases: pre-death, the actual death notification, follow-up, and grief.

The pre-death phase includes every factor that is a part of the death announcement. The individual or team that is tasked with making the death announcement assembles quickly. The facts of the death are reviewed and confirmed. The person or team immediately proceeds to the home of the family of the deceased or to another appropriate location where the family is gathered.

Although the mere presence of the team is enough to signal that something bad has happened, it is important that the team leader states that the team has come to discuss a serious matter. "Hello, are you Mrs. Jones? I am Captain Jonathan Forest from the police department. I have some extremely important information for you. May I come in?" If you are working with a team, introduce each of the team members. The pre-death phase of the death announcement process is a preparation phase. In this phase, the person or the team should assure privacy and attempt to get the person or people comfortable and preferably sitting. The team member tasked with doing so should cover the events that led up to the person's death. The team member discusses the accident or illness and confirms that the friend or loved one was, in fact, involved in the situation. The team member may say something like, "About an hour ago there was a very serious accident on route 35 near Franklinville. Your husband was involved in that accident. We are sure of this because of the license plate on the car and his driver's license."

The nature of the victim's injuries or resuscitative efforts should be described briefly. ("Your husband's car was very badly damaged.") It is important not to rush this information. Bad news should be given in small doses. Do not blurt out the information all at once. In most cases the family members give hints that they are ready for the next piece of information, saying, "Yes," "Okay," or "Go ahead." They may express feelings of dread and discomfort with the news so far. The feelings of the relatives or friends should be validated and their concerns or questions are addressed as they arise. Sometimes someone might ask if the person is dead before you think they are actually ready to hear that information. If the family members ask directly, respond by affirming that the person died as a result of the injuries he or she sustained; acknowledge that it is difficult and painful to deliver this news. Answer any questions that arise before moving on with the final announcement.

Finally, unless a team member has already done so, the designated team member makes the actual death announcement. The person making the announcement should summarize, in simple terms, what has been said so far. The actual announcement should avoid complicated medical terminology. Use clear words, such as "dead" or "died." Use the deceased's name throughout the announcement. ("Mrs. Jones, I am paramedic Susan Walsh. I was at the scene that Captain Forest just described to you. I treated your husband, Charles, at the scene. Mr. Jones was unconscious and he had very serious head injuries, as well as chest injuries. We were in contact with a physician at Union Hospital. I am very sorry to tell you this, but your husband, Mr. Jones, died as a result of his injuries.")

Accept and validate any expressions of emotion from the bereaved. The notification team should express sorrow and empathy for those who are suffering the loss of a friend or family member. Avoid trite statements and euphemisms such as, "He is in a better place now," "You know, you can grow stronger as a result of such a loss," or "At least the person isn't suffering any more." Such comments are counterproductive and generally cause people to feel worse about the situation. Answer all questions honestly.

The follow-up phase is a time for being present with the family members or friends and providing them with whatever comfort and support is possible. The individual or team making the death announcement should take a few minutes to validate feelings and ask if there is anything else the team can do to assist. The family members may ask you to call relatives, friends, or neighbors to assist them, or they might ask you to contact a clergy person. This is also the time to answer any additional questions. Family members often want to know if they will be able to see and touch the body. Normally this is permitted, unless the body is part of a crime scene. People may also request information on autopsies, organ donations, and other issues; address these concerns as needed and as appropriate. The team should be as helpful as possible and refer the bereaved to other resources as necessary, such as hospital personnel, the medical examiner's office, funeral homes, or crisis counseling centers.

Ordinarily, the team will accommodate requests to view the body. However, the team should be sure to prepare family members for what they are going to see. If there is substantial damage to the body, advise family members of that fact. You might say, "Mrs. Holt, I do not want to upset you, but before you choose to see your son's body, you need to know that the damage to his body is extensive. Do you really want to see it or would you prefer to just hold his hand? I will assist you as much as I can with your decision, but I think it is essential that you know how bad his condition is. Do you want me to describe some of his injuries before you decide?" Holding the deceased person's hand rather than viewing the entire body may be helpful for some family members. You should gently point out that young children might be overwhelmed by what they see and that it may not be in the best interest of children to see the loved one.

Even in cases of horrible disfigurement, many family members insist on seeing the body of a loved one. You should accompany family members when they view the body; most people react with strong emotions and physical reactions, including vomiting, dizziness, tremors, physical instability, or fainting. Be as supportive of the family members as possible. Help them to find a seat, get a drink of water, express your condolences, hold a hand, or put a hand on a shoulder or an arm around a shoulder. Do what you can until family members or friends arrive and take over these caretaking activities.

After a relatively brief time, they may develop some questions. They might ask if a suspect was arrested in a criminal case, if anyone else was injured in the accident, or what was done to save the person's life. Continue to answer questions as they arise. Sometimes silence in the face of suffering is the appropriate response. Your presence will often mean more than your words.

All emotional reactions should be supported, with one exception. It is unacceptable for people to engage in self-destructive behaviors or to harm others as a result of their anguish. Distraught family members might express a wish to die immediately, or they may express a direct threat against the person they feel caused the death of their loved one. The team must interfere with those manifestations of grief. You may have to assess for suicidal or homicidal ideation. If it appears that a person intends to carry out such threats, bring in the police to further assess the danger.

Grief is the last phase of the death announcement process. It will be characterized by:

- Shock and disbelief
- Crying
- Angry outbursts
- High anxiety
- Sadness
- Feelings of guilt
- Physical reactions such as nausea and lightheadedness

Offer your own expressions of sympathy and acknowledge the pain the recipients of the death announcement are experiencing. Do not leave the bereaved alone. Mobilize whatever resources are necessary to take over the care of the bereaved individuals or family members. Resources include clergy members, family, friends, and sometimes social services agencies. The best way to find out what resources are needed is to ask the family what would help them most. Provide the deceased's family members with as much information as necessary and answer any additional questions they may have. Once the bereaved feel that sufficient relatives or other resources have arrived to assist the family, the team begins the withdrawal process from the scene.

As the death notification team completes its work, it should leave communications open for further contact from the bereaved in the event they have more questions or concerns. Let the family know how to connect with the team members. Ask if the family members need anything else before the team departs and provide answers to any remaining questions. Express your sympathies and say goodbye to the family. The team then withdraws. It is essential that the team not discuss the situation with neighbors or the media.

Remember the primary goals of the process. A death notification should review the circumstances that led to the death and clearly state that a person has died. The death notification process focuses on assisting the bereaved with managing the details associated with the death. This includes notifying other family members and friends about the death, if requested. The notification process should also aim at guiding people who are in shock. Once the bereaved begin to make decisions and take actions that are in their own best interests, the notification team should reduce or relinquish their activities on behalf of the bereaved. Finally, the team should manage any medical conditions among the family members or friends that are exacerbated by the death announcement and should make appropriate referrals as needed.

Expected Death

Some people assume that an expected death—for example, a death that follows a long illness—should not cause a great deal of distress. That assumption is unsupported by actual experience. Instead of the concentrated shock associated with a sudden death, numerous smaller shock waves roll over the bereaved during a prolonged time frame. It is as if small bits of the person die over and over until the death is completed. As the person gradually dies, the relationships with that person also die, and each loss is mourned. Every small loss produces its own miniature grief reaction.

When a death is expected, people often, but not always, experience **anticipatory grief**, actively processing thoughts and feelings related to the loss of a person they love before the death has occurred. In most cases, anticipatory grief does not lessen the intensity of the grief response or short-circuit the grief process that occurs once the person actually dies. It may, however, have some benefits for some grieving people. For example, anticipatory grief may help bereaved people make more sense out of the death because it follows a long illness that gradually attacks the person's life functions and interpersonal relationships. Observers can see the dying process one step at a time. Shock is typically lessened when the death is expected, but the grief process is not necessarily modified in such situations.

The anticipatory grief associated with a potential loss causes enormous physical and emotional pain. It generates powerful, although fruitless, efforts to ward off the impending death. Eventually people may feel useless and defeated. By time the death occurs, the bereaved often feel emotionally exhausted and physically fatigued. They often react to the actual death with little in the way of outward displays of emotion. A limited expression of emotion at the time of the death does not, however, imply that the bereaved are not reacting with a deep sense of loss and inner emotional distress. The bereaved must still work their way through a grieving process. They need the kind of support that is described in this chapter. Information and emotional support are always the most crucial elements of death notification, even when the death is expected.

There are no specific guidelines that will fit every death notification situation. Emergency personnel see people in either the earliest phases of a death notification or the earliest stages of grief. Therefore, emergency personnel must adhere to basic principles of giving bad news and of managing early grief reactions. Get the facts before making a death announcement.

1. Give bad news in short, precise, and gently worded sentences.
2. Provide as much information as is available at the time of the announcement.
3. Use the name of the deceased person. Provide information of the circumstances of the death. Use the words *dead, died,* or *death.*
4. Express your concern and condolences.
5. Fulfill immediate requests of the bereaved to the extent possible.
6. Ask what the bereaved may need to assist them.
7. Assist the family members in mobilizing whatever resources they deem necessary. This includes relatives, friends, neighbors, clergy, and medical personnel.
8. Stay with the family until enough help arrives.
9. Determine if there is anything else that the family needs before you again express your condolences, say goodbye, and depart from the family.

Relating to Hospice Programs in a Death-Related Crisis

Hospice programs have been in operation for many years. Hospice workers assist people who are terminally ill and help prepare them and their families for an expected death. It is always a very wise decision to invite hospice personnel to an emergency services in-service training to inform operations personnel about what to expect when coming into contact with a dying person or a deceased person under hospice care (**Figure 8-3**). By explaining the condition and needs of a dying person, hospice personnel can pave the way for emergency personnel and ensure that their contact with the dead or dying is smooth and in concert with the procedures that have already been established in the days, weeks, or months leading up to the death. Preparation of emergency personnel for the impending death of a patient in the community can prevent unnecessary and emotionally distressing efforts to resuscitate the person when death occurs.

When called to confirm a death, emergency personnel should ask the family if the person was in hospice care. If the family confirms that to be the case, emergency personnel should ask if the hospice worker has been notified of the death. It is helpful for the emergency personnel to speak with the hospice worker to gain some insight into assisting the family members in the acute crisis stages of a death notification or confirmation. Ask the family for permission to discuss the situation with the hospice worker, because the hospice worker can often suggest specific guidelines that might help emergency personnel alleviate distress for the family. It is generally helpful for emergency personnel

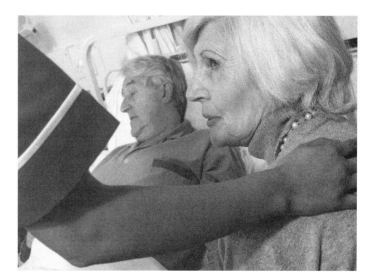

Figure 8-3 Hospice workers can be an invaluable resource when assisting the family of a recently deceased person.

to know the diagnosis or cause of death as well as the length of the illness and any special precautions that need to be taken in handling the body to confirm the death.

It is also helpful to ask the hospice personnel for guidance in assisting the family members. Many times hospice personnel have rehearsed the steps a family is to take after the death of the loved one. The family might forget these steps in the distress that follows the final loss. The informal partnership between hospice and emergency personnel can function as a powerful tool to confirm death, make appropriate death announcements, and provide immediate assistance to the family and friends of the deceased.

Sudden Death

Sudden death concentrates all of the intense emotions associated with a loss of a loved one into a compressed time frame. If the death was a result of violence, an accident, or a natural disaster, there may be many issues that complicate the grieving and recovery processes, including unanswered questions about pain and suffering and efforts to save the person. These questions often play out repeatedly and persistently in the minds of the surviving loved ones.

There are numerous powerful emotional reactions to sudden death. They include the following:

Psychological shock. Sometimes the physical manifestations of shock are so severe that medical intervention is required. Treat this condition just as you would physical shock. The signs and symptoms are identical. They include rapid heartbeat, profuse sweating, nausea, shallow breathing, pale face, and a drop in blood pressure. Treat symptomatically.

Numbness. The shock of the sudden death so seriously affects the person's mental and physical capacities that he or she is temporarily unable to feel anything or to react to the loss. People in this state are very emotionally vulnerable, and great care must be taken to guide them and keep them out of harm's way. Keep onlookers out of the area. Stay with the shocked and bereaved family members. Speak calmly, fulfill reasonable requests, and provide information. Express your care and concern.

Overwhelmed. Multiple, simultaneous feelings flood the person and cause him or her to be incapable of thinking clearly. The bereaved frequently have significant problems making decisions. Quieting the environment and reducing or eliminating stimuli are very important steps in helping the person regain some sense of control. Some people describe a sense of "drowning" in emotions. It is best to acknowledge how painful the situation must be for the person. This is an expression of sympathy for the person's distress.

Intense sadness. The deep sense of loss that accompanies the recognition that the person is gone forever can produce physical and emotional pain. Crying is very common. Acknowledge and validate feelings, provide for privacy and comforts, provide information, and offer consolation and guidance.

A flood of memories. Many people report a flood of memories of the loved one that race through their minds and deepen the sense of loss. Listen to them and ask about the loved one. Ask what the person was like in life. Make sure you have the trust of the person before asking such questions. Sometimes listening and being quiet will work well. You do not always need to be talking. Be supportive and sympathetic. That in itself is a good message.

Disturbing thoughts. Some people report that they have disturbing thoughts regarding the sudden death of a loved one. They imagine what the death would have been like, and they are horrified by what they imagine. For some that experience is as intense as if they had actually witnessed the death. The thing that helps the most is accurate information about the circumstances of the death.

Guilt. Family members and friends sometimes believe that they bear some responsibility for the death. They think that if they had done or not done something the person would still be alive. Much of the emergency services person's reactions will depend on how much they actually know about the circumstances surrounding the death. It is generally best to say something to the effect of, "It must be very painful for you right now. We often hear people say that they feel guilty about the death of a loved one. Over time they usually come to understand that they are not responsible for the death. I hope that happens in your case."

Anger. It is common for people experiencing a sudden death to feel angry toward the perpetrator or the cause of the death. Some are angry at the person who died. Sometimes they are angry at you for no other reason than you are there. Do not take the anger personally. You may say, "I know that you are very angry and upset right now, and that is normal. I would like to try to help you. What kinds of things can I do to assist you?" The worst thing you can do is try to argue with the emotions.

Worry. A sudden death throws people into situations that may threaten their security and financial welfare. They may have to take on unfamiliar responsibilities and more independent functions than they feel ready to manage. The future looks bleak and worries intensify. For a person struggling with intense worries, your best approach is to acknowledge that the situation is chaotic right now and that it will take some time to sort out. Grieving family members may need assistance from trusted people to assess their financial status. If family members express concern or worry about these matters, ask them who they might speak with and guide them to the appropriate resources.

Crisis intervention efforts in a sudden-death situation should aim at helping the bereaved take care of themselves and their family members, particularly children. Those who are grieving must be encouraged to establish reasonable patterns of eating, resting, sleeping, and accomplishing household tasks. Emergency personnel can remind family members that they need nourishment even when they do not feel like eating. In addition, family members need to be reminded that children need stability and as near-normal schedules as possible. Family members will have to deal with grief individually as well as within the family system. They will not all be feeling the same thing at the same time. Sometimes one family member becomes angry at the others because he or she is expressing different emotional reactions. One family member might remember a funny story about the loved one. Another family member thinks that the funny story is inappropriate and insensitive and blows up in rage at the person telling the story.

Crisis intervention workers should let family members know that everyone will handle grief in their own way and that each person's response should be accepted and valued. When you hear such tension in a family system, just tell the person who seems to be the family spokesperson how normal it is for family members to be at different levels of emotional reactivity. The spokesperson may quietly pass on such information to the other family members. Family members should be encouraged to talk to each other about their feelings and their thoughts. Again, have a discussion with the family representative and tell that person what to say to other family members. Many problems can be prevented if open communications in a family system are allowed and encouraged.

Family Reaction to Death

A family is a system. What affects one person in a family will have an effect, and often a dramatic effect, on other family members. A death in the family removes one part of the system. Each member of the family system must deal with the loss, work through the grieving process, adapt to life without the person, and find appropriate ways to remember the person. Faith and philosophical beliefs may have been challenged as a result of the death and now need to be repaired or restored. The family members must also construct a family life without the loved one. That requires working together to establish new routines that unite the family.

Emergency personnel and other crisis workers must keep in mind that family systems are complex entities. There are many issues to consider when outside resources are called in to a family to render assistance after the death of a family member. Here are a number of those issues.

Reactions of the family as a whole and of the individuals within the family will differ in timing, intensity, and, ultimately, their final resolution. Family reactions include disbelief, panic, numbness, as well as:

- Searching for a cause
- Seeking someone to blame
- Attempts to stay in control
- Attempts to maintain dignity
- Attempts to be brave in the face of loss
- Attempts to return to normal life pursuits
- Worry
- Overwhelming sadness
- Anger or rage
- Depression
- A sense of no feelings whatsoever
- Retreat from others and difficulties returning to normal functions

There may be significant variation within the family on the length of recovery time. Family members may search for meaning in their own ways and in their own time.

Religion and culture will have a considerable influence on the reaction of family members and individuals to the death. Sometimes religion and culture aid a grieving person. Unfortunately, in some situations, religious and cultural influences may impede a person's ability to work through the grief process. Each circumstance is unique, and it is difficult to predict the role of religion and culture in an individual's grief experience. It is best to avoid assuming that there are positive religious or cultural influences on the grieving process. Instead, crisis workers should ask the individuals involved in the loss if there are aspects of their religion or culture that might help them in their grief.

The greater the trauma associated with the death, the more difficult it may be for the family members to cope with it. If a death is seen as a relief from suffering for the deceased, it may be somewhat easier for the family members to adapt to the loss, but family members must come to that conclusion on their own. It is not helpful for emergency personnel to make statements about the dead person being relieved of suffering.

To help a family through a crisis after the death of a loved one, crisis workers and emergency personnel should provide as much comfort and support as possible. Crisis intervention personnel should unite the family in the same area unless they are resistant to that approach. Providing adequate information should be a high priority. Legitimate requests should be fulfilled if it is possible to do so. Help the family members to recognize and express their feelings. Assist the family members with making decisions: encourage family members to make decisions on urgent and crucial matters and to leave the less important decisions until the family is beyond the acute crisis phase. Call in the resources that the family members believe will be most helpful. Stay involved in helping a family until other appropriate assistance arrives to help the family.

Adult Reactions to Death

Humans respond in a wide variety of ways to the death of a loved one. The list below summarizes many of the primary reactions to death. Remember that these reactions can occur simultaneously, and they can occur in almost any order. It is not unusual for the various emotional states to be repeated several times.

- Shock
- Denial

- Feeling overwhelmed and lost
- Mental confusion
- Nausea
- Numbness
- Deep emotional and physical anguish
- Inability to make decisions
- Anger
- Sadness
- Depression

The aim in every case is to provide grieving people with information in small doses as long as they appear ready to receive it. As mentioned earlier in this chapter, people indicate that they are ready for the next piece of information when they nod their heads or say "okay," "yes," "I understand," or "go on." The family will remember kindness, understanding, and gentleness.

Children's Reactions to Death

Gentleness is of primary importance when dealing with a child's reaction to death. It is almost always best for a relative or a familiar person to announce a death to a child. Unfortunately, emergency personnel sometimes encounter a family that is severely emotionally distraught and incapable of announcing the death to their children. In such cases, doctors, nurses, police officers, or emergency medical personnel may be tasked with this uncomfortable assignment. They should concentrate on being well-informed about the circumstances of the death before approaching the child. Ask people who were at the scene what happened. Establish privacy for the child or children. Slow things down and proceed deliberately and carefully (**Figure 8-4**). Stop after every few lines and ask the child if he or she understands what you are saying. Do not hesitate to make the information simpler if the child is not getting it. Choose simple words and give small segments of information at a time. Ask the children if they understood everything so far, making sure to answer questions as you proceed. Once the final announcement of the death is made, be as supportive as possible.

You might start by saying "Your family asked me to speak with you about something very sad. Is it okay that I talk to you? What is your name? How old are you? My name is Mary. I am a paramedic. Do you know what a paramedic is?" Continue relaying information in words and language the child can easily understand, pausing frequently to ensure that the child is processing the information and to answer any questions he or she may have.

A child's reaction to death depends on how emotionally close the child was to the deceased and how involved the person was in the child's life. Other factors that affect a child's reaction are whether the person was sick, whether the child knew the person was sick and going to die, and the amount of time the child had to prepare for the death. Unexpected deaths are far more difficult for a child to comprehend and manage.

When presenting information, consider the child's age, maturity, and developmental level. Infants are more distressed by the level of grief reactions in the adults around them than they are by the actual death. It is usually best if a calm adult holds an infant child and walks with the infant, rocking gently. That task may fall to a paramedic or a police officer if the family is too distraught at the moment. When

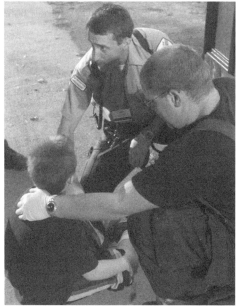

Figure 8-4 While discussing a death with a child, be sure to speak slowly and pause to ask the child if he or she understands what you are saying.

the adults calm down the infant may be transferred to the care of an adult family member. When infants and young children sense that the adults around them are upset and unhappy, they may become anxious and restless and require more attention. Preschoolers may believe that the death is temporary and that the person will live again soon. Let the family members intervene with the child. If you have to say anything, you should say something to the effect of, "No, once people die they cannot come back to life again." Children older than 5 years have a better understanding of death and are more likely to understand that it happens to every living thing and is a permanent condition. They also understand that death is caused by something. This age bracket can appreciate sincere expressions of sorrow for their loss. Sometimes it helps for the child to talk about their loved one. The most important thing in this case is sympathetic listening.

Most children feel sad, angry, and worried when an adult loved one dies. The death of a sibling or friend may intensify their feelings. Young children may react with anger and feelings of vulnerability. Anger is often displayed by loud, aggressive play. A child's anger may also be expressed by irritability or nightmares.

An anxious child may regress to baby talk, behaviors from earlier developmental levels, and demands on adults for food, attention, and physical contact. Young children may think that they caused the death because of some bad behavior. Many children feel unsafe after the death of someone they knew and they may become fearful.

Teenagers think about death in a similar manner as adults. They may be more aware of the feelings of others, or they may close others out of their lives. Often they have a very difficult time expressing their feelings in words. They will often hide or suppress their feelings so that they do not upset others. Sometimes they withhold their emotions to show their peers that they are cool, strong, and under control.

The circumstances of the death will have an influence on how a child of almost any age reacts to the death. Children have the least understanding of a sudden, unexplained, or traumatic death. Such deaths produce the highest levels of disturbance in children. Like adults, children often view sudden, unexpected deaths as unfair. Most children become seriously distressed if the adults in their world are unable to care for them because of their own grief affecting their ability to care for the children.

When helping children cope with the death of a person they love, be comforting and reassuring. Children need to know that they have not been abandoned and that there are adults who will continue to take care of them. Make sure that the child's environment is safe and secure. Make sure that caring family members will, in fact, be there to care for the children. Instruct adults to provide information about the death to the children and offer to assist them in discussion of the death. Allow children to express their thoughts and feelings while keeping discussions simple and basic. Teenagers may need considerably more information. Whatever discussions are held with children, they should be appropriate to the age of the children and not frighten or unnecessarily distress them.

Coping With the Loss of Children

There are few situations that are more difficult for emergency personnel and other crisis interveners than deaths of children. These situations demand extraordinary empathy and careful management of every aspect of the case, from the handling of the body of the deceased child through the death announcement and subsequent support of the family. What emergency personnel do and say in the time immediately surrounding the death of a child can have profound, long-term effects on family and friends. Grieving family members will value professionalism, concern, respect, dignity, care, and kindness.

When dealing with the death of a child, always be sensitive and caring in every action you take and in every word you speak. Without a basic understanding of the depth of loss associated with a child's death, crisis intervention personnel are handicapped in their ability to assist grieving people in their darkest moments.

Managing the aftermath of the death of a child can have extraordinary negative effects on emergency personnel and other crisis workers. They may experience <u>vicarious traumatization</u> by a child's death more so than by dealing with the death of most adults. Some may even develop various post-traumatic reactions such as depression, substance abuse, rage reactions, brief psychotic reactions, personality changes, and even PTSD. One of the best ways to manage the stress of a child's death is to use the services of a CISM team. Talk to someone. Do not let the distressing feelings fester and cause more disturbance as time passes.

There are many reasons why a child's death has a far greater impact on emergency and crisis support personnel than the deaths of adults. Adults always believe that children should outlive them. When that worldview is turned upside down by the death of young children, adults are grief stricken, confused, frustrated, fearful, and angered. They perceive those deaths as horribly unfair, and they often feel powerless and fearful about protecting children in their lives from a similar fate. Trained CISM team members can utilize supportive interventions for distressed emergency personnel.

A Word on Pets

Obviously, this chapter relates to death and <u>bereavement</u> in human beings. It would be a mistake, however, to discount the impact of the death of pets. The loss of a pet may be at least as distressing for some people as the death of a human loved one. In some cases, pets provide companionship for people who cannot get out easily or provide important services, as with guide dogs for people who are blind or who assist people who have other disabilities. Owners may have more contact with their pets than with other human beings, and the grief reactions for pets mirror those for human beings. Emergency and crisis intervention personnel should treat people who have lost a pet with the same respect and concern that they might express toward people bereaved by the loss of a human loved one.

Final Thoughts

Few crises will challenge emergency and crisis intervention personnel as seriously as death. In managing the death of others, emergency personnel may gain unexpected insights into their own deaths. As Leonardo da Vinci once said, "While I thought that I was learning how to live, I have been learning how to die."

Selected References

Carr A (ed): *What Works With Children and Adolescents? A Critical Review of Psychological Interventions With Children, Adolescents and Their Families.* London, England, Brunner-Routledge, 2000.

Connecticut Department of Public Health. Available at: http://www.ct.gov/dph/site/default.asp. Accessed July 20, 2008.

Eckstein M, Stratton SJ, Chan LS: Termination of resuscitative efforts for out-of-hospital cardiac arrests. *Acad Emerg Med,* 2005;12:65–70.

Gilbert KR: Anticipated losses and anticipatory grief: grief in a family context—HPER F460/F560. Available at: http://www.indiana.edu/~famlygrf/units/anticipated.html. Accessed July 20, 2008.

Greenberg LW, Ochsenschlager D, O'Donnell R, Mastruserio J, Cohen GJ: Communicating bad news: a pediatric department's evaluation of a simulated intervention. *Pediatrics,* 1999;103:1210–1217.

Iserson K: *Grave Words: Notifying Survivors About Sudden, Unexpected Deaths.* Tucson, AZ, Galen Press, 1999.

Koenig BA, Gates-Williams J: Understanding cultural difference in caring for dying patients. *West J Med,* 1995;163:244–249.

Miller JE: *Grief Tips.* Fort Wayne, IN, Willowgreen Productions, 1996.

Nardi TJ, Keefe-Cooperman K: Communicating bad news: a model for emergency mental health helpers. *Int J Emerg Ment Health,* 2006;8:203–207.

Rolland JS: Anticipatory loss: a family systems developmental framework. *Fam Process,* 1990;29:229–244.

Rolland JS: Helping families with anticipatory loss and terminal illness, in Wash F, Mcgoldrick M (eds): *Living Beyond Loss: Death in the Family,* ed 2. New York, NY, Norton, 2004, pp 214–236.

Schmidt TA, Harrahill MA: Family response to out-of-hospital death. *Acad Emerg Med,* 1995;2:513–518.

Shapiro ER: Family bereavement and cultural diversity: a social development perspective. *Fam Process,* 1996;35:313–332.

Shih FJ, Lai MK, Lin MH, et al: Impact of cadeveric organ donation on Taiwanese donor families during the first 6 months after donation. *Psychosom Med,* 2001;63:9–78.

Smialek Z: Observations on immediate reactions of families to sudden infant death. *Pediatrics,* 1978;62:160–165.

Smith TL, Walz BJ, Smith RL: A death education curriculum for emergency physicians, paramedics, and other emergency personnel. *Prehosp Emerg Care,* 1999;3:37–41.

Smith-Cumberland TL: *Course Lecture Notes on Death and Dying: Death Notification.* Baltimore, MD, University of Maryland Baltimore County, 1994, 2007.

Steinhauser KE, Christakis NA, Clipp EC, McNeilly M, McIntyre L, Tulsky JA: Factors considered important at the end of life by patients, family, physicians, and other care providers. *JAMA,* 2000;284:2476–2482.

Victim Service Network (2003). Available at: http://www.vs2000.org/denver/en/tech_asst_training/model/trauma.html. Accessed July 20, 2008.

Wash F, McGoldrick M (eds): *Living Beyond Loss: Death in the Family,* ed 2. New York, NY, Norton, 2004.

Prep Kit

Ready for Review

- Many people use the terms *bereavement, mourning,* and *grief* interchangeably. In reality, they are very different concepts.
- *Grief* is an intense sorrow or mental anguish and may include physical, social, behavioral, or cognitive aspects. Grief tends to be the more acute emotion demonstrated by family and friends following the death of a loved one.
- *Mourning* is a prolonged process during which one adapts to the loss of the loved one. This time is often influenced by one's culture, norms, or customs.
- *Bereavement* is a larger, broader state of loss and sadness that follows the death of a loved one. It includes the periods of grief and mourning.
- When facing our own mortality, we tend to go through a variety of phases as we move toward acceptance that we are going to die. It is common for individuals to deny the threat of death and even to try to bargain their way out of it through sacrifice or prayer. Many people express anger toward the situation. When one begins to accept that death is possible, the person will begin to grieve and experience great sadness and loss.
- Making a death notification to a family member is one of the most difficult tasks assigned to the emergency responder. However, learning and practicing the proper technique of death notification will enable the emergency responder to provide some comfort to the family. By contrast, haphazard and cold announcements can further confuse and traumatize loved ones of the deceased.
- There are four steps in making a death notification: pre-death, actual death notification, follow-up, and grief.
- Hospice personnel are experts in the area of managing dying patients. Progressive mental health professionals and EMS providers should actively seek out partnerships and training opportunities with hospice whenever possible.
- No two individuals or families respond to the death of a loved one in the same manner. Generally speaking, adults may express their grief in a variety of ways, including shock, fainting, denial, feeling overwhelmed, numbness, anger, or deep emotional and physical anguish.
- Children will react to death based upon their developmental age and knowledge of the death experience. Some families will ask you to tell a child while others will want to reserve that for a family member. Young children may appear unaffected by the death of a loved one, while adolescents will generally react much like adults.

Vital Vocabulary

anticipatory grief Actively processing thoughts and feelings related to the loss of a person before the death has occured.

bereavement A more generalized state of loss, sadness, grief, and mourning following the loss of a loved one.

grief The intense sorrow or mental anguish that occurs with one's death, which may include physical, social, behavioral, or cognitive aspects.

hospice A multi-disciplinary service program for the dying person and his or her family, which provides the support needed to keep the dying person comfortable and free from pain until the time of death.

mourning The process in which one adapts to the loss of an individual or loved one. Mourning is often affected by cultural customs, norms, and rituals.

validation The process or statements used in crisis intervention that acknowledge that the person's feelings or reactions are being heard and are acceptable given the current situation.

vicarious traumatization Vicarious trauma is a term used to describe the thoughts, feelings, and behaviors that can result from repeated exposure to the trauma of others.

Prep Kit | continued

Assessment in Action

Answer key is located in the back of the book.

1. You are watching the evening news and they are reporting a story about a car bombing in another country. You witness local citizens screaming, crying, and throwing themselves onto the ground. Others are grasping religious icons and holding them to the sky looking for guidance. These actions best exemplify which of the following concepts?

    A. Grief
    B. Mourning
    C. Sadness
    D. Bereavement

2. From the following list, select the best phrase when making a death notification.

    A. "Your wife is in a better place now."
    B. "God needed another angel."
    C. "Your wife has passed on."
    D. "I'm very sorry to have to tell you that your wife has died."

3. You respond to a residence where you are required to make a death notification to an elderly female about her husband of 54 years who died in his sleep during the night. Following your announcement, she falls over onto the sofa, begins crying, and screams that she can't live without him. She then gets up and runs into the kitchen as if looking for a knife to harm herself. Her reaction is best described as:

    A. mourning.
    B. depression.
    C. grief.
    D. bargaining.

4. A child's reaction to the death of a loved one is based upon which of the following factors?

    A. Age
    B. Maturity
    C. Developmental stage
    D. All of the above

5. A year ago, your partner, Louis, witnessed the death of a 3-year-old girl in a car crash. At the time, he kept telling you how his daughter had the same pink coat. In the past few months, you notice that Louis has become short and argumentative with patients, wants to obtain refusals, and prefers to drive. His wife tells you that he has had poor sleep and often wakes up with nightmares. You suspect which of the following?

    A. Depression
    B. Vicarious traumatization
    C. Prolonged grief
    D. Job "burnout"

Chapter 9

Crisis Intervention in Disasters and Other Large-Scale Incidents

History bears witness to the idea that disasters can set the stage for significant improvements in human experience. The Titanic's collision with an iceberg in 1912 took the lives of over 1,500 people; after that, passenger ships were required to have lifeboat drills and sufficient lifeboats for every person on board. Fire safety codes were changed dramatically after 492 people were killed in the Cocoanut Grove nightclub fire in 1942. After 11 people died in the 1996 collision of two trains in Silver Spring, Maryland, emergency exit release handles were mandated on the exterior of passenger train cars so that responding emergency personnel could access them quickly. Emergency exit windows were also made easier for passengers to open from inside the train (**Figure 9-1**).

It is dangerous for human beings to become complacent and think that just because nothing has gone wrong yet, nothing will go wrong in the future. We must remain vigilant for the signs of danger before they escalate into a disastrous situation. Prevention of catastrophic conditions is a primary goal, but we should also be prepared to manage disasters or other large-scale incidents should they develop.

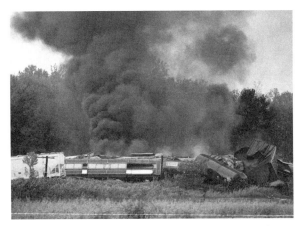 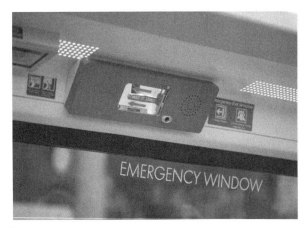

Figure 9-1 Disasters often lead to significant changes in safety precautions.

Psychological Effects

In the event of a large-scale disaster, it is easy to focus solely on managing physical injuries and to ignore the psychological effects of the situation. Because psychological trauma is not as easy to see as a broken arm, we may be predisposed to ignore it in times of crisis. Among the consequences of insufficient attention to the psychological reactions to disaster is the very real potential that emergency services organizations will be unprepared to deal with the majority of the victims they may encounter. Disasters often produce from 4 to 10 psychological casualties for every physically wounded or deceased casualty. In 1995, Aum Shinrikyo, a domestic Japanese terrorist organization, used Sarin gas to conduct five coordinated attacks on the Tokyo subway system. Twelve people were killed, 50 more were severely injured, and nearly 1,000 others experienced temporary vision problems. However, four times the number of wounded people sought immediate assistance from emergency services personnel or in the emergency departments of area hospitals. The overwhelming majority of these patients had no physical problems, but were obviously psychologically distressed. Government, emergency services, and hospital personnel were not adequately prepared to deal with this enormous surge in "unwounded casualties." The unwounded casualties represent a phenomenon called the iceberg effect. The part of an iceberg that is visible in the ocean is far smaller than the part that lays unseen below the water. Similarly, the obviously injured casualties in an emergency may be only a small fraction of the total number of people in need of psychological attention.

Among the many possible outcomes of exposure to traumatic events are depression, rage reactions, brief psychotic reactions, critical incident stress, personality changes, suicidal thinking, emotional withdrawal, deterioration in cognitive functions, physical manifestations of distress, and post-traumatic stress disorder (PTSD). Emergency services organizations and crisis intervention teams should take seriously preparations to manage the emotional needs of people affected by disaster. Good crisis intervention lowers the potential for both immediate distress and long-range psychological problems.

The Nature of Disaster

A **disaster** is any event that overwhelms the available emergency resources of a particular jurisdiction or community and causes the people providing emergency services to function at a less-than-optimal level of performance. Disasters can develop from many circumstances. They may be the result of natural causes, such as earthquakes, tornadoes, floods, ice and snow storms, strong winds, drought, wild fires, hurricanes, or tsunamis. There are about 200 significant natural disasters or near disasters in the world in an average year. Just as often, however, disasters are caused by human beings. Halifax, Nova Scotia, for example, was nearly wiped off the map in 1917 when two ships loaded with explosives collided. In 1947, Texas City, Texas, experienced a catastrophic ammonium nitrate explosion when incorrect fire suppression tactics for a ship fire were used. The Brooklyn Marine disaster in 1956 was either caused deliberately by disgruntled laborers or accidentally started by careless welding practices. Overcrowding and the resulting threats of disease, pollution, violence, war, terrorism, and the depletion of natural resources may all cause disasters. <u>Technological disasters</u> are disasters caused by human-made factors, including chemicals, utilities, buildings, bridges, planes, trains, buses, trucks, and ships. Crashes, explosions, fires, widespread poisonings, chemical leaks, and structural damage or collapse are but a few of the disasters that are possible as a result of human activity (**Figure 9-2**).

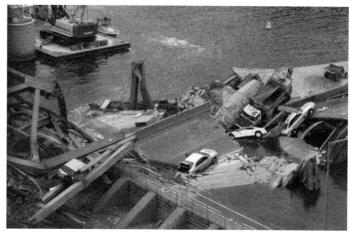

Figure 9-2 Technological disasters are disasters caused by human-made factors.

Psychological Stages of Disaster

In the 1970s, Dr. Calvin Fredericks, a mental health disaster researcher, identified specific psychological stages of many disasters. These stages are most likely to occur in disasters in which warnings have been issued, but some of the stages also have application to sudden, unexpected disasters. The specific stages of disaster are:

- Warning
- Alarm
- Impact
- Inventory
- Rescue
- Recovery
- Reconstruction

Each stage has its own prominent emotional states, and it is vital that emergency personnel know how to react and what to expect during each stage. Denial and anxiety begin as soon as the first distant *warnings* of disaster are announced. This is particularly so in threatening natural phenomena like tornados and hurricanes. People like to believe that nothing bad will happen to them or that they can survive the disaster unharmed. They may initially not want to take shelter or move out of the area. Other people may face difficulties in moving or taking shelter and so may hope to stay in place. However, once a warning has been given and repeated several times, even people who ignored the original warnings begin to grow more concerned about the approaching disaster. Your job as emergency personnel is to assist the authorities in convincing the population that the threat is real and people need to move out of the area or seek shelter. When people wait too long to protect themselves, they may lose their escape routes. They may then show up at your station requesting shelter and protection. Obviously this will complicate your work. As a disaster shifts from a distant potential to an imminent event, denial and anxiety do not disappear. They simply shift positions. Anxiety becomes prominent, and denial becomes secondary.

In the *alarm* phase, which is sometimes marked by sirens and other alert signals, the disaster is imminent and threatening, and anxiety becomes more focused, while denial, although still present, begins to fade. Denial tends to be a tenacious emotional state. Facing the facts of a situation and the fear that results is uncomfortable and people would rather believe that they are safe. Emergency personnel are most likely taking cover themselves in this phase. They face the uncomfortable decision of removing themselves from danger while the people who refused to evacuate earlier are now in a state of considerable threat to life and limb. Anxiety levels and feelings of guilt may rise for emergency personnel. There is also anxiety about what they may be facing after the storm passes.

When the *impact* of the disaster event occurs, there is another emotional shift. For example, that emotional shift occurs when the hurricane finally hits and then passes away. In this case, shock enters the psychological picture and may produce mental disorientation and, for many people, an inability to take immediate actions to help themselves. Specific fears replace vague anxieties. Denial, although far less prominent, still holds a place in the emotional reactions to the event and may drive people to do irrational things, such as taking excessive risks like climbing on top of significantly destroyed building structures without taking precautions.

Emergency personnel are going to be immediately busy in these circumstances. They will have rescue missions, and they will be treating the wounded and attempting to maintain civil order. It may not seem like crisis intervention, but every visible physical action emergency personnel take in the early stages of a disaster can be seen as reassurance to the community that emergency personnel are doing everything they can to help with the situation.

Once the threat posed by the disaster passes, people begin to assess their losses and review their available resources. This is the *inventory* stage. In the inventory stage, shock continues. As people survey the damages and begin to appreciate the losses they have encountered, numbness, apprehension, and fear become the strongest emotional states. Fear can become a significant driving force for people to take action. A strong presence of emergency personnel in the field is crucial to keep the people calm and under control. Give directions. Let people know where disaster relief agencies are setting up. Reassure people that help is mobilizing as quickly as possible.

After any disaster, especially tornados, hurricanes, and earthquakes, people try to help themselves and their families. This is the beginning of the *rescue* stage of the disaster, and it is characterized by altruistic feelings and people reaching out to help others. Family members and neighbors assist one another, even in difficult and dangerous conditions. Calls for assistance go out to the authorities beyond the affected community. Although apprehension continues, the first signs of relief arise. In some cases, the relief may be euphoric. The rescue stage is one of mixed emotions, including anxiety, relief, fear, shock, and disbelief. The most dangerous condition is severe emotional shock. A person may exhibit lowered blood pressure and, sometimes, cardiac symptoms. In many disasters, people die of cardiac arrest as a result of intense emotional distress. The arrival of emergency personnel and other resources may intensify feelings of relief during the rescue stage. A failure of emergency personnel to respond quickly, or not to arrive at all, can generate feelings of overwhelming anxiety, fears of abandonment, and depression. In some cases it can trigger panic or a riot.

The next phase of a disaster begins when the immediate dangers have subsided and at least fundamental resources like a food and water distribution system and a security perimeter have been established. This *recovery* stage should not be mistaken for a complete elimination of the effects of a disaster. It is a slow process that is subject to a variety of delays. After Hurricane Katrina in 2005, recovery efforts were delayed while rescues were still occurring (**Figure 9-3**). The area was so broad that it was difficult to establish security perimeters, and it was several days to a week before food and water could be assured to the population.

The first signs of the recovery stage are the establishment of safety and security in the disaster zone. Once perimeters are established, people begin to work on essential services such as food, water, temporary shelter, and latrine facilities. Many victims must be removed from the disaster zone to receive these services. That was certainly the case

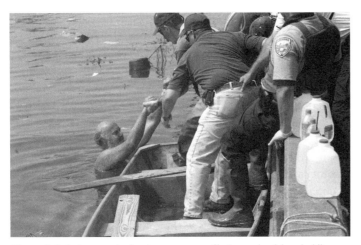

Figure 9-3 In large-scale disasters, recovery efforts may be delayed while rescues are still occurring.

in Hurricane Katrina. The prominent emotions typically are anxiety, relief, emotional numbness, fear, apprehension, and confusion. Emotional breakdowns are more likely to show up in this stage. More people who were not physically wounded will now be seeking evaluation by medics and treatment in emergency departments. Information, reassurance, and guidance, often provided by large-group Crisis Management Briefings (CMB), are going to be most helpful to the population.

The final stage of a disaster, *reconstruction*, is one in which a surprising array of negative feelings might arise. This is the rebuilding stage, and it is the longest. Even 3 to 4 years after Hurricane Katrina, rebuilding is still going on. People who are caught up in what appears to be an endless process of disappointments and frustrations lose patience and become depressed. Common feelings during the reconstruction period include frustration, grief, anger, disappointment, and feeling emotionally and physically overwhelmed. Although things are being rebuilt, there are delays, shortages, frustrations over unfulfilled government promises, disputes with insurance companies, and a host of other problems. People become distracted by their emotions. Injuries increase, as do illnesses. In the Texas City incident previously mentioned, blood pressure climbed and stayed elevated in most patients for almost a year after the explosion.

In the aftermath of disasters that have caused great losses, some people contemplate suicide. It is not unusual to find somewhat elevated suicide rates after tornadoes, hurricanes, floods, and earthquakes. People have lost almost everything they owned and the cost is far beyond what can be measured by means of a price tag. There are the emotional costs as well. Eventually, as things slowly progress, hope for a resolution of the disastrous situation may finally arise.

Psychological Reactions to Disaster

The psychological reactions to a disaster are many and varied. They can usually be sorted into five main categories: cognitive, physical, emotional, behavioral, and spiritual. Some reactions, such as agitation and distractedness during a disastrous event, are short-term and generally resolve with the passage of time or with a limited amount of emotional support. Some reactions and stress symptoms, however, do not resolve easily and eventually become manifestations of long-term psychological conditions.

Short-Term Reactions

- Worry and fear
- Bad memories
- Gastrointestinal symptoms (upset stomach and diarrhea)
- Sadness
- Mental confusion (feeling lost and disoriented)
- Feeling overwhelmed
- Acute emotional discharge or tirade
- Brief psychotic reactions
- Shock

In the Field

Psychological Stages of a Disaster

- Warning
- Alarm
- Impact
- Inventory
- Rescue
- Recovery
- Reconstruction

In the Field

Five Categories of Psychological Reaction to Disaster

- Cognitive
- Physical
- Emotional
- Behavioral
- Spiritual

- Difficulty solving problems and making decisions
- Acute cognitive impairment
- Dissociation (depersonalization and de-realization)
- Loss of appetite
- Lowered libido (sex drive)
- Headache
- Elevated blood pressure
- Rapid pulse
- Increased breathing rate
- Withdrawal from contact with others
- Hiding (particularly in children)
- Loss of self-confidence and self-esteem
- Guilt feelings
- Anger
- Frustration
- Irritability
- Feeling abandoned by God
- Loss of faith

The majority of the short-term reactions to disasters or other large-scale disturbing events are remarkably responsive to crisis intervention. Sometimes positive results begin to appear within a half hour. Not all of the reactions to crisis are completely resolved with crisis intervention, but the first steps toward recovery usually begin when properly trained emergency personnel and other crisis workers initiate crisis intervention services.

Short-term reactions can turn into longer-term or more serious reactions if they are not addressed early enough. Any symptoms that appear severe or incapacitating should be evaluated by medical and psychological professionals immediately. Information and guidance are the keys to dealing with the signals of distress. People need to know what is happening to them and why. They also need to know that the signals of distress are typical and not signs of abnormal conditions. It is reassuring to people to know that the majority of people recover fairly quickly from the distress experienced after a disaster. Crisis Management Briefings (see Chapter 5) are a remarkable tool and can be applied at almost any time during or after the disaster. They help to keep a constant flow of information and instructions going out to the victims. It is even possible to put such informational programs on television and radio to reach a broader audience. People should be warned that the normal symptoms of today may turn into the abnormal conditions of tomorrow if they are not resolved. If after about three weeks the symptoms do not subside noticeably, people should seek further evaluation from mental health resources.

Long-Term Reactions

- Chronic fear
- Depression
- Major depression (depressed mood with appetite disturbance, reduced libido, sleep disturbance, lethargy, helplessness, and hopelessness)
- Suicidal thinking
- Withdrawal from loved ones
- Anger
- Rage reactions
- Severe, debilitating guilt
- Excessive, prolonged grief (pathological grief)
- Psychosomatic problems or disorders
- Psychologically based sensory or motor dysfunction
- Memory dysfunction

- Recurrent disturbing thoughts
- Recurrent disturbing dreams
- Panic disorders
- Panic attacks
- Substance abuse
- "Burnout"
- An ongoing crisis of faith
- Loss of faith
- Complete withdrawal from religious practice
- Prolonged, debilitating stress reaction not meeting criteria for PTSD
- PTSD

Although spontaneous recovery is possible in some cases, many long-term reactions to disasters and other intense events require professional intervention from medical and psychological specialists. The difficult reactions do not simply disappear with the passage of time. The more prolonged, complex, and disruptive the long-term reactions, the greater are the needs for professional assistance.

Months after a disaster, emergency medical people might start seeing more people with nebulous complaints that do not have an immediate physical basis. That is a sign that things are breaking down for the victims. Ask people if they were living in the area when the disaster struck and what their experiences were during and after the disaster. You will be surprised how many people will find talking about their experiences uplifting and healing. Encourage people who are struggling months after a disaster to see their physicians and have themselves evaluated. It is best that depression be diagnosed and treated early. If there is a crisis counseling center or hotline, provide contact information to people who are still struggling.

A Planning Formula for Disasters: Target, Type, Timing, Themes, and Team

The reactions and needs of people who witness or work at the scenes of major events or who are victims of a disaster or other disturbing large-scale event may vary substantially. It can be very challenging for emergency operations personnel to know exactly what to do to assist people. There are, however, two extreme emergency responses that should be avoided at all costs. The first is to do *nothing* at all about obvious distress. The second is to do *too much*. Decision making in the midst of a confusing and chaotic condition is complicated by many factors. There are the usual dangers surrounding the actual incident, as well as the operational considerations. There are then the specific needs of individuals, the locations in which help is provided, and the difficulties of obtaining the right resources.

A simple planning formula may be very useful for emergency and crisis intervention personnel. The formula offered here is called the *five-T planning formula,* and it can help to organize an approach to assisting people during and after a large-scale event of virtually any magnitude. The five-T planning formula includes the following elements:

- Target
- Type
- Timing
- Themes
- Team

For operations personnel to respond appropriately to a disaster, they need to *target* who needs assistance and who does not. There are many potential targets within a large-scale event. Wounded victims, witnesses, unwounded survivors, emergency and disaster relief personnel, community members, children, the elderly, family members, the general public, and possibly other specific populations all have different needs and different issues. It is important that operations and crisis intervention personnel think in terms of psychological triage. People with different needs should be identified within specific categories to facilitate the provision of the proper support services in accordance with their needs.

The first step to managing the psychological aftereffects of a disaster is to call in a Critical Incident Stress Management (CISM) team. Team members have had extensive training and will be able to assess the various groups and divide them up into target populations. CISM team members also know how to identify the most serious cases and where to refer them to provide them with the best professional services.

The next step is to provide information to those who are doing reasonably well. That is typically all they need. There are just too many disaster victims, and you cannot reach them all. You must depend on adults to take care of children. Focus your energies on specific populations who can then assist others (**Figure 9-4**). For example, in a school setting, administration, faculty, and staff should be the focus of information from emergency personnel. They, in turn, will put their energies into managing classes, clubs, and athletic teams.

Finally, refer anyone for further evaluation who appears seriously distraught or dysfunctional. The referral resource will determine if someone needs counseling.

Crisis intervention and emergency personnel must select the best *type* of support services and not implement a one-size-fits-all philosophy. Some people need their safety and security issues addressed immediately. Others need shelter, rest, food, and water. Still others will need individual crisis intervention. Sometimes people need group crisis support as described in Chapter 5. Family support and referrals are also important in disasters. The list of potential services is long, and will depend in part on the resources in each community. Simply start any conversation with people who have called for assistance with a question: "What do you need most right now? How can we best help you?" If injuries are the first concern, treat the injuries. If the person does not need transfer to a hospital, then you must find out what other needs the person has. When you cannot manage their requests, you may either involve other resources or refer them to medical, legal, psychological, or social resources.

Timing refers to the right time to provide whatever support services are deemed necessary. Support that is initiated too early, when people are still involved in the immediate threat, will be rejected as unimportant under the circumstances. Assistance that is delayed will often be viewed as too little and too late. Always consider when the assistance would be most effective, given the current circumstances. Experience indicates that most people will tell you what they need during a disaster. If they do not bring it up, ask them. In the huge Missouri River and Mississippi River floods in 1993, the only way authorities were able to determine what types of support people needed was to send case workers out to farms and communities and knock on doors. Once the questions were asked, people opened up, described their experiences, and eventually told the case worker what they needed most.

Theme is a very broad concept. It refers to the current threat, the causes of the crisis reaction, the conditions under which the crisis intervention services would be applied, schedules, and any circumstances that would influence decision making or the resources needed to provide help. It also means any other issue, concern, or consideration related to the event and to the people in need of assistance. Themes are present in and influence all of the other aspects of the five-T planning formula. Crisis and emergency personnel must do their best to gather as much information as possible about a situation and the people who are involved to ensure that the very

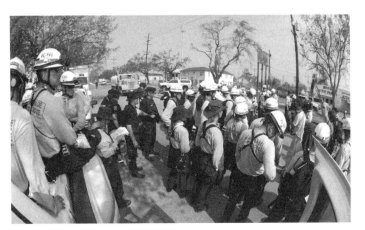
Figure 9-4 Focus your energies on specific populations who can then assist others.

best services are selected and presented at the right time to ensure the greatest potential for a successful intervention.

When many themes are present in a disaster response, emergency personnel may need to slow down and decide which themes are high priority and which are less important. Decisions need to be appropriate for the high-priority themes. Theme issues need to be satisfied in the planning process according to their urgency and their power to disrupt or enhance whatever you choose to do.

> ## In the Field
>
> **Five-T Planning Formula**
> - Target
> - Type
> - Timing
> - Themes
> - Team

The *team* aspect of the formula is the resource or resources needed to effectively render assistance. In some cases, only one person may be required to provide assistance to an individual or to a family affected by a disaster. In other cases, an entire team of people will be required to provide the assistance. Themes will dictate whether a single person or a whole team is required. Obviously, only people who are properly trained in crisis intervention should be selected to provide crisis support.

The five-T planning formula helps emergency personnel and crisis workers intervene strategically. In the 1993 Station nightclub fire in Rhode Island, 100 people died and more than 200 were injured. The scene was chaotic and horrifying for all involved. The fire fighters, police officers, and emergency medical personnel were shocked and overwhelmed by the speed and devastation of the fire, the extensive loss of life, and the serious injuries sustained by people in the nightclub during the fire. That brief description highlights numerous target groups. There are the bereaved families, injured people, fire fighters, law enforcement officers, emergency medical personnel, spectators, and media. The type of threat was a major fire.

There were numerous themes. The fire moved extremely rapidly and did not allow much time for escape. The participants were mostly older teens and young adults. They were in the club for an entertaining evening. Sub-themes included facts such as siblings who had come to the nightclub together and people who were celebrating birthdays. Many in the crowd mistakenly thought the fire was part of the show and were therefore reluctant to leave when the fire began. Another theme is that the fire came under legal scrutiny quickly. All of those themes and sub-themes mean that a CISM team has much to consider before instituting a crisis support program.

One of the first decisions is determining the types of interventions to be offered and the timing of those interventions. The different target populations have quite different needs. It is essential that the right help be provided at the right time, under the right circumstances, and by the right people. The bereaved will need immediate crisis support, but over time they may need bereavement support groups and possibly grief therapy. Fire fighters will need a Rest, Information, and Transition Session (RITS) during the incident, followed by individual support, a group Critical Incident Stress Debriefing (CISD) in about a week, and additional individual support services. Some of the fire fighters might have difficulty recovering from the event and might require a referral for professional assistance. Police officers who provided perimeter control will have different needs than those who tried to pull people from the burning building. EMS crews who dealt with the dead and wounded will need separate assistance, because their views and their issues will vary from those of fire fighters and police officers.

The last link in the five-T planning formula is the team or the resources required to provide the right support. The crisis team must match the needs of the target populations. Who should work with the spectators? Who would be best to work with the survivors? Which police officers on the CISM team have the most experience with multi-victim events?

The five-T planning formula helps emergency response personnel to mobilize an entire community to take effective actions that will enhance community recovery in the aftermath of an overwhelming event.

Psychological Triage

Triage should first place people into large categories and subsequently into smaller subcategories. For example, at a disaster there will be responders and community members. The main categories are easily identifiable with the use of those two labels, but we cannot stop there. Subcategories are necessary to further develop the best intervention plan. Under the broad category of responders are, of course, emergency personnel such as police, fire, rescue, organized search units, the National Guard and other armed forces units, and emergency medical personnel. But there may also be responders from the Federal Emergency Management Agency, the Red Cross, the Salvation Army, the National Association of Victim Assistance, and a wide range of faith-based organizations. Various other support services may also respond to the large-scale event. There may be construction workers and other volunteers who help remove debris, find missing people, or clean up the disaster site.

There are several subcategories within the category of community members. There are both wounded and unwounded survivors. Family members of those who experienced the disaster may quickly congregate in or near the disaster area. There may be bereaved people who have experienced the death of a loved one. Community members might include property owners who have sustained losses. There may be witnesses who saw or heard distressing events, but who were not otherwise directly impacted by the event. There might also be community members who live in the vicinity of a disaster and are generally upset but who have not been personally affected by the situation.

Once the target populations are categorized and sub-categorized, emergency and crisis intervention personnel can select the best intervention tactics and develop a plan for applying the various support services at the most appropriate times. **Table 9-1** provides a side-by-side guide of suggested interventions for the two main categories of people (responders and community members) involved in a disaster or other large-scale event. Note that support services for one category sometimes are identical with those for the other category. In most cases, however, there are substantial differences in the types of interventions to assist people through the acute stages of the incident.

Lists of crisis interventions should not be viewed as stagnant and fixed. Crisis intervention is a dynamic field that can easily adjust to challenges as long as crisis workers are thoughtful and flexible. Adjustments may be required within the large categories, especially when support services are provided to people in the various subcategories suggested in the preceding paragraphs.

Please note that the CISD, a small-group crisis intervention tactic for homogeneous groups of emergency personnel, was never intended for use as a crisis intervention tactic for individuals, nor was it intended for use with <u>heterogeneous</u> (mixed) <u>groups</u> such as disaster victims. It has almost no place on the list of crisis intervention tactics for community members during and after a disaster. It should only be used for homogeneous groups such as emergency personnel, military units, and others who are interacting as unified groups. To be a <u>homogeneous group</u>, the members must have a common history, have similar goals and objectives, be known to each other, and have shared time together in similar activities.

With emergency personnel, the focus or theme of crisis intervention must be:

1. *Maintain operational functions.* Emergency personnel have a job to do, and crisis intervention must never interfere with those jobs. In fact, crisis intervention should enhance job performance, not detract from it.
2. *Alleviate acute distress* by cutting down on auditory, visual, and olfactory stimuli.
3. *Enhance unit cohesion* by helping the group members listen to and understand more clearly what their colleagues are experiencing.
4. *Enhance unit performance* by helping individuals understand that they are part of a team and have obligations to support their fellow workers.
5. *Prevent dysfunctional stress* by helping emergency personnel understand that the majority of their stress reactions are quite normal and healthy and that most people will recover from them in a reasonable time frame.

Table 9-1 Matching Crisis Support Services to the Target Populations

Time Frame	Responders	Community Members
1 to 3 hours	• **Brief** before deployment • Mobilize CISM team • Link CISM to command • CISM **assessment** team • Develop CISM **strategic plan** • Provide **consultation to command** • **Assist individuals** as required	• **Evacuate** from danger • **Regroup** families/friends • **Guide** and direct • Set up gathering points • Establish **safe shelters** • Provide **food and fluids** • Provide **security** • Provide **information** • **Calm distress**
3 to 12 hours	• Provide **Rest, Information, and Transition Sessions (RITS)** to operations personnel who are being released from the scene after first exposure • **Assist distressed** individuals as necessary • Provide **command consultations** • **Food** and fluids • Brief newly arrived operations personnel before deployment • Develop CISM **plan** for next operational period • Use the **"five-T" planning** formula • Continue **RIT sessions** until all operations personnel on the first exposure to the incident are processed through the RIT • **Immediate small-group support** for homogeneous work units with a particularly distressing experience	• Move to shelters • Provide **essential services** • Provide **information** • **Reconnect** people with family, friends, and neighbors • Provide **Crisis Management Briefings (CMB)** • **Assist individuals** as necessary • **Instill hope** • **Assign helping roles** for those who can manage those roles in shelters • Begin the process of assisting people to exit shelter care as soon as they establish other **alternatives to the shelter**
12 to 24 hours	• Initiate **Crisis Management Briefings** for operations personnel who are new to or re-entering the scene and provide updated information • Continue **command consultations** • **Assist individuals** if necessary • Cease RIT programs and **use CMBs** after work shifts and pre-shift briefings	• Implement programs to **occupy children** in shelters • Use **periodic CMBs** to provide updated information • **Guide** shelter occupants **to** various **resources** • **Psychological first aid** to assist individuals and to determine their specific needs
24 to 72 hours	• **Brief** before each deployment • **Individual support** as required • Ensure **rest, food,** and **fluids** are available • Provide information and **support** to the **families** of operations personnel • Continue **respite centers** • **Monitor well-being** of operations personnel • Use **CMBs** as necessary • Provide **command consultations** • Assess for significant stress reactions • **Work site visits** by CISM team members • Have **chaplain services** available • **Immediate small-support** for homogeneous groups of operations personnel exposed to highly distressing situations during disaster relief work	• Use CMBs to community members • **Connect** people to appropriate resources (Federal Emergency Management Agency or Red Cross) • Assistance in **finding the missing** • **Assist the bereaved** • Provide for **prescriptions** and replace lost glasses • Assess for medical problems • **Assess** for development of **significant mental deterioration** • Offer **spiritual support** • **Set goals** for leaving shelter • **Arrange site visits** if family members or property owners need that to facilitate their recovery or to deal with grief • **Promote self-efficacy**

(Continued)

Table 9-1 (Continued)

Time Frame	Responders	Community Members
72 hours to end of disaster	• Individual support • Briefings as necessary • CMBs as necessary • Family support • Chaplain services • Disengagement from operations • Handout materials • Rest and recovery time • Referrals if required	• CMBs to update information • Individual psychological first aid • Preparations for exit from shelter and return to "normal" life functions • Referrals for professional care if required
After the disaster	• Individual support • Post-disaster education • Powerful Event Group Support for homogeneous groups of operations personnel (also known as Critical Incident Stress Debriefing–CISD) • Post-Action Staff Support for the CISM team • Additional referrals if required • Review experiences for lessons learned	• Individual support • Informational flyers • Follow-up on referrals • Psychotherapy for those who need it • Some group work may be helpful only for homogeneous groups • Ongoing support groups • Follow-up services as required

The focus of crisis intervention with community members (actual victims, witnesses, and family members) should be:

1. *Promote a sense of safety* by moving people out of the danger zone and reducing the stimuli that are bombarding them.
2. *Promote calming* by speaking in a controlled voice and by giving adequate stress-related information and specific guidance.
3. *Encourage self- and community efficacy* by reuniting common groups such as families and encouraging them to care for one another during the emergency situation. Encourage people to perform tasks as they are able to do so; this will help them feel effective and in some degree of control.
4. *Connect people to their natural support systems and resources.* Make sure that neighbors, friends, and relatives are reunited as early as possible in a disaster.
5. *Instill and maintain hope.* Let people know that they are going through a very bad situation but that most people do recover from such things and continue on with happy and productive lives.

The choice of the most helpful *types* of interventions must match the needs of the *target* populations. Those interventions must be applied at the right *time* and be in accordance with the *themes* associated with the distressing event. Finally, the most appropriate resources from crisis *teams* must conduct the interventions carefully to achieve the maximum benefit.

The following sections discuss some challenging large-scale situations. The management of those situations will rely heavily on the information presented up to this point in this chapter.

Terrorism

Terrorism can have an enormous debilitating impact on large segments of a population. The explicit goal of terrorism is to create fear, uncertainty, feelings of futility, and helplessness as a coercive or punitive force. Terrorism may be designed to break the will of the enemy to resist.

As with other large-scale events, there is an iceberg effect with terrorism. Physical death, injuries, and destruction are only the tip of the iceberg. Behind those visible horrible effects, there is even more widespread devastation in the form of psychological toxicity.

Psychological toxicity occurs when people lose hope and self-confidence, become anxious and depressed, feel hopeless, and wish to give up. Psychological toxicity intensifies as innocent people are killed or maimed. The unpredictability and undetectable nature of the attacks increases their psychological power. When terrorists claim moral justifications to defend their acts, people may react with profound mental confusion and emotional shock, because such justifications can challenge core belief systems.

There are several important and powerful tools necessary for managing a terrorism event from a psychological perspective. The first tool is the truth. People can usually handle bad news as long as the truth is presented in a careful and professional manner. The truth should be spoken consistently, and inadvertent errors must be corrected immediately. As circumstances change and the course of action is altered, people should be informed of those changes in a timely and efficient manner.

Information is one of the most powerful tools for assisting a population traumatized by a terrorist incident. Information can guide and direct people, encourage them to avoid danger zones, and enable them to take positive actions that are important for their survival. Accurate information lowers anxiety and calms distressed people. Information helps people unite and form a common bond with others in the community, and it instills hope and courage to continue resistance in the face of extraordinary distress.

Incidents Involving Children

Situations involving children are among the most challenging and emotion-provoking large-scale events. We relate personally and strongly to children, because most of us have important children in our lives. It is uncomfortable for us when the young and the innocent are victims of tragedies. It is, however, very important that we not allow the personal emotions stimulated by the distressed, injured, and deceased persons to interfere with our ability to assist them through a crisis.

Children's reactions to traumatic events may be immediate or delayed, depending on the age of the child and the circumstances of the traumatic event. Performing triage and determining the target of crisis intervention are crucial. Not all children are alike in their reactions. Children who are 5 years old and younger often suffer from a fear of separation from parents. They may cry, whimper, scream, experience immobility, or wander aimlessly. It is not unusual to see trembling, terrified facial expressions and excessive clinging to parents. Some children regress to younger behaviors, such as thumb sucking, bed-wetting, and fear of darkness. Parental reactions heavily influence a child's reaction. Likewise, other adults can also influence the reactions of children to disaster. Emergency workers must remain calm and in control of themselves and must express themselves in ways that suggest confidence (**Figure 9-5**).

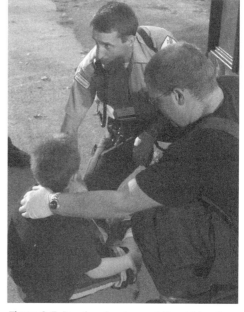

Children who are 6 to 11 years old may withdraw from contact with others. Sometimes their behavior becomes disruptive. Children in this age bracket often find it difficult to pay attention. Schoolwork often deteriorates in the weeks and months after the disaster. Sleep disturbances, irrational fears, regressive behaviors, refusal to go to school, angry outbursts, and fighting with others are common reactions to distressing disasters. Some children complain of vague physical complaints, such as stomach aches and headaches, without any medical basis for such complaints. Some children in this age group will become depressed, anxious, and guilt ridden, while others will experience emotional numbing.

Figure 9-5 Remain calm when assisting children in a disaster situation.

Some of the symptoms described may also appear in adolescents who are 12 to 17 years old. These children may also experience symptoms common to adults. Symptoms include flashbacks, emotional numbing, and avoidance of anything that reminds them of the traumatic event. Depression, substance abuse, peer conflict, and antisocial behaviors also occur. Withdrawal from contact with others and social isolation may accompany guilt feelings, suicidal thinking, mental confusion, and sleep disturbances, along with anger, rage, and desire for revenge. School shootings are an example of a disaster situation that puts emergency personnel into close contact with teenagers. The calm, professional approach by emergency personnel may be very reassuring to teenagers. Teens will try to model their own behavior on what they have witnessed (ie, confident and thoughtful emergency personnel).

Some adolescents will lose trust in the adults around them. Children who are victims of abuse and neglect, have a history of previous disturbing traumas, or have existing mental health problems are generally more vulnerable to disaster-related traumatic events. Children without adequate family support will have the greatest difficulty recovering from a traumatic event.

As with adults, always be truthful with adolescents. They need to know your word is good and that what you tell them is accurate and current.

Assisting Children in Need

To assist children in a disaster or other large-scale event, begin interventions as quickly as possible once they are out of immediate danger. Ensure safety and prevent further exposure to disturbing sights and sounds. The media can make things worse for children, so keep the media away. Move children to safety zones away from the scene of the disaster. Someone, preferably a family member if one is available, should stay with distressed children. Stay with children who are experiencing acute distress or intense grief. They may exhibit signs and symptoms such as panic feelings and panic attacks, trembling, severe agitation, rambling speech, becoming mute, strange behaviors, loud crying, rage reactions, and immobility. Remain with severely distressed children until calm is restored.

Children and their parents or other relatives need clear, precise, and short instructions and directions. Provide reassurance, appropriate hugs, and concerned support to the distressed children. Reunite children with their family members as soon as possible. Engage parents in the care of their own children and of children without parents in the immediate vicinity.

Explain what happened in the event as simply and as clearly as you can. Never force a discussion about the traumatic event, but allow children to discuss it if they wish. You will usually only have enough time for such discussions while you are awaiting the arrival of parents who must travel some distance to be near their children. Accept and validate children's feelings. It is natural for them to be upset. Reassure them that things will gradually return to normal over time.

Without rushing, but as soon as reasonably possible, children should be returned to as normal a school program as is possible under the circumstances. The child should eventually be able to view the disaster as a temporary disruption in his or her life. In most cases, emergency personnel will not be involved in the child's life long enough to see the positive results described here, but the honesty, confidence, and professionalism of emergency workers may serve as a substantial positive influence for distressed children.

Children often imagine that they are at fault for the tragedy. Reassure them that this is not the case. Provide accurate information about how the event occurred.

Encourage parents to restore normal family schedules as much as possible, but have flexibility as well. It will take some time for things to return to normal. Although this is not something a paramedic, police officer, or fire fighter would have any control over, it is not unusual for parents to ask emergency personnel for some guidance and information regarding these issues. Suggestions for parents may include:

- Do not criticize children when they display regressive behaviors. Kindness, understanding, and concern will go far to extinguish those behaviors.

- Do not establish expectations that children should be brave or tough. They may be sad and anxious, and that is expected and understandable.
- Let children have a say in schedules, meals, and what they want to wear. That gives them a sense of control.

Assist parents, teachers, and other adults who care for children. If they can be calmed down and given specific, practical information regarding the management of the crisis, children usually follow the lead of the adults and become calmer and more controlled. Children can be assisted either individually or in groups as needed.

If homogeneous groups of children (homeroom classes, athletic teams, and clubs) need group support, it may be provided by means of group discussions or activities. The leaders of group intervention programs, such as class discussions, should be experienced in group work and the sessions should not be too long or delve too deeply into the emotions of the group members. On occasion, emergency personnel have been invited into such discussions. Emergency personnel who are members of CISM teams are more likely to encounter discussions like these.

Some periodic discussion is important, but do not overdo it. Any child who does not wish to participate in a class discussion about a school tragedy should be allowed to go to another place, such as the school library, during the discussion. Finally, it is very helpful to hold informative meetings with parents to provide them with guidance on helping their families to recover from the tragedy. Except in prolonged sheltering situations, emergency personnel are unlikely to play key roles in the discussions described here. There are over 500 CISM teams who serve emergency personnel in the United States alone. It is advisable that members of the closest CISM team be involved in such discussions. They have received training to manage the emotions that might arise during those meetings.

Search Operations

It is becoming increasingly common to activate a CISM team in the early stages of a search operation. The team responds, and a key CISM team leader is placed within the command sector of the incident command system to act as an advisor and to coordinate CISM resources should they be required during or after the search. Although not considered a disaster according to most definitions, a large-scale search-and-rescue operation may escalate into a challenging event that may stress and strain the lost person, search personnel, the family of the missing person, and the community. Even in cases of a successful live find, the victim may be extremely stressed and may benefit from support from a crisis intervention–trained emergency services person.

As in other large-scale incidents, there are several main categories of people who may need CISM assistance. Support programs should be in place to assist people in the different categories: the lost person, the family, the community, and the response personnel.

The Lost Person

People get lost for many reasons. However, there are some typical psychological and physical conditions that are likely to contribute to the crisis.

Psychological conditions include being mentally distracted or inattentive to details in the environment. Emotionally upset or despondent people are more prone to get lost. When people are upset, they often do not pay attention to their surroundings and they can get disoriented and lost easily. If a person is unprepared for and unfamiliar with an area, getting lost becomes a distinct possibility. Feelings of overconfidence, rejection, fear, guilt, anger, revenge, and frustration, along with a diminished self-image, can all contribute to a person becoming lost.

There are numerous medical conditions that may contribute to a person getting lost. Dyslexia, hypothermia, heat exhaustion, fatigue, physical and emotional stress, alcohol and substance abuse, dehydration, physical injury, and reactions to medication all play a role in becoming lost.

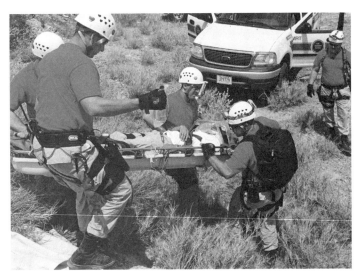

Figure 9-6 Once a person who has been lost for a period of time has been found, he or she will often need psychological first aid.

Once found, the subject of the search will usually need some psychological first aid (**Figure 9-6**). Here are some suggestions that may be helpful in restoring the person's psychological well-being.

First, assess and treat medical conditions immediately. Ensure the physical safety of the found person and treat the person as needed for hypothermia or hyperthermia. Dehydration, cold, heat, high altitude, injury, and toxicity can all cause further mental deterioration. A shocked, very silent, and withdrawn person is the highest priority for immediate evacuation from the scene. Although providers often tend to pay attention to noisy, hysterical, or acting-out victims, they are actually a secondary priority. It is better that they are expressing themselves (although they tend to interfere with the operations) than to be extremely silent and withdrawn. Keep someone with them to help keep their agitation under control. Those who seem to be doing fine at the scene are the third priority for evacuation. Being a third priority, however, does not imply that they should be ignored.

Second, when possible, speak directly to the person once he or she has been rescued. Direct communication is the best means of assessing the condition of the person. Listen carefully to the victims if they are conscious and able to speak. They need opportunities to express themselves. They often need to tell their story. Gently touch a distressed person on the shoulder or hand if they seem receptive to such contact.

Third, accurate, current, and timely information is extremely important to the well-being of victims. Keep yourself calm and your voice soothing and reassuring. Bring them up-to-date. Provide bad news in the field about a friend or colleague who did not fare as well as the person you are assisting *only if the person is medically stable*. Give bad news gently and carefully. Do not rush or delay the information unnecessarily, but give bad news in brief segments, not all at once. The person hearing bad news needs a little time to absorb it piece by piece. Periodically reassure people that they are safe now, especially if they become agitated. Do not tell victims that they are "lucky" or that it could have been worse. Those sorts of statements almost never console and usually anger a distressed person.

Fourth, establish a private area for the victims as soon as possible. Reconnect people with their family and friends. Provide for medical, social, religious, psychological, shelter, food, and other needs as they arise.

Children are the most vulnerable to psychological harm during a stressful search operation or a disaster. Special care should be afforded children. They need plenty of reassurance and sometimes physical contact.

Assisting the Lost Person's Family

Search operations personnel are either very busy or very tired during a search mission. The last thing rescuers want to hear is that they need to take care of the lost person's family and friends. A local CISM team can be enormously helpful in alleviating that burden. The local CISM team should send two or three team members to the search base camp to advise and guide the command staff and to provide crisis support services to the family when that is needed. CISM team members can also be helpful in interviewing distressed family members and friends to obtain further details about the missing person.

Assign a competent family liaison to function as an intermediary among the command and plan sectors and the loved ones. Provide family members and friends with information on the search actions taken so far and the plans for further action. When family members and friends are reasonably well-informed, they tend to remain cooperative and supportive of search personnel. Provide regular briefings to the family members so that the family members know what is going on during a particular shift and when they might expect the next update of information. If appropriate information is not shared with the family and friends, the relationship with search personnel will deteriorate and problems will arise.

All information should follow the *ACT* rule. That is, make sure the information is *accurate, current,* and *timely.* Accurate information helps keep people calm and lowers anxiety. It also generates hope in the family members and friends. Ask the family members and friends what they need most. Offer suggestions if appropriate. Brief family members first before announcements are made to the public. If there is bad news, be kind and gentle, and do not push too fast.

Protect the family members and friends from further stress such as the press, curiosity seekers, gory sights and sounds, and exposure to any particularly disturbing aspects of the incident. It is best to keep the family and friends of the missing person separated from the operations personnel. Families often exert excessive pressure on the search personnel.

If it is at all possible, engage family members in activities that keep them occupied and feeling as if they are making a contribution to the effort. They might search outbuildings like sheds or barns, a campground, a playground, or a known gathering place. They will probably need some instructions and direct supervision to carry out these tasks. Encouraging the family and friends to cooperate with the investigators on the search can also be helpful.

Mobilize resources such as the Red Cross or clergy members to assist the family and friends. Reconnect group members in the same area. There should be one recognized meeting spot for family members so they know where to go each time they arrive at the search base camp. Protect family members from exposure to weather conditions.

Manage the needs of family members and friends as they arise. Use appropriate touch if they seem receptive. Maintain professionalism, however, and do not become too closely involved with the family members. Search personnel cannot afford to become too enmeshed in the family they are trying to serve.

Listen carefully to close friends and family. They may offer a new insight into the lost person even after being interviewed several times. They also need opportunities to express themselves. Provide accurate, current, and timely information, along with reassurance. Do *not* tell them that everything will be okay. You cannot guarantee that. Keep yourself calm and your voice soothing, and strike a balance between being reassuring and avoiding false hope.

Children are the most vulnerable to psychological harm during a stressful search operation. Special care should be afforded children, especially siblings or immediate family members of the lost person. Do not discount children's thoughts. They often know something about a sibling or a friend that may help the search personnel.

Assisting the subject of a search and the person's family can be both challenging and gratifying. The energy expended on such support will go far in maintaining a positively motivated search operation. Having a CISM team involved throughout the operation can reduce the stress on operations' personnel, family, and the missing person.

Wildfires

Wildfires are among the most dangerous of natural disasters. During the Yellowstone National Park fires in 1988, over 9,000 fire fighters and about 4,000 military personnel worked for months to contain destructive fires that affected more than 793,000 acres. Although no fire fighters were killed, there were two civilian fire-related deaths outside the park. Bringing that many fire fighters together creates a virtual city in itself.

Many psychosocial needs can arise during a wildfire. People need information, leadership, guidance, and emotional support for the most threatening experiences. Long deployments, such as those in wildland firefighting operations, generally have a negative impact on family and social life. Tensions arise and frustrations may be expressed in multiple ways. Crisis intervention teams may be instrumental in maintaining a healthy, functional firefighting force. Needless to say, the general community may also benefit from crisis support services.

The value of a well-trained CISM team will be immediately apparent in wildfires that result in injuries or deaths to fire service personnel. Crisis teams may be instrumental in making death or injury announcements, in supporting family members of injured or deceased fire fighters, and most especially in providing a wide range of support services to the emergency operations' personnel experiencing the losses.

Civil Disorder

Few large-scale incidents have the inherent dangers for emergency personnel that come with civil disorder incidents. Any authority figure, including emergency medical personnel, may find himself or herself under threat and duress. The highest priority must be given to ensuring one's safety and that of one's colleagues. It is better to withdraw and request police assistance than to face an angry mob as a single unit.

Community leaders should be brought together. Appropriate leaders should prepare and present calming statements and appropriate guidelines as quickly as possible. Coordinating these efforts is not a function of emergency personnel at the street response level, but commanders, supervisors, and CISM teams can and should encourage those efforts. Appropriate leaders should tell citizens what is happening and should advise citizens to return to their homes if possible. Clear messages should be distributed via every form of media available. If there are grievances, spokespersons should be selected to meet with community leaders and appropriate authorities as quickly as possible.

While negotiations are underway, people should be discouraged from gathering in large groups and should be cautioned that law enforcement personnel cannot allow lawlessness to continue without a response. Do not make that statement as a threat, but as a calm statement of fact. These statements are best delivered by law enforcement supervisors.

Post-Action Staff Support

After any intense Critical Incident Stress Management team action, as is the case in disasters, CISM staff members should be given the means to unwind and put the situation behind them. The Post-Action Staff Support program was designed to facilitate a CISM team's return to normal. The program is made up of many support services. One of those is a semistructured discussion of the experiences of helping others in a critical incident. The process is quite simple, and most CISM teams know how to conduct the conversation. The point to be made here is that recovery from a traumatic experience should include the CISM team that provided support services during the event. They should go over their experiences and the lessons they learned from helping people during the difficult situation. Failure to organize proper support services for a CISM team may impair their capacity to assist in future events.

Final Thoughts

The tremendous aftereffects of exposure to large-scale events and disasters often leave people with powerful visual, auditory, tactile, and olfactory impressions and engraved mental images. David McCullough, in his book on the Johnstown Flood in 1889, states that virtually all survivors had a permanent mental picture of some aspect of their experience. They carried those images to the very end of their lives and often spoke of them in incredible detail.

Crisis intervention services will not erase such powerful memories and mental representations. They can, however, make those images somewhat easier to tolerate. It is not the goal of crisis intervention to erase the mind or cure the wounded soul but to make the chaos and turmoil of a crisis more bearable.

Selected References

Boscarino JA, Adams RE, Figley CF: A prospective cohort study of the effectiveness of employer-sponsored crisis intervention after a major disaster. *Int J Emerg Ment Health,* 2005;7:31–44.

Crocker LG: *Diderot, the Embattled Philosopher.* New York, NY, Free Press, 1966.

Faberow NL, Frederick CJ: *Training Manual for Human Service Workers in Major Disasters.* Rockville, MD, National Institutes of Mental Health, US Department of Health, Education and Welfare, 1978. DHEW publication (ADM) 77-538.

Federal Emergency Management Agency (FEMA) Emergency Management Institute: *National Incident Management System (NIMS), An Introduction IS-700 Facilitator Guide.* Emmitsburg, MD, US Department of Homeland Security, Federal Emergency Management Agency, 2004.

Frederick CJ: Crisis intervention and emergency mental health, in Johnson WR (ed): *Health in Action.* New York, NY, Holt Rinehart & Winston, 1977.

Frederick CJ (ed): *Aircraft Accidents: Emergency Mental Health Problems.* Washington, DC, National Institutes of Mental Health, US Department of Health and Human Services, 1981.

Gibson M: *Order From Chaos: Responding to Traumatic Events.* Bristol, England, The Policy Press, University of Bristol, 2006.

Goenjian AK, Karayan I, Pynoos RS, et al: Outcome of psychotherapy among early adolescents after trauma. *Am J Psychiatry,* 1997;154:536–542.

Hobfoll SE, Watson P, Bell CC, et al: Five essential elements of immediate and mid-term mass trauma intervention: empirical evidence. *Psychiatry,* 2007;70:283–315.

McCullough D: *The Johnstown Flood: The Incredible Story Behind One of the Most Devastating Natural Disasters America Has Ever Known.* New York, NY, Simon & Schuster, 1987.

Mitchell JT: *Group Crisis Support: Why It Works, When and How to Provide It.* Ellicott City, MD, Chevron Publishing Corporation, 2007.

Mitchell JT: Search psychology: tools for efficient search operations, in Stoffle R (ed): *Management of Land Search Operations.* Olympia, WA, Emergency Response International, 2007.

Myers D, Wee D: *Disaster Mental Health Services: A Primer for Practitioners.* New York, NY, Brunner-Routledge, 2005.

National Incident Management System Integration Center: *National Incident Management System (NIMS–National Standard Curriculum Training Development Guidance–FY07).* Washington, DC, US Department of Homeland Security, FEMA, 2007.

National Incident Management System Integration Center: *NIMS Guide.* Washington, DC, US Department of Homeland Security, FEMA, 2007.

National Incident Management System Integration Center: *NIMS Training.* Washington, DC, US Department of Homeland Security, FEMA, 2007.

National Incident Management System Integration Center: *Welcome to the National Incident Management System Integration Center.* Washington, DC, US Department of Homeland Security, FEMA, 2007.

National Institutes of Mental Health (NIMH), Office of Communication and Public Liaison: *Helping Children and Adolescents Cope With Violence and Disasters, Fact Sheet.* Washington, DC, National Institutes of Mental Health, 2001.

National Wildfire Coordinating Group: A history of the Incident Command System (ICS), in *NWCG Incident Command System (ICS) National Training Curriculum.* Available at: http://www.nimsonline.com. Accessed July 20, 2008.

Smith EM, North CS: Posttraumatic stress disorder in natural disasters and technological accidents, in Wilson JP, Raphael B (eds): *International Handbook of Traumatic Stress Syndromes.* New York, NY, Plenum Press, 1993, pp 405–419.

US Department of Homeland Security: *National Incident Management System.* Washington, DC, US Department of Homeland Security, FEMA, 2004.

The White House. Homeland Security Presidential Directive/HSPD-5. Available at: http://www.whitehouse.gov/news/releases/2003/02/20030228-9.html. Accessed August 25, 2008.

Yehuda R, McFarlane AC, Shalev AY: Predicting the development of posttraumatic stress disorder from the acute response to a traumatic event. *Biol Psychiatry,* 1998;44:1305–1313.

Prep Kit

Ready for Review

- A disaster is any event that overwhelms the available emergency resources of the system and causes them to function at a less than optimal level of performance.

- Following a large-scale disaster, it is easy to identify the physical injuries of victims. However, it is important to remember that psychological changes will also affect those involved. Common reactions are depression, anger, increased stress, personality changes, suicidal thinking, deterioration in cognitive functioning, and PTSD.

- Dr. Calvin Fredericks outlined seven psychological stages of a disaster: warning, alarm, impact, inventory, rescue, recovery, and reconstruction. The emergency responder should recognize that each stage is associated with different emotional reactions, such as anxiety, denial, or shock.

- When the emergency responder evaluates patients who have been exposed to a disastrous event or trauma, remember that reactions may vary substantially. Most reactive symptoms can be classified into five categories: cognitive, physical, emotional, behavioral, or spiritual.

- The five-T planning formula can be used to organize assistance to individuals during and after a large-scale disaster. The five elements are target, type, timing, themes, and team.

- Psychological toxicity occurs as a result of ongoing terrorist events such as bombings. Individuals lose self-confidence, become anxious, depressed, and hopeless, and eventually want to give up.

- Disastrous events involving school-age children are very difficult to manage. Meeting physical needs of those involved is a priority at the onset of the event, but it is difficult to predict how these events, such as a student-involved shooting or a tornado that hits a school, will affect involved children in the years to come.

- The search for a lost individual can be either extremely rewarding or tremendously devastating. Search maneuvers can last for hours or days, resulting in both physical and psychological stress of families and rescuers. These events often require both short- and long-term follow-up psychological services for emergency responders.

Vital Vocabulary

disaster Any event that overwhelms the available emergency resources of a particular jurisdiction or community and causes them to function at a less than an optimal level of performance.

heterogeneous group A group made up of "mixed" members who do not have the same background, perceptions, or objectives surrounding an event.

homogeneous group A group made up of similar members with similar backgrounds, such as police, EMS, or military personnel. A homogeneous group should also have similar experiences, goals, and objectives.

Post-Action Staff Support A program of support for CISM personnel who have assisted others in the aftermath of a traumatic event such as a disaster.

psychological toxicity A term used to describe when people lose hope and self-confidence, become anxious and depressed, feel hopeless, and wish to give up.

technological disaster A disaster that results secondarily because of something that humans have created.

Assessment in Action

Answer key is located in the back of the book.

1. You are part of a disaster response team that arrives three days after a devastating tornado. You find individuals starting to make their way back into their neighborhoods. You witness families surveying the damage to their homes, looking for heirlooms, and trying to understand how this could have happened to them. Many appear to be crying and numb.

According to Fredericks, this psychological stage of a disaster is known as:

A. alarm.
B. rescue.
C. inventory.
D. recovery.

2. There are five categories in which individuals who have psychological reactions to a disaster will respond. From the following list, select the one that is NOT one of those reactions.

   A. Affective
   B. Spiritual
   C. Emotional
   D. Cognitive

3. Depression, suicidal thinking, burnout, and PTSD are all examples of what type of psychological reaction to a disaster?

   A. Long-term
   B. Short-term

4. A person who loses hope and self-confidence and often becomes anxious or depressed following a disaster or act of terror is experiencing which of the following conditions?

   A. Haplessness
   B. Grieving
   C. Psychological toxicity
   D. Sensory dysfunction

5. You are involved in a prolonged search for a lost 10-year-old child with mild autism who wandered away from his family while camping in the national park. After a 2-day search, the child is found safe under a pile of brush. He is cold and scared but otherwise uninjured. From the following list, select the one item that you would NOT do as a crisis responder when interacting with this patient.

   A. Periodically reassure him that he is safe now and that you are there to help him.
   B. Provide a quiet place for him and his family to reunite.
   C. Address any medical illness or injury first.
   D. Tell him that his parents are very upset and threatened never to go camping again.

Developmental Disorders Diagnosed in Infancy, Childhood, and Adolescence

As an emergency responder, you will often come in contact with children with both medical and psychological problems. Disorders commonly diagnosed during infancy, childhood, or adolescence vary in nature from impaired cognitive functioning to psychosocial conduct (**Figure 10-1**). It is important to keep in mind that some of these disorders can be found in adults and not just in children or adolescents.

Background

There are many developmental disorders that affect the way a child relates to his or her social and learning environment. Many of these conditions can affect cognition, adaptation, behavior, conduct, and social interaction. Disorders diagnosed during infancy, childhood, or adolescence may be linked to external problems such as trauma, abuse and neglect, physiological conditions, or other psychological events during the developmental stages. The *DSM-IV-TR* describes many disorders commonly diagnosed during infancy, childhood, or adolescence, but the seven categories most likely to be seen in the prehospital environment are:

- Mental retardation
- Pervasive developmental disorders
- Childhood disintegrative disorder
- Rett's disorder
- Attention-deficit/hyperactivity disorder (ADHD)
- Conduct disorder
- Oppositional defiant disorder
- Separation anxiety disorder
- Reactive attachment disorder

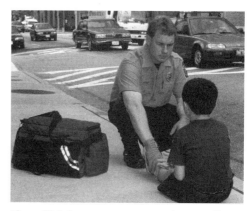

Figure 10-1 As an emergency responder, you will often come in contact with children with both medical and psychological problems.

Assessment

When responding to calls involving children with developmental disorders, the emergency provider should be prepared to thoroughly assess both the scene and the patient. In some cases, your services will be requested by law enforcement to provide transport to a child. It is important to guarantee the security of responders on every call.

Special consideration is necessary when obtaining information and performing the physical examination in cases involving childhood developmental disorders. Bear in mind that children and adults with these disorders will often have language impairments and will struggle to communicate with you. Patience and reasoning are helpful skills when interviewing these patients. It is best to have a parent or guardian present to bridge the communication gap between the child and emergency responder. In many situations, parents will be able to calm and reassure the child as well as provide you with the information needed for your assessment. However, if the patient has been diagnosed with conduct disorder or oppositional defiant disorder, it might be suitable to have the parent or guardian removed in order to obtain an accurate patient history, depending upon the child's age. In most cases, simply asking the parent to step out for a few minutes will suffice. In escalated situations in which yelling, threats, or violence are present, it may be necessary to ask law enforcement to remove the parents. Children with some of these disorders have a higher incidence of drug abuse and early sexual activity and will often hide this information from their parents. Removing the parents from the situation may help you gather information vital to the care of your patient. If at any time you feel that your safety is in question, remove yourself from the scene and request police assistance. In some situations with older adolescents who have a diagnosis of conduct or oppositional defiant disorder, police should be automatically requested, given the potential violent nature of some disorders. Likewise, police should be involved any time there is a physical altercation, threat of suicide, or actual suicide attempt.

Assessment tools such as the pediatric assessment triangle are useful for evaluating children before the emergency responder touches the patient physically (**Figure 10-2**). The pediatric assessment triangle evaluates a child's appearance, work of breathing, and circulation. It is worthwhile to use familiar assessment tools, such as SAMPLE and OPQRST, to obtain useful information regarding the patient. Likewise, the SEA-3 mental status exam can be used to assess the mental state of the patient and possible neurological deficits.

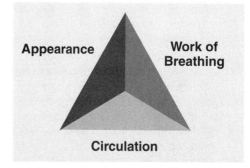

Figure 10-2: The pediatric assessment triangle.

Pediatric Assessment Triangle

- **Appearance:** What is the general appearance of the child, caregiver, and environment? When not associated with trauma, patients with many of these childhood-onset disorders will be found either with a scared or desperate look because of interactions to which they are not accustomed. Note how the child interacts with the caregiver and determine if it is a positive or negative relationship. If you suspect stress, consider having your partner talk to the parents or caregiver apart from the child.
- **Work of Breathing:** Is the child having difficulty breathing? Observe the respiratory pattern as the child converses with his or her caregiver before you begin to talk with the child. Some children with separation anxiety or reactive attachment disorders will exhibit worsened respiratory conditions in order to seek attention.
- **Circulation:** What is the color of the skin? Can you see any circulatory compromise, including bleeding? Is there any sign of accidental or intentional injury that could result in shock?

SAMPLE History

- **Signs and symptoms:** Disorientation and wandering thoughts can be observed. Children with separation anxiety disorder may experience or describe symptoms such as headaches and nausea.
- **Allergies:** Allergies to food, medications, and environmental factors are all possible.
- **Medications:** Patients may be taking medications such as Adderall® for ADHD, mood stabilizers, or tranquilizers.
- **Pertinent past medical history:** Patients may have multiple overlapping conditions. For example, a child diagnosed with a **pervasive developmental disorder (PDD)** may also suffer from **mental retardation**. Be sure to ask lots of questions about developmental status, previous medical events, and whether the patient has ever demonstrated violence toward self or others.
- **Last oral intake:** Parents will often provide this information. Evaluate the current eating habits of all children to be sure that they are receiving proper nourishment, and do not forget to inquire about drug or alcohol consumption.
- **Events leading to illness or injury:** Patients with these disorders will generally be found in the care of a parent or guardian or living in group homes. It is important to note the physical surroundings, including sensory stimulation, because light and loud noises can trigger seizures. With patients diagnosed with behavioral disorders, it is important to ask about drug use prior to the call for help. Also, if possible, attempt to determine whether a family disagreement brought about or contributed to the event.

Common Disorders Affecting Prehospital Care

Mental Retardation

Mental retardation is commonly associated with a below-average adaptation and learning of basic motor and communicative skills. The principal criteria for mental retardation include onset before the age of 18 years and decreased levels of general intellectual functioning with limitations in adaptive functioning. *General intellectual functioning* refers to the aptitude that can be assessed through individual intelligence tests that yield an IQ.

Adaptive functioning is a measure of how effectively the person can perform everyday tasks. Skills involved in adaptive functioning include, but are not limited to, communication and social interaction abilities, fine motor skills, and occupational skills.

The etiology of mental retardation has not been clearly defined, but it is believed to have biological and psychosocial components. Major factors contributing to mental retardation include:

- Heredity
- Maternal (and possibly paternal) age at conception
- Problems associated with pregnancy
- Maternal substance abuse
- Medical conditions
- Environmental influences
- Other mental disorders

Classification of Retardation

A person diagnosed with mild mental retardation will generally have an IQ level range of 50 to 70. This population is often referred to as *educable*, because they have minimal sensorimotor and intellectual impairments. Children with this condition are often indistinguishable at early ages and are able to develop social and communicative skills. The first sign of mild retardation is often poor academic performance and a slower understanding of school material as the years progress. Adults with mild mental retardation can acquire many or most of the basic daily life skills to support themselves and are able to live independently or in communities with minimal supervision.

In moderate mental retardation, the IQ levels range from 35 to 50. Patients develop some communication skills during early childhood, but lack the intellectual capacity to progress past about a second-grade level of academic knowledge. Adolescents with moderate mental retardation struggle to acclimate with their peers and have difficulty developing further social interaction abilities. Adults are able to adapt to the community with some degree of supervision in both living and work settings.

The IQ scale levels for severe mental retardation range from 20 to 35. A person with severe retardation will have a diminished vocabulary and limited communicative skills. Because of the elementary-level capability to self-support, individuals typically live in supervised communities or with their families.

When a person has been affected by a neurological condition since childhood and has an IQ level below 20, he or she is diagnosed with profound mental retardation. The neurological condition often affects the person's sensorimotor functioning, including visual, motor, and auditory functions. Individuals tend to have other medical conditions, such as cardiovascular and musculoskeletal problems. Self-inflicted injuries may result from compromised neurologic functioning. Profoundly retarded patients are dependent on caregivers and usually live in group homes or with their family, where they have constant monitoring.

Emergency personnel are rarely called to the scene strictly for the care and management of a person with mental retardation. Most often, you will be called to evaluate a person who is experiencing illness, trauma, or another psychological reaction and care may be complicated by their developmental disability. These individuals can exhibit signs of stress, anxiety, and panic under what most of us would consider normal circumstances.

OPQRST

- **Onset:** The time of onset is usually gradual, unless there is seizure activity, which could be a sudden onset.
- **Provocation:** Did the symptoms start after taking any medication? Determine whether there was external stimulation, like flashing lights, that may have caused the child to feel overwhelmed or that provoked seizure activity.
- **Quality:** What emotions does the child exhibit towards his or her caregiver?
- **Radiation:** Is the child's deviant attitude affecting others apart from his or her caregiver? Teachers, classmates, and friends are often affected by the child's behavior.
- **Severity:** It is a good idea to use a system such as the FACES pain rating scale **(Figure 10-3)** to assess for pain or discomfort when dealing with children.
- **Time:** How long has the child been acting unusual?

Pervasive Developmental Disorders

Pervasive developmental disorder (PDD) is a broad descriptor for conditions that affect a person's intellectual, adaptive, and social capabilities. The disorders in this category affect a person as a child and require clinical attention.

Children diagnosed with <u>autism</u>, or autistic disorder, are affected in three specific areas: social interaction, communication, and abnormal patterns of behavior. In order for a person to be

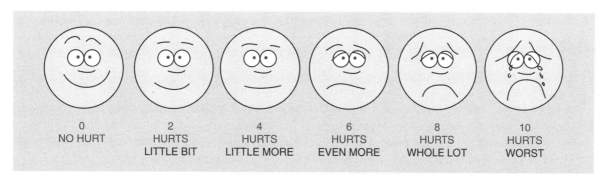

0	2	4	6	8	10
NO HURT	HURTS LITTLE BIT	HURTS LITTLE MORE	HURTS EVEN MORE	HURTS WHOLE LOT	HURTS WORST

Figure 10-3 The Wong-Baker FACES rating scale. Reproduced with permission from Hockenberry MJ, Wilson D, Wikelstein ML: *Wong's Essentials of Pediatric Nursing,* ed 7. St Louis, MO, Mosby, 2005, p 1259. Copyright, Mosby.

SEA-3

- **Speech:** The flow and organization of the patient's speech may be affected by the levels of linguistic impairment and mental retardation. Some patients will speak in codes or with body language.

- **Emotions:** What emotions does the patient convey? Some patients will prefer solitary activities and express little emotion. Others will exhibit anger, disgust, defiance, or fear. Children diagnosed with reactive attachment disorder might show inappropriate affection to you.

- **Appearance:** What does the patient look like physically? Is there any evidence suggesting self-inflicted injuries?

- **Alertness:** Because children with these disorders may not be good at assessing time, evaluate orientation to person, place, and things (such as a toy) and take into consideration that a child's orientation and judgment will be different from an adult's. Observe the patient's attentiveness to the whereabouts of his or her caregiver to assess alertness in a child.

- **Activity:** What is the patient doing when you first see him or her? Does the patient demonstrate repetitive stereotypical movement indicative of autism disorder?

given a diagnosis of an autistic disorder, he or she must exhibit the criteria defined by the *DSM-IV-TR* prior to the age of 3 years old. It is estimated that 75% of children diagnosed with autism also meet the criteria for moderate retardation, according to the *Journal of the American Academy of Child and Adolescent Psychiatry*. Children with autism may have higher levels of cognitive ability that are not related to intellectual functioning. The increased level of cognition may hamper the child's ability to express himself or herself to others.

Children with autism will rarely take the initiative to start a conversation with others, and prefer individual activities rather than interacting with peers. Patients tend to fix their attention to specific objects or topics in a repetitive manner. When the child is in his or her personal zone, you will observe an extreme sensitivity to sensory stimulation and specific motor movements such as finger tapping or a rocking motion. People with autism may be more comfortable if they can follow an exact routine that does not vary from day to day. Changes in the pattern can create confusion and extreme distress that may hamper your ability to care for the child in an emergency.

Assessing the child with autism can be very difficult, because of the child's unwillingness or inability to communicate on a one-to-one basis. Because these individuals may have restricted speech, communication skills, and social impairment, taking a history may be difficult or impossible. You will have to gather information from family members and from your observations. The child may resist your efforts to provide first aid, and you may require the assistance of a parent. In many cases, family members are stressed when caring for children with these severe mental disorders. It is important to provide empathetic support to parents and caregivers in these situations.

In Asperger's disorder, or **Asperger's syndrome**, the child exhibits similar behavior to autism, but the individual has little or no delay in language development and suffers from social interaction detriment. Language, curiosity, and cognitive development mature as expected. The child often develops a highly developed vocabulary with a limited ability to use language in a social context. There are many behavioral factors that influence the way children with Asperger's interact with their peers. An extreme focus on irrelevant details may cause a lack of searching for spontaneous pleasure. The attraction to details often causes the child to have focused, repetitive language. Motor skills may be uncoordinated and repetitive. Patients may only be able to maintain an attention span of a few minutes before they turn away and focus on something else.

Individuals with Asperger's disorder can be challenging to interview, but will generally have better communication skills than those with autism. It is not common for emergency personnel to be sent to evaluate a patient solely because the patient has Asperger's. More commonly, you might be called by family members who feel distressed because they are unable to get the child to go to school or attend to assigned tasks. The result is often a stressed family dynamic and one that is in need of prolonged intensive case management by a social worker or support group.

In **childhood disintegrative disorder**, also known as **dementia infantilis** or **Heller's syndrome**, there is a decline in the child's language, social, and motor skills after the first two years of normal development. This sudden deterioration can present at any time before the age of 10 years. It is thought to be caused by damage to the central nervous system. As the central nervous system continues to develop, the areas of communication and fine motor skills regress, causing the impairments observed in childhood disintegrative disorder. As with autism, children struggle with adaptive functioning and social interactions. Children illustrate specific repetitive movements like those with autistic disorder. A unique trait to childhood disintegrative disorder is the possibility for a loss of bowel or bladder control and elevated electroencephalographic activity in the brain, resulting in an increased probability of seizures requiring emergency care.

Rett's syndrome is a disease process found only in females. It is characterized by the undeveloped physical appearance of the child's head and extremities after 5 months of normal development and the lack of psychomotor control. It also affects language and social interaction. Even though there is a lack of social development, the affected child can adapt and learn enough social skills to interact with her peers.

The impaired growth of their hands and feet often causes gait or walking problems and uncoordinated fine-motor movement like writing. Some visible signs that can occur because of the psychomotor retardation include scoliosis or curvature of the spine, seizures, and abnormal breathing patterns. Additionally, patients will often suffer from gastroesophageal reflux disease, resulting in the regurgitation of acidic stomach contents into the esophagus.

Based on these presentations, the prehospital care provider should suspect calls involving falls, spinal cord injuries, seizures, shortness of breath, and gastric distress such as heartburn or esophageal bleeding. Each of these conditions would be managed according to your level of training and local protocol. Good supportive care is needed for both the patient and the family.

Attention-Deficit/Hyperactivity Disorder

Attention-deficit/hyperactivity disorder (ADHD) is a neurodevelopmental disorder affecting the individual's attention span, impulsivity, and activity levels. The first signs indicative of ADHD are typically seen during the early school years when overall academic performance declines. A person with ADHD will have a short attention span while avoiding most activities or tasks that require mental concentration. ADHD also includes levels of hyperactivity in which the person affected feels restless and is always moving. The patient may also display impulsiveness to do or say things that are socially out of place. The etiology of ADHD is not fully understood, but numerous studies show that heredity plays an important role.

In the predominantly inattentive type of ADHD, a person's mind easily wanders. People suffering from the inattentive type of ADHD tend to be careless, unorganized, and easily distracted. In a classroom setting, they will have a hard time focusing on the lecture and can easily be distracted by the minimal activity around them. Often they will leave a task unattended to follow a different task.

The hyperactive-impulsive type of ADHD involves excessive uncontrollable physical movements and impatience. A hyperactive person cannot stand or sit calmly for long periods of time and will move often. Movements can vary from standing up for a walk to excessive tapping of the finger or leg. It is important to note that this behavior of restlessness is normal in most toddlers and adolescents and may not be a symptom of ADHD.

The urge to talk will often force children suffering from ADHD to interrupt a conversation. Impulsive behavior can consist of verbal or physical impatience. Those affected with this condition will normally have a hard time listening and respecting other people's personal space. Impulses can also lead to dangerous activities to satisfy a certain pleasure. For example, a teenager might feel the need to drive fast to meet his or her need for stimulation and spontaneous excitement or impatience toward other drivers.

The most common subtype of this disorder is the combined type. The combination includes inability to pay attention, hyperactivity, and impulsiveness. Generally the symptoms last for at least 6 months and affect the person's life at school or work. Prehospital emergency personnel will rarely get dispatched strictly for a child with a complaint of ADHD. However, children suffering from ADHD tend to get picked on at school and may be involved in altercations with other students. They also tend to be sent to the principal's office for disrupting the classroom environment. This can result in great frustration and in some cases may result in physical conflicts with parents or authority figures.

Another concern is overdose of prescription medication used to control ADHD. These overdoses can be accidental or purposeful. Patients with ADHD are usually managed with <u>amphetamine derivatives</u> such as Adderall or methylphenidate (Ritalin). At toxic levels, extreme tachycardia and life-threatening cardiac dysrhythmias can develop.

Conduct Disorder

<u>Conduct disorder</u> is a term used to define various levels of misbehaviors against others. These misbehaviors can be aggressive or nonaggressive and may include physical harm, vandalism, self-inflicting harm, forceful sexual behavior, and stealing. Conduct problems often create social problems with school, work, or social environments. Conduct disorders are usually associated with drugs, alcohol, smoking, and early exposure to sexual behavior. Children suffering from conduct disorder will often have low self-esteem and below-average performance in school.

Children affected with this disorder often blame others for their misconduct. There are four major categories of misconduct: (1) aggression to people or animals, resulting in physical harm, such as bullying in school or stealing something with a confrontation; (2) destruction of property, such as setting a building on fire deliberately; (3) defiance against the rules; and (4) misleading or stealing.

Conduct disorders can be further subdivided according to the severity of the misbehaviors and the age of onset. There are three levels of severity: mild, moderate, and severe. Additionally, there are two subtypes based on the age of onset: childhood and adolescent onset. In the childhood-onset type, the person is diagnosed before the age of 10 years old. This type is more predominant in male children. Behaviors tend to be more persistent, with physical and aggressive elements, and children are at a higher risk of developing antisocial personality disorder as adults. Children who demonstrate the patterns for conduct disorder after the age of 10 years are diagnosed with the adolescent-onset type. This type is less aggressive and physical than the childhood-onset type, and patients tend to have normal relationships with others.

Given the nature of this disorder, emergency responders may be called to the scene to care for an adolescent with some form of physical trauma. It is common for patients to be involved in fights, bullying, and sexual assault. In addition to rendering proper care to the patient, be sure to provide thorough documentation, as many of these incidents will be crime scenes.

Oppositional Defiant Disorder

<u>Oppositional defiant disorder</u> is often diagnosed when the child displays behaviors out of normal conduct but does not meet all of the criteria for conduct disorder. This disorder includes behavior that is negative, hostile, irritable, defiant, and disobedient. The onset of oppositional defiant disorder is gradual.

Children with this condition are often stubborn and resistant, and they like to argue with authority figures. The authority figure is generally a person the child knows well. Hostile behavior can include foul language and verbal threats. Because children with oppositional defiant disorder often choose to test the limits of people with whom they are familiar, their misbehavior can be limited to a home setting.

During the school years, children may have low self-esteem and get frustrated easily. The defiant nature of their conduct often provides challenges in their academic, social, and working interactions. Unfortunately, individuals with this disorder will often anger quickly and will easily become confrontational.

It is important for you, the provider, to be aware that patients diagnosed with oppositional defiant disorder will often be misleading during assessment, especially in the presence of parents or other authority figures. Be careful not to show any signs of taking sides with either the parent or the child. Remember that your job is to provide emergency care in an unbiased manner and document only your objective findings.

Separation Anxiety Disorder

Separation anxiety disorder is a condition in which a person feels extreme levels of anxiety when he or she is removed from a person to whom he or she is emotionally attached. In most cases, parents are the center of attachment for children with this condition. In order to be considered a disorder, the anxiety attacks must affect the child's academic and social functioning. The level of anxiety exhibited by the child is usually inappropriate and excessive relative to the child's age group.

The emergency responder often separates children and parents during the care phase in emergency situations. You will need to do this for a variety of reasons, including getting a more thorough history about the child or protecting the parent from seeing invasive treatments that might be disturbing to the parent. However, in cases in which a child is diagnosed with separation anxiety, it is generally recommended that the child and parent remain united if possible. By separating the two, you will see an escalation of anxiety as well as a stimulation of the sympathetic nervous system, which can result in the unnecessary increase in heart rate, respiratory rate, and blood pressure (**Figure 10-4**).

Children diagnosed with this disorder are often attached to their parents and fear losing them if separated. The child often seeks full attention from his or her parent for reassurance that he or she has not been forgotten. This can be extremely stressful for the parents, so this may be a situation in which you technically have two patients—the child and the parent.

The affected child will often fear traveling alone or physically leaving his or her parents out of fear of getting lost and not returning to his or her parents. This concern for separation and getting lost prevents the child from participating in social activities with other peers such as school field trips and sleepovers. In order to prevent separation, children will fake illness to stay home. Should you be called to the home to evaluate the child, use standardized assessment tools and make a treatment plan based on your findings. When in doubt, consult medical direction or a supervisor for advice

Reactive Attachment Disorder of Infancy or Early Childhood

Reactive attachment disorder is a mental disorder associated with unsuitable social interaction because of pathogenic care. In other words, the child lacks the social skills needed to differentiate between appropriate and inappropriate behavior because of insufficient interaction with the caregiver. Parental neglect often leads to the potential for reactive attachment disorder.

Prehospital Management

Providing care for children is always a challenging task. Unlike adults, a child's condition can degrade rapidly, and children usually cannot express with detail what they are experiencing. It is up to you as the provider to use your assessment tools to obtain

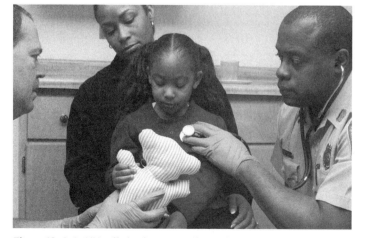

Figure 10-4 A child suffering from separation anxiety may make providing care difficult.

a good history and commence adequate treatment. In most situations, parents or caregivers can provide the best information on how to treat the child. Usually the parents or caregivers have been informed of the complications of their child's condition and often can aid you in determining a course of treatment.

Many patients with developmental disorders are protective of their personal space and do not interact well with strangers. It is important to respect that space by slowly approaching the patient and introducing yourself. Use simple language and conversation to begin building trust with the patient. As part of that process, you can explain to the patient why you are there, how you are going to conduct yourself, and why it is necessary for the patient to assist you.

It is important to perform a thorough physical examination on the patient to determine if injuries are self-inflicted or from another mechanism. Patients diagnosed with pervasive developmental disorders will often develop a stereotypical motor movement that may include self-inflicting injuries such as repeatedly biting themselves or hitting their head against the floor. These injuries usually are not life threatening; however, they should be treated if possible and if the child allows it. Most of the time, the child will allow the parents or caregivers to make contact. Ask the caregiver to assist you in your physical examination and treatment of any small injuries.

Treating adolescents with behavioral problems can be difficult and may require that you call for extra resources. Patience is critical with aggressive adolescents. Patients with oppositional defiant disorder will challenge you and may behave inappropriately when you are performing your assessment. Most adolescents will generally submit to your requests after the target of aggression has been removed. Many patients who have been diagnosed with a behavioral problem will feel invulnerable and perform dangerous activities to defy the rules. It is important to note if such an activity was the cause for the call and, if so, treat accordingly. Realize that although you may have been called to a high school to treat an adolescent who was involved in a fight, he or she may also have psychological issues as the underlying cause of the initial confrontation. It is very rare for an adolescent to become aggressive to the point of needing physical restraint. If patients do need to be restrained, be sure to involve law enforcement whenever possible and to follow your local protocol regarding the proper technique for securing a child.

Pharmacological Considerations

There are two major types of medications commonly used in children with developmental disorders: amphetamine derivatives and mood stabilizers.

In children with ADHD, stimulants known as amphetamine derivatives, such as Adderall® and Ritalin®, stimulate the central nervous system to regulate neurotransmitters such as dopamine and norepinephrine. This helps children with ADHD concentrate on their daily activities.

This particular type of drug has a high potential for abuse, both by prescription and illicit users. A child overdosed on stimulants will often exhibit shaky motor movement, hyperactivity, fever, muscle pain, and headaches. While adolescents enjoy the high it gives them, they will often combine it with alcohol, a depressant, to temper the effects. This combination can be life threatening, as it stresses the cardiovascular and central nervous systems. Patients may present with tachycardia, respiratory depression, altered mentation, or coma. Aggressive advanced life support protocols and transport to the closest medical facility should be initiated.

Mood stabilizers for children's disorders can be divided into four classifications: lithium, anti-seizure medication, antidepressants, and neuroleptics.

Lithium has been used for over 50 years to treat individuals with bipolar disorder. It is an alkali metal that is chemically similar to sodium. It is not common to find children on lithium; however, it may be used if other types of medications fail to help the patient. A major difficulty with lithium is that its effective level is very close to its toxic level; it is necessary to monitor drug levels carefully.

The two most common anti-seizure medications used in children are divalproex sodium (Depakote®) and carbamazepine (Tegretol®). It is important to remember that just because the patient is on an anti-seizure medication does not necessarily mean the patient has a seizure disorder. These particular drugs are given also to assist in stabilizing neurotransmitters and can even be given in the treatment of migraine or cluster headaches.

More commonly you will find your patients on one or more of the following two classifications of medications. Antidepressants such as fluoxetine (Prozac®), paroxetine (Paxil®), sertraline (Zoloft®), and citalopram (Celexa®) are often used with children with mental disorders. In addition to treating chemical and psychological depression, they serve to generally stabilize the overall mood of the patient. In recent years, there has been some research and antidotal reports of suicide, particularly among adolescents taking some brands of antidepressants. While little is known about the cause at this point, the emergency responder should always assess for suicidal ideation or previous attempts.

Neuroleptics or antipsychotics are relatively new in the treatment of these disorders. Neuroleptics such as risperidone (Risperdal®), olanzapine (Zyprexa®), and clozapine (Clozaril®) are commonly used; however, like many medications, they can have strong side effects. Some of the more severe side effects are weight gain, resulting in the onset of diabetes mellitus; muscle twitching; failure of the temperature-regulating mechanism in the brain, resulting in high fever; and lower seizure threshold for those patients with a history of epilepsy or other seizure disorder.

Final Thoughts

It does not matter how long you have been in EMS—the management of children is always difficult and stressful. The children who have been discussed in this chapter have difficulties with communication and understanding. Your patience and empathy will help lead you to a successful resolution of the presenting problem. That said, it is important for you to remember that dealing with children can also create stress in your own life. Do not be afraid to reach out and talk with someone when you feel that your life has been affected by your work. It only shows your strength as a professional.

Selected References

ADD ADHD Advances. Mood stabilizers. Available at: http://addadhdadvances.com/moodstabilizers.html. Accessed January 29, 2008.

American Psychiatric Association: *Diagnostic and Statistical Manual of Mental Disorders, Fourth Edition, Text Revision (DSM-IV-TR)*. Washington, DC, American Psychiatric Association, 2000.

Answers.com. Asperger's disorder and Asperger's syndrome. Available at: http://www.answers.com/topic/asperger-s-syndrome?cat=health. Accessed January 29, 2008.

Lord C, Volkmar F: Genetics of childhood disorders XLII: autism, part 1: diagnosis and assessment in autistic spectrum disorders. *J Am Acad Child Adolesc Psychiatry*, 2002;41:1134–1136.

Pollak A, Elling B, Smith M (eds): Nancy Caroline's Emergency Care in the Streets. Sudbury, MA, Jones & Bartlett Publishers, 2008.

The Science of Mental Illness. Glossary. Available at: http://science.education.nih.gov/supplements/nih5/mental/other/glossary.htm. Accessed January 29, 2008.

Steiner H (ed): *Handbook of Mental Interventions in Children and Adolescents: An Integrated Developmental Approach*. San Francisco, CA, Jossey-Bass, 2004.

Prep Kit

Ready for Review

- When evaluating children with developmental disorders, it may be difficult to communicate effectively. Often, a parent or friend may provide you with a detailed history of the patient. Using standardized models such as the pediatric assessment triangle, SAMPLE, OPQRST, and SEA-3 will make assessing these patients easier.

- Many children with developmental disorders will be on complex regimens of strong drugs such as antidepressants, antipsychotics, and anti-seizure medications. Beware of the possibility that drug interactions may be the cause of the current complaint.

- Children with oppositional defiant disorder are often confrontational and may behave inappropriately in your presence. A calm, non-threatening approach will be the most effective in assessing these patients. However, remember that your safety is always paramount.

- The diagnosis of mental retardation is somewhat misleading because of the wide range of disability that patients may present. Patients with mild retardation are often good historians and able to understand what is occurring. On the other hand, people with severe retardation are challenged to complete daily living tasks without extensive guidance and structure.

- Children diagnosed with one of the pervasive developmental disorders present with deficits in their intellectual, adaptive, and social capabilities. Many of these patients will have difficulty communicating effectively with emergency responders. Extra effort may be required to obtain a correct and thorough history from family or caretakers.

- Attention-deficit/hyperactivity disorder is a neurodevelopmental disorder affecting the individual's attention span, impulsivity, and activity level. Rarely will this condition be the presenting problem for the emergency responder. However, should the child be involved in physical trauma, such as a bicycle crash, inattentiveness could be easily confused with the early signs of altered mental status or shock.

- Children with conduct disorder may present to the emergency responder as the result of a fight, self-inflicted injury, or drug overdose. In addition to providing empathetic care for the patient, be careful that the patient does not attempt to physically assault you. Remember that if the patient feels that he or she will be in trouble for his or her behavior, he or she may try to escape, even if it is from a moving vehicle.

- It is not uncommon for emergency responders to separate parents and children, particularly in the case of trauma. However, for children with separation anxiety disorder, removing the parents can elevate the child's anxiety and fear level beyond that of the average child.

Vital Vocabulary

adaptive functioning A measure of how effectively the person can perform everyday tasks. Skills involved in adaptive functioning include, but are not limited to, communication and social interaction abilities, fine motor skills, and occupational skills.

amphetamine derivative Drugs that are chemically similar or that produce similar effects to that of amphetamines. These drugs stimulate the central nervous system, resulting in elevated blood pressure, heart rate, and other metabolic functions.

Asperger's syndrome A developmental disorder, usually diagnosed in childhood, characterized by impairments in social interactions and repetitive behavior patterns.

attention-deficit/hyperactivity disorder (ADHD) A condition characterized by an impaired ability to regulate activity level (hyperactivity), attend to tasks (inattention), and inhibit behavior (impulsivity).

autism A disorder that typically affects a person's ability to communicate, form relationships with others, and respond appropriately to the environment. Some people with autism have few problems with speech and intelligence and are able to function relatively well in society. Others are mentally retarded or mute or have serious language delays. Autism makes some people seem closed off and shut down; others seem locked into repetitive behaviors and rigid patterns of thinking.

childhood disintegrative disorder A condition occurring in young children that is characterized by normal development in the first several years of life, followed by a marked developmental regression (a child who previously had been speaking in sentences becomes totally mute); various autistic features develop. Also known as dementia infantilis or Heller's syndrome.

combined type A form of ADHD in which the individual exhibits signs of both the predominantly inattentive and hyperactive-impulsive types of ADHD. The individual will present with the inability to pay attention and hyperactivity-impulsiveness.

conduct disorder A personality disorder of children and adolescents involving persistent antisocial behavior. Individuals with conduct disorder frequently participate in activities such as stealing, lying, truancy, vandalism, and substance abuse.

dementia infantilis See childhood disintegrative disorder.

Heller's syndrome See childhood disintegrative disorder.

hyperactive-impulsive type A form of ADHD in which the individual exhibits excessive uncontrollable physical movements and impatience.

mental retardation A condition in which a person has an IQ that is below average and that affects an individual's learning, behavior, and development. This condition is present from birth.

mood stabilizer A psychiatric medication used to treat mood disorders, particularly bipolar disorder, in which patients experience wide-ranging mood swings from mania to depression.

oppositional defiant disorder A disruptive pattern of behavior of children and adolescents that is characterized by defiant, disobedient, and hostile behaviors directed toward adults in positions of authority, lasting at least 6 months.

pervasive developmental disorder (PDD) A group of disorders seen in children characterized by delays in the development of socialization and communication skills.

predominantly inattentive type A form of ADHD in which the person's mind easily wanders and the person pays little or no attention to his or her surroundings.

reactive attachment disorder A mental health disorder in which a child is unable to form healthy social relationships, particularly with a primary caregiver.

Rett's syndrome An inherited developmental disorder observed only in females that is characterized by a short period of normal development, followed by loss of developmental skills (particularly purposeful hand movements) and marked psychomotor retardation.

separation anxiety disorder A child's apprehension associated with separation from a parent or other caregiver.

Assessment in Action

Answer key is located in the back of the book.

1. The mental health disorder present since birth that is diagnosed during childhood and is based upon the measurement of the IQ is called:

    A. pervasive developmental disorder.
    B. mental retardation.
    C. Rett's syndrome.
    D. childhood disintegrative disorder.

2. The class of medication commonly given for the treatment of ADHD is:

    A. monoamine oxidase inhibitors.
    B. tricyclic antidepressants.
    C. amphetamine derivatives.
    D. neuroleptics.

Prep Kit | continued

3. You are dispatched to the home of a 3-year-old girl who has fallen and hit her head. It appears that the child's only injury is a small half-inch cut over her eyebrow. The bleeding is easily controlled with a direct-pressure dressing. A decision is made to transport the child for the sake of the parent's comfort that everything is going to be alright. En route to the hospital, the mother tells you how the child was perfectly normal for the first two years but now seems to be going "backward" with her speech and learning. She also tells you that she was nearly toilet trained and now is unable to hold her bladder or bowels. You suspect what condition might be present in this child?

   A. Childhood disintegrative disorder
   B. Oppositional defiant disorder
   C. Autism
   D. None of the above because you suspect a closed head injury

4. You are dispatched to the local high school for a 16-year-old male who has been arrested by the school resource officer (police) after verbally and physically assaulting the school principal. In order to break up the fight, the student was pepper sprayed and is now being taken to the hospital for follow-up. Police inform you that this young man has a history of "trouble" and tends to "test his boundaries" with authority figures. You also find out that he comes from a troubled home. From the following list, select the mental disorder that may apply to this student.

   A. Autism
   B. Oppositional defiant disorder
   C. Asperger's syndrome
   D. Conduct disorder

5. You are dispatched to a residence where a family fight has just occurred. Upon arrival, police tell you that Stephen is a 15-year-old who has been in trouble since the age of 12 years, when he first tried to break into a car. Since that time, he has developed a pattern of lying and stealing from friends and family. He was recently suspended from school because of skipping class and constantly disrupting the classroom. Tonight his father came home and found him in his bedroom with his girlfriend with the door locked, smoking marijuana. A fight developed and police have placed him under arrest and want him taken to the hospital for evaluation and drug testing. Given his history, you suspect which of the following mental disorders?

   A. Pervasive developmental disorder
   B. Reactive attachment disorder
   C. ADHD
   D. Conduct disorder

Delirium, Dementia, and Amnestic Disorders

This chapter deals with conditions of the mind that tend to alter one's ability to think clearly. Responders are often called to assist patients who present with altered mental status (AMS). AMS can be caused by many different medical and psychological conditions (**Figure 11-1**). The EMS provider will need training, clinical expertise, and patience when evaluating individuals experiencing a state of confusion. Through a combination of classroom and field experience, emergency personnel will be better able to determine whether a particular patient's condition is treated as emergent or further follow-up is indicated.

Background

The *DSM-IV-TR* states that <u>delirium</u> is "characterized by a disturbance of consciousness and a change in cognition that develops over a short period of time." Generally speaking, delirium is not actually a disease, but a syndrome or presentation of conditions such as confusion, attention deficit, difficulties with thought processes, and hallucinations. Most cases of delirium are acute, have a recent onset, and have a specific cause.

By contrast, the *DSM-IV-TR* classifies <u>dementia</u> as a condition with "multiple cognitive deficits that include impairment in memory."

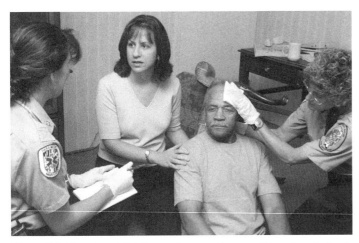

Figure 11-1 Altered mental status can be caused by many different medical and psychological conditions.

Dementia is not a disease but a group of drastic personality, mood, and behavioral changes resulting from brain impairment and the loss of memory. Dementia occurs when various parts of the brain that involve learning, language, decision making, and memory become affected by infections or diseases. Scientists do not fully understand many of the causes of dementia.

<u>Amnesia</u> is defined as a pathological absence, impairment, or loss of memory. It can be caused by a variety of conditions affecting the brain, but is usually the result of either severe emotional or brain trauma. There are two common types of amnesia seen in the prehospital environment. <u>Retrograde amnesia</u> is diagnosed when the patient cannot remember some things prior to a point in time; <u>anterograde amnesia</u> is diagnosed when the patient has difficulty remembering new things that occur after a specific time or event.

Assessment

The assessment process of a patient with AMS is not always clear or easy to accomplish. AMS presents in many forms that can often lead the emergency responder on a variety of assessment pathways. Delirium, dementia, and amnesia share some signs and symptoms, and there are signs and symptoms that are very specific to each condition. A thorough and detailed history should lead you in the correct direction.

Begin by getting a thorough medical and trauma history from the patient and family members present. Try to elicit details surrounding head trauma, diabetes, alcohol or substance use and abuse, cancer, Alzheimer's disease, and other medical conditions. Ask those present if the current presentation is normal or different from what they see on a regular basis. Have the patient or a family member describe to you what a normal day is like for the patient. If it is now different, what has changed? The use of SAMPLE and OPQRST questioning at this point will assist you in gathering information.

Common signs and symptoms of delirium, dementia, and amnesia are changes in cognition, memory, and orientation. Although these items alone will not tell you the patient's underlying condition, they are the foundation of the history-gathering process. It is not unusual for patients suffering from these disorders to repeatedly ask the same question. As a result, much of the interview will be based on repetition and reorientation. It is common to find patients with altered mental status and confusion. Be sure to ask questions that will demonstrate their thought processes. For example, you can ask them to tell you the meaning of a simple proverb, such as "a rolling stone gathers no moss," and carefully observe their reaction.

In the Field

You may want to ask ...

- Does the patient have a history of head trauma? Diabetes? Alcohol or substance use or abuse? Cancer? Alzheimer's disease? Other medical problem that we should know about?

- Tell me what your normal day is like. What do you do from the time you get up until you go to bed?

- Has that daily routine changed recently?

- Is the patient acting different today from how the patient normally acts?

- Does the patient hear voices in his or her head?

- Does the patient receive signals or messages from someone?

- Ask family members or caretakers if the patient makes up stories to fill in for missing memory.

The term <u>cognition</u> is used to describe one's mental function and processes. In assessing the patient, emergency personnel can use questions to evaluate the ability to comprehend, make decisions, and demonstrate memory.

Asking questions such as "Where are you now?" and "Do you know who I am and why I'm here?" can help build patient rapport and evaluate the patient's level of comprehension. Simple math problems can also be very useful in evaluating the patient's ability to process information. The serial-7 test is easy to administer and provides useful information about higher-level thought processes. Simply ask the patient to start with the number seven and continue to add seven, resulting in the series 7-14-21-28-35-42-49. Failure to accomplish this task suggests diminished cognition that should be documented and reported to medical staff.

To test memory, tell the patient that you are going to give him or her three simple items to remember, and in approximately one minute, you are going to ask the person to repeat them back to you. A chair, pen, and table are common items that are easily remembered by a person with good cognitive skills. Document the result of this test in your patient care report. (For example: "Three items were listed for the patient to remember. Following additional questioning, the patient was able to recall all three items [or could only remember two of the three items].")

Historically, the standard test for orientation is person, place, and time (ie, Can patients explain to you who they or others are, where they currently are located, and the time or date of the day?). However, many providers have found that the use of time is not a reliable indicator of orientation. The reality is that many people under normal conditions cannot accurately tell you the date or time. Instead, the use of a thing or event will likely be more accurate. Asking the patient what happened to him or her, why help was called, or who is the current president of the United States may provide a more valid response from the patient.

If your system requires that you use time, you could use an alternative approach such as "Can you tell me if it's morning, afternoon, or evening?" It should be noted that whenever questions such as these are used, the provider must be able to validate the correct answer. Always document any answer that is not appropriate.

Delirium

Delirium is identified by the *DSM-IV-TR* as a mental disorder resulting from variations that occur to a person's level of consciousness and changes in emotion, behavior, and mental functioning. It is most commonly caused by physical disease, cerebral trauma, or drug effect. The emergency service provider will witness patients with delirium due to a variety of medical conditions, such as diabetes or exposure to drugs, alcohol, or toxins (**Table 11-1**). Fever, heat exposure, hypothermia, altitude sickness, or trauma can also cause delirium. A patient suffering from delirium might seem confused and distressed. The person may act

---

SAMPLE

- **Signs and symptoms:** Confusion, disorientation; confabulates or makes up a story to fill in gaps in memory.
- **Allergies:** Allergic reactions can occur with any medication, many of which will cause confused states.
- **Medications:** Cholinesterase inhibitors commonly used for the treatment of Alzheimer's disease include tacrine (Cognex), donepezil (Aricept), galantamine (Reminyl), rivastigmine (Exelon), or memantine (Namenda) (**Figure 11-2**).
- **Past medical history:** Medical history will vary. If the patient has dementia, then there may be a history of confusion and symptoms associated with organic brain syndromes. If it is acute, suspect a medical condition such as alcohol withdrawal or diabetes.
- **Last oral intake:** Dependent upon the situation; if the patient is an alcoholic, last intake is important information.
- **Events leading up to today's event:** Assess to determine if EMS was called for an acute or chronic condition. What happened today that required an EMS response?

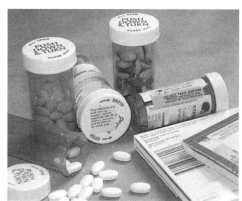

Figure 11-2 Cholinesterase inhibitors are commonly used for the treatment of Alzheimer's disease.

OPQRST

- **Onset:** When did the symptoms begin? Sudden onset or chronic condition?
- **Provocation:** What happened today to trigger someone to call EMS?
- **Quality:** How pervasive or significant are the patient's feelings and emotions at the time of assessment?
- **Radiation:** Is the state of confusion being experienced by the patient radiating out to family members, neighbors, or others? Has it affected important components of the patient's life, such as employment, or simply the ability to live alone?
- **Severity:** On a scale of 0-10, how severe is the distress today for the patient? For family or others involved?
- **Time:** How long have the symptoms lasted since the time of onset? Is there a need for the patient to be transported for lifesaving intervention? Has the time arrived for family members to request that a symptomatic family member be evaluated for some complication of an organic brain syndrome?

strangely and may not recognize familiar faces or things. You will have to rule out many causes of this altered mental status, based on your other medical training. It is always important to remember that no matter how confusing a scene may be, the management of life-threatening illness and injury takes precedence over psychological presentations.

Alcohol Withdrawal and Delirium Tremens

One specific type of delirium that is common in the prehospital environment is delirium tremens or simply "the DTs." Alcohol withdrawal syndromes can range from mild symptoms to full-blown DTs. The DTs are the result of withdrawal in a person who is chronically and chemically dependent on alcohol. Because of the nature of the addiction, alcohol withdrawal can be life threatening and the patient may experience seizures, coma, and death.

Alcohol is a central nervous system depressant. For the person who is addicted to alcohol, the brain's neurotransmitters have worked for years to compensate and maintain a normal level of stimulation. When the person stops drinking, the sympathetic nervous system is no longer being suppressed. As a result, numerous neurotransmitters in the brain that have worked against the depressive agent now overload the brain (**Table 11-2**). Seizures can occur as a result (**Figure 11-3**). Aggressive advanced life support care must be provided to stop the seizures and maintain the patient's airway and cardiovascular status.

Patients presenting with acute DTs might develop seizures due to alcohol or chemical withdrawal. Emergency responders should be knowledgeable about local protocols, which may include the pharmacologic sedation of the patient to prevent or treat seizures.

Dementia

Dementia presents as a gradual decline in mentation and cognitive function (**Table 11-3**). Generally speaking, there is a loss of alertness and a decline in memory, particularly recent memory. Thorough questioning of the patient can investigate events of the far, intermediate, and recent past.

Prehospital providers should resist the notion that dementia is strictly a disease of the elderly; although dementia is more common after the age of 65 years and the incidence increases greatly after the age of 75 years, the condition may be seen in younger patients, particularly those with chronic conditions. Human immunodeficiency virus (HIV) disease, cerebral trauma, Alzheimer's disease (AD), and Parkinson's disease are all possible causes of dementia.

Dementia patients often present with some unusual characteristics not generally seen in the delirium patient (**Table 11-4**). Patients with chronic changes in mentation, such as Alzheimer's disease, will often invent

SEA-3 for Delirium, Dementia, and Amnesia

Speech: Able to speak; however, note any confusion.

Emotion: May present with a normal affect, or anxiety or anger may be present.

Appearance: Varies depending on the degree of confusion. May present as normal or altered. Patients may be wearing inappropriate clothing for the seasonal temperature.

Alertness: Generally alert but commonly confused. May not be oriented to person, place, or event.

Activity: Activity varies for patients with dementia or delirium. The range of sedation to agitation may be exhibited. Note that medications can alter activity levels.

Table 11-1 Medical Conditions Associated With Delirium

System	Disorder
Central nervous system	Head trauma
	Infection (meningitis, encephalitis, HIV, or neurosyphilis)
	Seizures and post-seizure confusion
	Vascular disorders (stroke or bleeding after head injury)
	Degenerative disease (dementia)
Metabolic causes	Kidney failure
	Liver failure
	Anemia
	Low blood sugar
	Dehydration
	Vitamin deficiency such as B_{12}, folate, or thiamine deficiency
	Electrolyte imbalance
Cardiac and respiratory system	Myocardial infarction (heart attack)
	Congestive heart failure (heart failure)
	Cardiac arrhythmia (irregular heart rhythm)
	Shock
	Respiratory failure
	Decreased oxygenation
Systemic illness	Infections (urinary tract infection or pneumonia)
	Postoperative state
	Tumor (cancer)
	Severe trauma (fractures)
	Temperature dysregulation (hypothermia/heat stroke)
	Sleep deprivation

Source: Compton, 2007.

information to replace memory gaps. This process, known as <u>confabulation</u>, is common in the elderly with chronic dementia. The prehospital provider may be led to believe that the patient actually lived in a faraway land or held a job that did not exist. Every effort should be made to validate the patient's statements and confirm his or her responses. Even if you discover that the statements are false, continue with a caring and empathetic approach and assess the patient as well as you can under the circumstances.

Dementia patients may also demonstrate aphasia, agnosia, and apraxia. <u>Aphasia</u> is when language function is defective or absent and the patient has difficulty in speaking or expressing

Table 11-2 Timing of Alcohol Withdrawal Syndromes

Syndrome	Clinical Findings	Onset After Last Drink
Minor withdrawal	Tremulousness, mild anxiety, headache, diaphoresis, palpitations, anorexia, and gastrointestinal upset	6 to 36 hours
Seizures	Generalized, tonic-clonic seizures, and status epilepticus (rare)	6 to 48 hours
Alcohol hallucinosis	Visual, auditory, and/or tactile hallucinations	12 to 48 hours
Delirium tremens	Delirium, tachycardia, hypertension, agitation, fever, and diaphoresis	48 to 96 hours

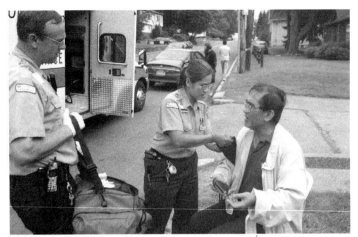

Figure 11-3 Seizures can occur as a result of severe alcohol withdrawal.

words that make sense to the listener. Aphasia is a common neurological presentation that can be seen with dementia, stroke, or other types of cerebral dysfunction. In some patients, you may find that they seem to know what they want to say but are unable to communicate with you. The appropriate course of action is to tell the patient that you are trying to help and that you recognize he or she is having difficulty communicating.

Agnosia is a patient's failure or inability to identify or recognize common objects or people. This is an easy sign to validate. Ask the patient to verify the name of a loved one, neighbor, or caregiver who is present. As with aphasia, patients will present as frustrated or confused as to why they cannot answer your questions. Supportive questioning and compassionate care are paramount in these situations.

Apraxia is a complex condition that many EMS providers have likely witnessed in patients without knowing what to call it or how to identify it. Apraxia is the inability of the patient to perform purposeful tasks or to manipulate objects in the absence of paralysis. Several types of apraxia exist.

Ideational apraxia is commonly seen in patients with dementia. It is an impairment that results from a loss of the understanding of how to use a familiar object or how to perform a task as it needs to be conducted. For example, in order to fry an egg, there is a specific order in which the task needs to be completed. One would begin by going to the refrigerator, getting the egg, selecting a pan, and so forth. The patient with ideational apraxia, however, may know how to get the egg from the refrigerator but might not know how to get the egg out of the shell. Likewise, the patient may be able to perform each task individually but not be able to put them in the proper order to complete the process. It may appear as though the patient simply has forgotten how to conduct the task.

The other types of apraxia—ideomotor, amnestic, buccofacial, and kinetic—are various motor function or speech disorders caused by illness or injury to the brain. Patients with ideomotor apraxia are unable to respond and perform a requested task, such as "Show me how you brush your teeth," or "Wave goodbye." Amnestic apraxia is seen in patients who cannot perform a function simply because they cannot remember how to accomplish the task. Patients who cannot perform skilled movements involving the tongue, lips, and mouth (in the absence of paralysis) have what is

Table 11-3 Common Signs and Symptoms of Dementia

Mild Symptoms	Moderate Symptoms	Severe Symptoms
• Memory lapses • Inability to perform everyday tasks • Confusion and disorientation in familiar surroundings	• Language disturbances • Needs help with bathing, grooming, and hygiene • Inability to recognize family and friends • Disturbing behavior (aggression)	• Slowed or incomprehensible speech • Loss of bladder/bowel control • Increased or total dependence on caregiver

Source: Compton, 2007.

commonly known as <u>buccofacial apraxia</u>. <u>Kinetic</u>, or <u>limb</u>, <u>apraxia</u> is similar to buccofacial apraxia, except that the patient is unable to perform skilled movements with his or her extremities.

When called to the scene of a patient who is exhibiting confusion or neurologic deficits, your knowledge of confabulation, aphasia, agnosia, and apraxia will prove useful in ruling out true neurologic crises such as stroke. It should be noted that the presentations listed in this section are not in themselves emergencies—they are signs of an underlying central nervous system dysfunction. Continuous re-evaluation and documentation is very important as you make your care transition to the emergency department or the patient's family physician.

Non reversible Dementias

<u>Alzheimer's disease (AD)</u> is the most common form of dementia among older patients. This form of progressive dementia, named for Alois Alzheimer, begins gradually and develops over a period of several months or years. AD is a diagnosis by exclusion, meaning that all other possible causes have been ruled out.

The disease results from a loss of nerve cells in specialized areas of the brain that deal with cognitive functions, especially those cells that release the neurotransmitter acetylcholine. Alzheimer's disease affects the parts of the brain that control thought, memory, and language.

Table 11-4 Delirium Versus Dementia

Feature	Delirium	Dementia
Onset	Develops suddenly	Develops slowly
Course	Fluctuating; most cases resolve with correction of the underlying medical condition	Chronic and progressive
Duration	Days to weeks	Months to years
Cause	Frequently caused by medical illness and drugs	Usually caused by Alzheimer's disease or other neurodegenerative diseases
Level of consciousness	Fluctuating levels of consciousness with decreased attention	Normal until late stages
Distinguishing feature	Predominantly affects attention	Predominantly affects memory
Memory	Trouble processing new information and inability to recall recent events	Gradual loss of recent memory in mild to moderate stages; eventual loss of remote memory in severe stage
Language	Slow and often incoherent	Difficulty in finding the right word
Sleep	Reversed sleep-wake cycle	May have insomnia
Other associated symptoms	Disorientation, visual hallucinations, agitation, apathy, and withdrawal	Disorientation and agitation
Treatment and outcome	Involves immediate workup and treatment of underlying medical condition; potentially reversible	Involves non-emergent medical workup and treatment; not reversible

Source: Compton, 2007.

Patient symptoms begin with changes or loss of memory of recent events or the names of people they know. As the disease progresses, it is common for patients to have problems recognizing family members, which often causes great emotional stress in loved ones. It is not unusual for patients to forget how to dress themselves or how to perform normal activities such as eating or going to the bathroom.

In the later stages, patients may use surprisingly vulgar language, become aggressive and anxious, and frequently wander away from their home or nursing facility. Remember that these patients and family members will need your compassion and understanding during these times. It should be noted that currently there is no cure for Alzheimer's disease; however, new medications are being developed to slow the progression of the symptoms.

Calls involving the evaluation and care of a patient with any form of dementia or Alzheimer's disease can be very challenging. Depending on the progression of the disease, patients can present as slightly confused or completely disoriented and aggressive. Often times, patients have wandered away from a residence or nursing home facility. As a result, they may have been lost in the outside environment for hours or even days.

Because AD patients are poor historians, you will have to make decisions based on whatever information is available. Sometimes that information is minimal and your skills as an emergency responder will be put to the test. You will need to attempt to gather information without upsetting the patient and while recognizing that the patient may be uncooperative. The patients may present with signs of trauma, altered mental status, dehydration, malnutrition, diabetes, hypo- or hyperthermia (depending on the temperature), or coma. Always be prepared to provide oxygen, intravenous fluids for rehydration, and a glucose and cardiac evaluation.

Vascular dementia, also known as multi-infarct dementia, is the second most common type of dementia after Alzheimer's disease. It can be caused by a cerebrovascular accident or stroke or a series of small strokes, commonly called transient ischemic attacks. As a result of multiple vascular injuries, the brain's cognitive sites experience deterioration and lose function.

The research on this particular type of dementia is limited. Studies have noted that the incidence of dementia following a stroke ranges from 6% to 32% over a period of 3 months to 20 years. Additional research indicates that those patients with a history of left-hemisphere strokes have a higher incidence of developing dementia.

Patients with confusion and altered mentation, with or without traditional signs of stroke, may be providing you information about the circulation and function of their brains. If the patient has vascular dementia and classic stroke presentation, you would expect facial droop, paralysis on one side, and difficulty speaking, among other signs of neurological deficits. In accordance to local protocols, these patients should be quickly assessed, given oxygen and supportive care, and rapidly transported to a primary care hospital or stroke center.

Dementia with Lewy bodies is the most common dementia syndrome associated with Parkinson's disease. Parkinson's disease is a condition in which the part of the brain that controls muscle movement fails, due to a breakdown of the dopamine-producing neurons. These patients present with trembling of hands, arms, legs, jaw, and face; stiffness of the joints; slowness of movement; and poor balance and coordination. Unlike Parkinson's disease, dementia with Lewy bodies presents not only with a lack of muscle coordination, but with a progressive form of dementia. Patients with dementia with Lewy bodies may have persistent, clear visual hallucinations and altered mental status with a diminished cognition. In the prehospital environment, evaluate the patient using the standardized SAMPLE, OPQRST, and SEA-3 assessment tools, documenting the neuromuscular presentation and alterations in mentation.

Reversible Dementias

Not all dementias are permanent. There are other types of non-Alzheimer's dementias that can present acutely and be treated if they are diagnosed in a timely manner. These dementias are collectively called the <u>reversible dementias</u>. For example, in those patients with alcoholism, adverse reactions to prescription medication, depression, or vitamin B12 deficiency, traditional treatment modalities would correct the underlying condition and reverse the dementia.

Amnestic Disorders

The term *amnesia* is one that you may be very familiar with simply by watching television. It is often used in the news or on a show as an alibi for a criminal. As a result, many individuals may not believe that amnesia is a valid and serious mental health condition. Nothing could be further from the truth. In fact, some patients' amnesia is so debilitating that they are unable to live alone and require assisted living facilities.

Amnesia is defined as a pathological absence, impairment, or loss of memory that can be caused by various problems affecting the brain, but is usually the result of either severe emotional or brain trauma. It is important to note that not all forms of brain trauma are limited to actual physical trauma, such as hitting one's head against a windshield. Trauma may also be due to a medical or metabolic issue or substance use. The degree of amnesia or impairment is based on the area of the brain that is affected.

Amnesia often interrupts one's ability to learn new information. It may also impair the recall of previously learned information, making it difficult for the individual to remember important dates, events, or tasks. Amnesia is commonly classified as being either retrograde or anterograde. Amnesia as the average person thinks of it is retrograde amnesia, meaning that the patient cannot recall parts of the past. This is commonly seen in patients who sustain concussions at the scene of a car crash. When asked what happened, they may reply "I don't remember" or ask how they got there. It is common for the individual to repeatedly ask the same questions. The emergency responder should provide the same answer each time to help reorient the patient to person, place, and event. Reassure the patient that he or she is safe and that you are there to provide care.

Anterograde amnesia occurs when the individual is unable to retain new memories or to learn new bits of information. This is a common condition associated with brain injuries. Anterograde amnesia will not be the cause of your primary response. It is a symptom of a more severe central nervous system disorder. This is a common condition seen with patients with a history of brain insults due to lesions, trauma, or years of substance abuse. Anterograde amnesia may make gathering a complete history particularly difficult, but it is important to maintain a calm, understanding demeanor in an effort to reassure the patient.

Amnestic Disorder Due to a General Medical Condition

Conditions that commonly cause amnestic disorder include cerebrovascular accidents (stroke), tumors, vascular diseases affecting blood flow to the brain, or head trauma. In these cases, the medical emergency or trauma will be the primary presentation. This amnestic diagnosis is given once the patient has been stabilized and is in rehabilitative care.

Substance-Induced Persisting Amnestic Disorder

In the prehospital setting, every emergency responder or mental health professional has cared for an intoxicated patient who, upon questioning, does not remember many of the evening's events. Usually, when the blood alcohol level returns to zero, the patient's cognition returns to normal. However, in the case of substance-induced persisting amnestic disorder, this memory disturbance persists beyond that of the normal duration of substance intoxication or withdrawal. A permanent injury occurs over time due to severe structural and chemical changes within the brain tissue itself.

Chronic alcohol abuse, long-term use of sedative, hypnotic, or anti-anxiety drugs, and toxins can be responsible for substance-induced persisting amnestic disorder. Some examples of toxins reported to cause amnesia include carbon monoxide, mercury, lead, industrial solvents, and organophosphate insecticides. You may not recognize the cause of this patient's amnesia unless someone is there to provide you with a history, or an obvious event has occurred such as someone spraying insecticides on a garden.

Korsakoff's syndrome is a permanent amnesic disorder that follows an acute onset of Wernicke's encephalopathy. Wernicke's is a neurological condition that results from the presence of alcohol in the absence of vitamin B1 or thiamine. Thiamine is a vitamin normally absorbed from foods such as bananas, whole grain breads, spinach, beans, pork, beef, and nuts. As the result of a poor diet, malabsorption, and increased loss of the water-soluble vitamin (as a result of increased urine output), the brain fails to receive the needed thiamine and brain changes and lesions develop. Wernicke's encephalopathy can also be seen in patients with anorexia nervosa and acquired immunodeficiency syndrome, in dieting individuals, and in those undergoing prolonged intravenous feeding without proper vitamin supplements, gastrointestinal surgery (including bariatric surgery), and dialysis. The patient will present with a series of neurologic symptoms such as abnormal eye movements, confusion, and uncoordinated movement, especially gait ataxia (staggering walk). If treated with high doses of thiamine, Korsakoff's syndrome may be prevented, although not in all cases.

Prehospital Management

Field management for the patient with any type of delirium or dementia tends to focus on maintaining a safe and calm environment. Patients with altered mental status are often scared and confused; thus, the EMS provider should make every effort to create a controlled and safe environment.

The majority of patients with delirium and dementia will be calm and easy to manage, but there is always the possibility that they will exhibit some anger or hostility and may ultimately become violent. Should this occur, physical restraints may be used, based upon local protocols. Some EMS systems will have provisions for advanced life support providers to administer a chemical restraint agent such as haloperidol. The EMS provider should have the involvement of local law enforcement officials and must have a thorough understanding of how to properly restrain patients.

SAFER-R Field Intervention

Stabilize: Create a calm environment by presenting a professional demeanor. Offer words of support that will make the patient and family feel safe.

Acknowledge: Assess and recognize the current situation by gathering information.

Facilitate: Understand the situation by determining if cognitive processes are intact or disturbed. Begin thinking about what type of help the patient and family needs.

Encourage: Continue to build rapport with the patient and family by attempting to reorient the patient and move him or her toward transportation and definitive care.

Recovery: Reinforce treatment and transportation plan with the patient.

Referral: Assist the family by suggesting community contacts such as the Department of Social Services or Alzheimer's support group.

Pharmacological Considerations

Confusion is one of the most common side effects of some over-the-counter and prescription medications. Additionally, homeopathic remedies are becoming an increasing problem, because many patients do not tell their traditional health care providers that they are taking them. Two common examples of herbal remedies are Ma Huang and herbal ecstasy. Ma Huang is another name for ephedra and can cause severe tachycardia. Herbal ecstasy is a combination of kola nut, nutmeg, and ginseng and can cause a person to present with hallucinations, nausea, vomiting, tachycardia, and hypertension.

Over 250 medications list confusion as a side effect. When assessing the patient, a thorough medical and pharmacologic history is paramount. Certain classes of medications are known to cause confusion or delirium-like symptoms, particularly in elderly patients, and medications such as sleep aids, antihistamines, analgesics (pain), and benzo-diazepines (sedatives) are commonly prescribed to this population.

> ## In the Field
>
> ### Tips for Crisis Response
>
> Always use caution with patients with an altered mental status. Confusion can result in patients becoming aggressive or hostile toward loved ones or emergency responders.

Treatment modalities will be based upon your assessment and field diagnosis. In a case in which confusion or delirium is caused by hypoglycemia, the treatment would be glucagon or intravenous dextrose. Altered states caused by the injection of illicit drugs such as heroin, may call for the administration of naloxone (Narcan®), a narcotic antagonist.

Patients with acute alcohol withdrawal may require aggressive management such as airway devices, suctioning, and intubation, and providers should administer diazepam (Valium®) to control the seizure activity. The administration of thiamine is recommended prior to giving dextrose in patients who you suspect may be suffering from Wernicke's encephalopathy or in those with a history of chronic alcoholism.

Final Thoughts

The assessment of patients exhibiting dementia, delirium, and amnesia is a challenge for even the most experienced prehospital providers. As a slow-onset, chronic condition, dementia does not necessarily require immediate intervention. Delirium, on the other hand, is often the sign of an acute, life-threatening illness that needs a rapid response. A detailed survey and history will help you to differentiate between benign symptomatology and a neurologic crisis.

Local protocols will dictate your response for these patients. Generally, treating the patient in a calm, reassuring, and respectful manner will accomplish your task of getting the patient to the hospital safely. In patients with more severe conditions involving the central nervous system, aggressive treatment is warranted.

Selected References

American Psychiatric Association: *Diagnostic and Statistical Manual of Mental Disorders, Fourth Edition, Text Revision (DSM-IV-TR)*. Washington, DC, American Psychiatric Association, 2000.

Behavenet Inc. Available at: http://www.behavenet.com/. Accessed May 15, 2008.

CME: continuing medical education. Available at: http://www.mhsource.com/demconsult/index.jhtml. Accessed April 1, 2007.

Compton MT, Kotwicki RJ: *Responding to Individuals With Mental Illnesses*. Sudbury, MA, Jones & Bartlett Publishers, 2007.

eMedicine from WebMD. Available at: http://www.emedicine.com/neuro/topic438.htm. Accessed May 15, 2008.

Helpguide.org. Available at: http://www.helpguide.org/elder/vascular_dementia.htm. Accessed May 15, 2008.

MedlinePlus, National Library of Medicine and National Institutes of Health. Available at: http://www.nlm.nih.gov/medlineplus/parkinsonsdisease.html. Accessed May 15, 2008.

Mosby's Medical, Nursing, and Allied Health Dictionary, ed 4. St Louis, MO, 1994.

Stedman's Medical Dictionary for the Health Professions and Nursing, ed 5. Baltimore, MD, Lippincott Williams & Wilkins, 2005.

Thomas JA, Woodall SJ: *Responding to Psychological Emergencies: A Field Guide*. Clifton Park, NY, Delmar Learning, 2006.

UpToDate Inc. Available at: http://www.UpToDate.com. Accessed May 15, 2008.

WebMD. Available at: http://www.webmd.com/alzheimers/guide/alzheimers-dementia. Accessed May 15, 2008.

WrongDiagnosis.com. Available at: http://wrongdiagnosis.com. Accessed April 1, 2007.

Prep Kit

Ready for Review

- Delirium and dementia are often confused, although they are very different conditions. Delirium is a disturbance of consciousness and change in cognition that develops acutely with a specific cause such as alcohol withdrawal, altitude sickness, or heat exposure. Dementia is a slow-onset, chronic condition that results in multiple cognitive deficits, including memory impairment. HIV, brain trauma, Alzheimer's disease, and Parkinson's disease are common causes of dementia.

- Patients with a history of chronic alcohol abuse can be in physical danger if they suddenly are deprived of alcohol. The uncontrolled cessation of alcohol can result in a condition known as delirium tremens or the "DTs." The DTs are a response to the body's need for the drug of alcohol and can result in altered mental status, seizures, coma, and death if not treated in a hospital or medical detoxification unit.

- Evaluating the patient's thought process, or what is known as cognition, is a very important assessment tool. Asking patients to complete simple mental tasks such as counting backwards or answering questions about specific events is a good way to assess an individual's cognitive ability.

- Apraxia is a common sign demonstrated by patients with delirium, dementia, and amnestic disorders. This chapter discusses four types: ideomotor, amnestic, buccofacial, and kinetic. These impairments are easy to evaluate and document simply by asking a few questions or having the patient attempt to complete simple tasks.

- Alzheimer's disease is the most common form of dementia among the elderly. It is a progressive form of dementia that destroys the individual's ability to remember, think, and use language properly. The disease results from a loss of nerve cells in the brain that release the neurotransmitter acetylcholine.

- Amnesia, or the loss of memory, can have many causes, such as emotional distress, stroke, or brain trauma. Commonly two types of amnesia are recognized. Retrograde amnesia means that the individual cannot remember parts of the past. Anterograde amnesia occurs when the person cannot retain new memories or information.

Vital Vocabulary

agnosia The inability to identify or recognize familiar people or objects.

Alzheimer's disease (AD) A disease process that results from a loss of nerve cells in specialized areas of the brain that deal with cognitive functions, especially with those cells that release the neurotransmitter, acetylcholine. It is the most common form of dementia among older patients.

amnesia A pathological absence, impairment, or loss of memory.

amnestic apraxia A condition in which patients cannot perform a function simply because they cannot remember how to accomplish the task.

anterograde amnesia A condition in which the individual is unable to retain new memories or to learn new bits of information.

aphasia The inability to produce or comprehend language.

apraxia An inability to perform useful tasks or conduct object manipulation even though the patient is not paralyzed.

buccofacial apraxia The inability to perform skilled movements involving the tongue, lips, and mouth (in the absence of paralysis).

cognition The mental process of gaining knowledge and comprehension, including aspects such as awareness, remembering, perception, reasoning, judgment, and problem solving.

confabulation The fabrication of events, facts, or experiences to fill in gaps in memory.

delirium A disturbance of consciousness and a change in cognition that develop over a short period of time.

delirium tremens (DTs) A syndrome resulting from the withdrawal of alcohol.

dementia A condition with multiple cognitive deficits that include impairment in memory.

ideational apraxia An impairment that results from a loss of the understanding of how to use a familiar object or to perform a task.

ideomotor apraxia A form of apraxia in which one is unable to respond and perform a requested task.

kinetic apraxia A condition in which the patient is unable to perform skilled movements with the extremities (in the absence of paralysis).

limb apraxia See kinetic apraxia.

multi-infarct dementia See vascular dementia.

Parkinson's disease A condition in which the part of the brain that controls muscle movement fails because of a breakdown of the dopamine-producing neurons. Patients will present with trembling of the hands, arms, legs, jaw, and face, stiffness of the joints, slow muscle movement, and poor balance and coordination.

retrograde amnesia A condition in which the individual is unable to recall parts of the past.

reversible dementia Specific types of dementia that can be reversed if they are diagnosed and treated in a timely manner.

vascular dementia A degenerative cerebrovascular disease that leads to a progressive decline in memory and cognitive functioning.

Assessment in Action

Answer key is located in the back of the book.

1. Ms. Jones is an 85-year-old female in the local nursing home. According to the staff, she has been confused for the past hour. She does not know where she is, cannot tell you who she is, and does not recognize her nurse. Normally, she is an active patient who is alert and oriented to person, place, and event. As part of your differential diagnosis, you suspect all of the following conditions EXCEPT:

   A. hypoglycemia.
   B. stroke.
   C. delirium.
   D. dementia.

2. When visiting with your grandfather, you notice that he begins to tell you stories about how he was a space engineer and helped to build the space shuttle in the 1980s. However, you know that your grandfather worked as a farmer for his entire life. The space engineer story is best described as:

   A. confabulation.
   B. renal disease.
   C. agnosia.
   D. aphagia.

3. You give a patient three objects to identify. After much thought, the patient is unable to recognize what they are. This best exemplifies:

   A. delirium.
   B. confusion.
   C. apraxia.
   D. agnosia.

4. Delirium tremens is a potentially life-threatening condition that results from acute withdrawal of alcohol in the addicted patient.

   A. True
   B. False

5. In assessing a patient, you note that he is unable to smile or stick out his tongue when asked. This change in neuromotor response is known as what type of apraxia?

   A. Ideomotor
   B. Amnestic
   C. Buccofacial
   D. Kinetic

Chapter 12

Substance-Related Disorders

Introduction

If you have been working in the prehospital environment for any period of time, you have had patients who were taking drugs that affected their behavior. This chapter will discuss four components of substance-related disorders: intoxication, abuse, dependence, and withdrawal. Many of the drugs discussed will present as though your patient has a mental disorder, when in fact the symptoms are chemically induced.

Background

Substance-related disorders are set apart from other mental disorders inasmuch as they are defined by cause rather than by a set of symptoms. The symptoms of substance-related disorders are caused specifically by the use of a substance, not by a general medical condition or a mental disorder (**Figure 12-1**). For example, individuals experiencing a substance-induced perception disorder, such as <u>hallucinations</u> from taking lysergic acid diethylamide (LSD), may not believe the perception represents external reality. They may recognize that they are "seeing" things, but they are aware that the visions are drug-induced. If an individual believes the perception does represent external reality, a psychotic disorder such as schizophrenia is more likely to be an appropriate diagnosis.

The *DSM-IV-TR* organizes substances into 11 categories. Examples of each of the following will be given and discussed in this chapter.

- Alcohol
- Amphetamines or similarly acting sympathomimetics
- Cocaine
- Caffeine
- Cannabis
- Hallucinogens
- Inhalants
- Nicotine

- Opioids
- Phencyclidine (PCP) or similarly acting arylcyclohexylamines
- Sedatives, hypnotics, or anxiolytics (anti-anxiety medications)

The diagnostic criteria for substance-related disorders are extremely complex, multi-layered, and confusing, even for the most experienced of mental health practitioners. Understanding substance-related disorders requires mastering four key concepts: *substance dependence, substance abuse, substance intoxication,* and *substance withdrawal.*

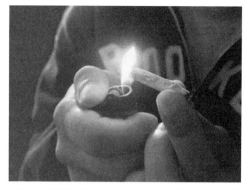

Figure 12-1 Prehospital personnel must be prepared to recognize and treat substance-related emergencies.

Substance <u>dependence</u> is generally diagnosed when an individual continues to use a substance despite adverse physiological changes and negative life events, such as developing severe health problems or losing a job. The emergency responder will be able to see many of the symptoms of dependence. The patient will often report <u>craving</u> or a strong drive to use a substance, along with increased tolerance and unsuccessful attempts at discontinuing use of the drug. <u>Tolerance</u> is when a higher amount of a substance is required to produce the effect previously induced by a lower dose of substance. The patient may demonstrate withdrawal symptoms that vary according to the substance used. Some of the more common withdrawal symptoms are nausea, vomiting, headaches, muscle tremors, and possibly seizures.

Substance <u>abuse</u> is diagnosed when an individual continues the use of a substance despite significant impairment or distress caused during or shortly after the use of a substance. A diagnosis of substance abuse differs from substance dependence in that abuse does not require any level of tolerance or withdrawal symptoms. An easy-to-understand example would be a college student who experiments with alcohol during his or her first year by attending fraternity parties for the first few weeks of school. The student is unable to wake up for an 8:00 am class Thursday mornings because of a severe hangover. As a result, the student fails the class because of poor participation and missing two examinations.

The principal feature of substance <u>intoxication</u> is reversible maladaptive behavior (eg, belligerence or impaired social or occupational functioning) caused by ingestion of or exposure to a substance. The specific clinical symptoms are determined by myriad factors and vary among individuals. Factors that may affect the presentation of intoxication are the substances involved, the dose, the individual's tolerance, the frequency of use, and even the individual's expectations of the substance and the environment in which it was used. In the above example, the college student's activities of getting drunk on Wednesday nights exemplifies the definition of intoxication. It should be noted that for most substances, including alcohol, one can take too much of the drug, resulting in an overdose or toxic level of the chemical in the bloodstream.

Substance <u>withdrawal</u> occurs and is diagnosed when ceasing or reducing prolonged or heavy substance use causes maladaptive behavior. Commonly, individuals with substance withdrawal will experience a great urge to use the substance in order to alleviate their symptoms. Symptoms of substance withdrawal may start as soon as a few hours after the last dosing. Some of the slower-acting substances may produce withdrawal symptoms that last for days. Patients with withdrawal symptoms are truly medically sick, and, in some cases involving drugs such as barbiturates and alcohol, may even die when the drug is suddenly taken away. In most situations, nausea, vomiting, sweating, muscle aches, and spasms are seen.

The Mental Disorder and Medical Overlap

Although dependence, abuse, intoxication, and withdrawal may occur with many substances, some of these states do not cause clinically significant symptoms that would require the

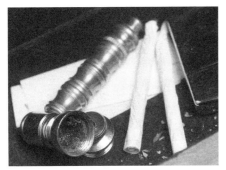 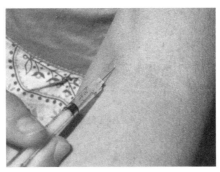 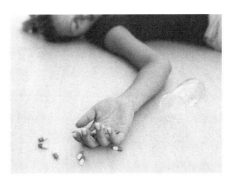

Figure 12-2 The route of administration is an important factor in determining the effects of the substance.

disorder to have a category of its own. For example, nicotine may cause symptoms that would be diagnosed as nicotine dependence or nicotine withdrawal; however, no clinically significant symptoms were observed in order to justify a separate diagnosis of nicotine abuse or nicotine intoxication.

Substance-related disorders can lead to emergency medical situations (eg, overdose, stimulant-induced cardiac arrhythmias, stroke, or respiratory arrest) caused by the physiologic effect of the substances abused. Often the medical emergency will be the result of a violent act committed in an attempt to obtain a substance, especially with cocaine, methamphetamines, and heroin. Sometimes the emergency will be due to an irrational action such as trying to fly while under the influence of a hallucinogen. According to the *DSM-IV-TR*, approximately one half of all highway fatalities involve either a driver or a pedestrian who is intoxicated.

Substance-related disorders rarely develop overnight and may be challenging to diagnose in the prehospital environment. The diagnosis of a substance-related disorder requires a physical examination and detailed history from the individual and will often require obtaining additional information from alternative sources such as a spouse, relatives, medical records, prescription drug containers, or close friends. When available, laboratory test results can be helpful in making the definitive diagnosis.

The route of administration is an important factor in determining the effects of the substance (**Figure 12-2**). Routes of administration involving rapid absorption (eg, intravenous, smoking, or snorting) have a higher likelihood of creating substance dependence. Because of the rapid delivery of the substance to the central nervous system, these routes of administration are also more likely to lead to an overdose. The route of administration may lead to additional medical conditions. Intranasal administration (snorting) may lead to erosion or perforation of the nasal septum. Sharing needles for intravenous administration of substances may lead to a variety of infections and maladies such as HIV infection, hepatitis, cellulitis, and bacterial endocarditis.

In the Field

Prescription psychiatric medications often present with unusual side effects. Remember that medications taken by your patients may produce any of the following conditions: delirium, amnesia, psychosis, depression, anxiety, sleep disorder, or sexual dysfunction.

The class of the substance may also affect the speed of onset. Rapidly acting substances such as diazepam (Valium®) and alprazolam (Xanax®), which are normally used as sedatives or **anxiolytics**, are more likely to lead to substance dependence or abuse than a slower-acting anticonvulsant such as phenobarbital.

The duration of the effect is another important factor in determining which disorder a substance may induce. Relatively short-acting substances have a higher potential of leading to substance dependence or abuse, while longer-acting substances cause prolonged withdrawal symptoms. For example, the onset time for the withdrawal symptoms of heroin is short, but the withdrawal symptoms of methadone last longer.

Although not very common in the prehospital environment, laboratory tests may prove helpful in determining which substance is causing a disorder. Because street drugs are often contaminated with other substances, a toxicology screening may be the only method of discovering what caused the disorder. Laboratory testing of blood or urine may also assist in discerning a particular substance out of a group of substances that have a similar syndrome.

Assessment

In the prehospital environment, treatment will revolve around alleviating the symptoms of the substance-related disorder, but a diagnosis of the specific syndrome or the appropriate toxic syndrome will allow caregivers to take better care of the patient. Toxidrome groups such as central nervous system (CNS) stimulants (amphetamines and cocaine), opioids (heroin and oxycodone), and CNS depressants (alcohol and some inhalants) allow you to sort substances according to their common signs and symptoms (**Table 12-1**).

A thorough physical examination will allow the provider to observe the physical signs and symptoms that are often the first clues to a substance-related state. The key to the successful examination will be your ability to be professional and use nonjudgmental questioning to build trust. While talking with the patient, scan the scene for additional information. For example, where was the patient found? How was the patient dressed? Were any drug paraphernalia present? Was the patient wide awake and anxious or sleepy and sedate? Are the pupils dilated or constricted?

Table 12-1 Signs and Symptoms of Substance Intoxication and Withdrawal			
	Intoxication	**Withdrawal**	**Substance**
Appearance and behavior	Incoordination, unsteady gait, strong odor, impairment in attention or memory, or stupor or coma	Hand tremor, sweating, hallucinations or illusions, agitation, anxiety, and rarely grand mal seizures	Alcohol, inhalants, and sedatives, hypnotics, or anxiolytics (anti-anxiety)
	Emaciated appearance, picked raw skin, hyperactivity, psychomotor agitation or retardation, perspiration or chills, grandiosity, and coma	Depression, fatigue, and anhedonia (absence of pleasure)	Amphetamines and cocaine
	Restlessness, nervousness, excitement, rambling flow speech		Caffeine
	Grand mal seizures (overdose)		
	Sweating, tremors, incoordination, and labile (free and uncontrolled) mood		Hallucinogens
	Vein sclerosis (tracks) and puncture marks	Dysphoric or unpleasant mood, muscle aches, goose bumps, sweating, or fever	Opioids

(Continued)

Table 12-1 (Continued)

	Intoxication	Withdrawal	Substance
Head, ears, eyes, nose, throat	Slurred speech, nystagmus (involuntary movement of the eyes), blurred vision, or diplopia (double vision)		Alcohol and inhalants
	Pupillary dilation, septal erosion, sinusitis, or dry mucosa		Amphetamines and cocaine
	Blood-shot eyes		Cannabis
	Pupillary dilation (possibly with blurring of vision)		Hallucinogens
	Pinpoint pupils	Lacrimation (watery eyes) or rhinorrhea (runny nose), pupillary dilation, and yawning	Opioids
Respiratory	Respiratory depression		Amphetamines and cocaine
	Chronic cough, or chronic obstructive pulmonary disease		Cannabis and nicotine
	Respiratory depression		Opioids
Cardiovascular		Tachycardia	Alcohol
	Hypertension or hypotension, tachycardia or bradycardia, tachypnea, chest pain, and cardiac arrhythmias		Amphetamines and cocaine
	Tachycardia or cardiac arrhythmia		Caffeine and hallucinogens
	Hypotension		Opioids
Gastrointestinal	Nausea, vomiting, and abdominal pain	Nausea or vomiting	Alcohol and caffeine
		Nausea or vomiting, diarrhea	Opioids

Source: Adapted from Pollak AH, Elling B, Smith M (eds) *Nancy Caroline's Emergency Care in the Streets,* ed 6. Sudbury, MA, Jones & Bartlett Publishers, 2008.

The presence of empty pill bottles, cans of spray paint, needles, tourniquets, spoons, or candles suggests different ways that drugs were introduced into the patient's body. An individual who smokes substances such as marijuana or tobacco (nicotine) will have an increased likelihood of laryngopharyngeal pathologies indicated by chronic cough and respiratory disorders. Individuals who use substances such as heroin intravenously may have <u>vein sclerosis</u> (tracks) and puncture marks on their extremities. Be mindful of the fact that intravenous substance users may be infected with bloodborne diseases such as hepatitis and HIV. If intravenous substance use is suspected, be sure to don proper personal protective gear (**Figure 12-3**).

Inhaling a substance often leads to nasopharyngeal pathologies such as <u>septal erosion</u>, sinusitis, dry mucosa, or post-nasal drip. Substances that are ingested orally often lead to gastrointestinal pathologies such as nausea, vomiting, and abdominal pain.

Some substances share the same toxidrome, and similar symptoms therefore will be present. An increase in blood pressure, respiratory rate, heart rate, and body temperature, along with dilated pupils and agitation, can be seen in intoxication with amphetamines or cocaine. Intoxication with a sedative, **hypnotic**, or anxiolytic (anti-anxiety) medication will present with a decrease in blood pressure, respiratory rate, pulse, and body temperature.

As discussed in other chapters, the use of the standardized SAMPLE, OPQRST, and SEA-3 evaluation tools will assist you in gathering information. Once you begin delving deeper into your patient's history, you may find that substance dependence and abuse are often associated with a variety of general medical conditions.

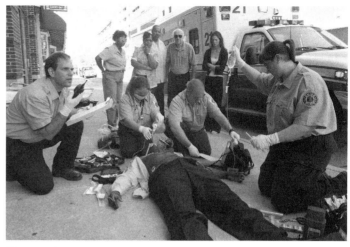

Figure 12-3 If intravenous substance use is suspected, be sure to don proper personal protective gear.

Substance-Related Disorders

Alcohol-Related Disorders

Alcohol is a CNS depressant and is one of the most commonly used substances in the United States. According to the *DSM-IV-TR*, most adults in the United States have had some experience with alcohol, and a large number of those individuals have admitted to having a negative life experience because of alcohol intoxication (injury while driving under the influence or missing work because of a hangover). Signs of tolerance or withdrawal are a mark of alcohol dependence. Most alcohol abuse is diagnosed when the recurrent use of alcohol is established but no signs of tolerance or withdrawal are observed.

Alcohol intoxication is diagnosed when some of the following signs are observed while or shortly after alcohol consumption: clinically significant maladaptive behavior, slurred speech, incoordination, unsteady gait, **nystagmus** (rapidly oscillating eye movements not controllable by the patient), impairment in attention or memory, or stupor or coma. Alcohol withdrawal will present with tachycardia, insomnia, hand tremor, sweating, nausea or vomiting, hallucinations or illusions, agitation, and anxiety. Occasionally grand mal seizures occur 12 to 24 hours after the cessation or reduction in prolonged or heavy use of alcohol.

In the prehospital environment, the misuse of alcohol can result in both medical and psychosocial problems. For some individuals, the chronic use of alcohol can result in family dysfunction, the loss of income or employment, or legal problems. Prolonged or heavy use of alcohol may also cause many medical problems or may exacerbate existing ones. In general, gastrointestinal symptoms such as nausea, vomiting, and abdominal pain are common with alcohol-related disorders. Low-grade hypertension is a general sign of alcohol use, and prolonged use may cause tingling, numbness, and muscle weakness because of alcohol-induced peripheral neuropathy. Memory or cognitive disruptions may be present in severe cases of intoxication or withdrawal.

SEA-3 Assessment for Substance-Related Disorders

Speech: The speech patterns of patients will vary according to the degree of intoxication and type of substance taken. Patients can be somewhat sedate and lethargic with depressants or excited with stimulants.

Emotion: Patients may exhibit any number of emotions from sad and crying to happy and laughing. Patients on hallucinogens may be scared because of the particular hallucinations or other sensations they are experiencing.

Appearance: It is not uncommon to find substance-related emergency patients soiled with urine and feces, especially if they have an altered mental status. Some who attempt to cover up their addiction may wear many layers to cover up track marks.

Alertness: Alertness will depend on the substance taken. Patients range from alert and oriented to person, place, and event, to disoriented, to comatose, to dead in the case of overdose.

Activity: Activity levels will vary according to the class of drug taken. For example, patients intoxicated with depressants will be sedate and present with a low activity level or may be sleeping. Patients on heroin, cocaine, or amphetamines will be anxious and present with increased muscle activity.

It is important to remember that the smell of alcohol alone does not mean that the patient does not also suffer from other medical illnesses. It is common for patients with mental disorders such as depression, bipolar disorder, or schizophrenia to self-medicate with alcohol. In some cases, psychiatric medications mixed with alcohol can cause drowsiness or sedation, hallucinations, or gastrointestinal upset.

Amphetamine-Related Disorders

Amphetamines (or amphetamine-like substances) are stimulants that may be illicitly used for their stimulating and euphoric effects. In some forms, amphetamines may be legally used as appetite suppressants or diet pills. Amphetamines can be prepared in several forms and may be absorbed through different routes. Amphetamines may be ingested orally when in pill or capsule form, while crystals may be inhaled intranasally or smoked in order to achieve faster absorption.

Chronic stimulant users (speed freaks or tweakers) are recognizable because of their wild-eyed, nervous, or jittery appearance. A thin or emaciated body and picked-open raw skin is common. Individuals with amphetamine dependence will often exhibit aggressive and violent behavior and may require the presence of law enforcement in order to be restrained (**Figure 12-4**). Intense anxiety as well as paranoia and psychotic episodes are common.

Amphetamine intoxication generally begins with a feeling of a euphoric high and then shifts to hypervigilance and impaired judgment, accompanied by a myriad of physiological signs and symptoms. The physiological signs of stimulant (eg, amphetamines or cocaine) intoxication are due to their <u>sympathomimetic</u> effects and may include tachycardia or <u>bradycardia</u>, pupillary dilation, elevated or lowered blood pressure, perspiration or chills, nausea or vomiting, evidence of weight loss, <u>psychomotor agitation</u> or <u>psychomotor retardation</u>, muscular weakness, respiratory depression, chest pain, cardiac arrhythmias, confusion, seizures, dyskinesias (disorganized muscle movements), dystonias (abnormal muscle tone), or coma. Signs of depression, fatigue, and inability to feel pleasure (<u>anhedonia</u>) related to the cessation of substance use may lead to a diagnosis of amphetamine withdrawal. Signs of amphetamine withdrawal may last several days to weeks and may be accompanied by suicidal thoughts. Be vigilant for your safety in these situations, as suicidal patients may also be homicidal if they believe that you may disrupt their plans.

Cocaine-Related Disorders

Cocaine is extracted from the leaves of the coca plant (*Erythroxylum coca*). Different preparations of the plant have different onset times and vary in potency. Powdered cocaine is a hydrochloride salt that can be dissolved and injected or snorted intranasally. Crack cocaine is sold in the form of small rocks that have not been neutralized by some form of acid to make the hydrochloride salt. Crack has a relatively low vaporization point, and the vapor is inhaled for its rapid onset of effect. The effect of cocaine is relatively short-lived; thus, individuals with cocaine dependence expend great sums of money in a short period of time in order to maintain a high. Individuals with cocaine dependence often resort to acts of crime or prostitution in order to obtain funds.

Because cocaine, like amphetamine, acts as a stimulant, the signs of cocaine intoxication are similar to the signs of amphetamine intoxication. The symptoms of cocaine withdrawal have a faster onset and shorter duration than amphetamine withdrawal because of the short half-life of cocaine.

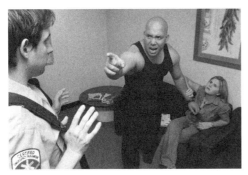

Figure 12-4 Individuals with amphetamine dependence will often exhibit aggressive and violent behavior.

Caffeine-Related Disorders

Caffeine is a stimulant commonly found in coffee, tea, some sodas, anti-drowsiness pills, and chocolate. Although widely used and legal, one can actually overdose on caffeine. Alhough this is rare, a dose exceeding 10 grams (an average coffee contains 100 mg/8 oz) has been shown to cause grand mal seizures and may lead to respiratory failure, cardiac dysrhythmia, or death. Potentially fatal comorbid conditions such as cardiac conditions or anorexia can also lead to life-threatening reactions.

A diagnosis of caffeine intoxication is advised when at least five of the following symptoms appear during or shortly after consuming caffeine: restlessness, nervousness, excitement, insomnia, flushed face, diuresis, gastrointestinal disturbance, muscle twitching, rambling flow of thought and speech, tachycardia or cardiac arrhythmia, periods of inexhaustibility, or psychomotor agitation. Common prehospital scenarios include individuals who are living on caffeine and getting little sleep or college-age students who attempt to stay awake for extended periods of time.

Cannabis-Related Disorders

Cannabis is the most commonly used illicit substance in the United States. Various parts of the cannabis plant can be prepared in several different ways in order to produce the array of substances, including marijuana and hashish. The active ingredient in cannabis related substances are termed cannaboids. The main active ingredient in cannobis is delta-9-tetrahydrocannabinol, or THC. Legally synthesized THC is sometimes used to relieve the adverse symptoms of chemotherapy in cancer patients and anorexia in individuals with acquired immunodeficiency syndrome.

As tolerance develops, cannabis dependence may cause significant distress as an increasing amount of time and resources are used each day for the attainment and consumption of cannabis. A decrease in goal-oriented activities and a chronic cough are also associated with cannabis dependence. Symptoms of cannabis withdrawal, such as tremor and sleep disturbance, have been observed, but, according to the *DSM-IV-TR*, their clinical significance is uncertain.

Cannabis intoxication begins with a euphoric high and may be accompanied by inappropriate laughter. Bloodshot eyes, increased appetite (munchies), and slight tachycardia may occur within 2 hours of cannabis use. THC is fat soluble and consequently may be released in the body unexpectedly while fat deposits are metabolized.

Cannabis smoke is highly irritating to the nasopharynx and bronchial lining and may induce chronic cough and other symptoms of nasopharyngeal pathology such as sinusitis, pharyngitis, and bronchitis with persistent cough. Emphysema and pulmonary dysplasia (change in lung tissue) may occur with chronic heavy use. Cannabis smoke is also known to carry relatively large amounts of known carcinogens.

Generally speaking, prehospital intervention is rare for someone strictly using cannabis. These individuals usually present with non–life-threatening symptoms and do not require medical care unless the drug was tainted by another chemical.

Hallucinogen-Related Disorder

Substances that induce perceptual changes (eg, hallucinations or delusions) in a state of full alertness are dubbed hallucinogens. Examples of hallucinogens are LSD, methamphetamine (ecstasy), mescaline (peyote), and psilocybin (mushrooms). Perceptual changes from hallucinogens may vary from seeing shapes and colors to ideation of superhuman abilities and senses. Most hallucinogens are ingested, although some may be smoked or injected. An individual with hallucinogen dependence is highly prone to injury and trauma because of irrational actions such as driving under the influence or trying to fly while hallucinating. The physiological signs of hallucinogen intoxication include tachycardia, pupillary dilation (possibly with blurring of vision), sweating, tremors, incoordination, and <u>labile mood</u>.

Inhalant-Related Disorders

Inhalants include substances such as gasoline, glue, paint thinner, spray paint, and spray propellants. Inhalants reach the bloodstream and the brain quickly and therefore have a rapid onset

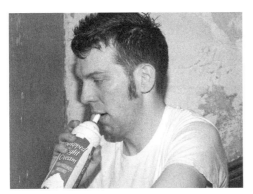

Figure 12-5 Inhalants reach the bloodstream and the brain quickly and therefore have a rapid onset.

(**Figure 12-5**). Although inhalant withdrawal has not been established as clinically significant, inhalant dependence may still be diagnosed in an individual who spends a substantial amount of time using inhalants and is experiencing negative life changes as a consequence.

Because most inhalants act as CNS depressants, the symptoms of inhalant intoxication are similar to those of alcohol intoxication and include dizziness, nystagmus, incoordination, slurred speech, unsteady gait, lethargy, depressed reflexes, psychomotor retardation, tremor, generalized muscle weakness, blurred vision or diplopia (double vision), stupor or coma, or euphoria. Inhalants may also cause hallucinations or delusions and therefore increase the risk of injury.

Because inhalants are legal and relatively easy to obtain, they have an appeal to adolescents, who commonly use them in a group setting. The process of breathing the inhalant is known as *huffing*. Because of their route of absorption, inhalants may pose a threat to the airway of a user. Chronic use of inhalants is known to cause the permanent loss of some mental functions such as hearing, fine motor skills, and equilibrium.

Strong odors coming from the clothes of an individual, along with a possible rash or paint around the nose and mouth, and general breathing difficulty may indicate the use of inhalants. Be aware that inhalants may be present in an industrial work environment and could be absorbed unintentionally. In these situations, always consider your own safety first and consider the use of respiratory protection or even calling for the hazardous materials team. When caring for an individual with inhalant intoxication, first remove the patient from the toxic environment and supply him or her with a high concentration of oxygen.

Nicotine-Related Disorders

Nicotine is legal and is most commonly found in tobacco cigarettes. Nicotine can also be found in chewing tobacco, nicotine gums, and transdermal nicotine patches. Nicotine dependence has a high comorbidity with other mental disorders, particularly schizophrenia; as with alcohol, there may be some attempts at self-medication. The signs and symptoms of nicotine withdrawal are severe, and sustaining full remission is difficult and may require multiple attempts. The smell of smoke, signs of chronic obstructive pulmonary disease, burned or stained fingers, and excessive skin wrinkling are a few easily detectible signs of smoking.

Opioid-Related Disorders

Opioids are a class of substances used for their analgesic, anesthetic, antidiarrheal, and cough-suppressing qualities. Prescription opioids include naturally occurring opioids or opiates (morphine and codeine) and synthetic opioids such as hydromorphone (Dilaudid®), methadone, oxycodone, meperidine (Demerol®), and fentanyl.

The most commonly used illicit opioid is heroin. Heroin is usually injected, but it may also be smoked or snorted. The pattern of opioid usage in individuals with opioid dependence is likely to become the center of daily activities for that individual. According to the *DSM-IV-TR*, drowsiness, slurred speech, and impairment in attention or memory shortly after substance use are the principal signs of opioid intoxication. The physiological signs of opioid intoxication are hypotension, respiratory depression, and pinpoint pupils. Depending on the opioid used, nausea, vomiting, and constipation may occur as well.

Opioid withdrawal can be caused by the cessation of opioid use or by the administration of an opioid antagonist such as naloxone (Narcan®). The *DSM-IV-TR* states that the following signs may be present with opioid withdrawal: dysphoric mood (feeling sad or down), nausea or vomiting, muscle aches, <u>lacrimation</u> (increased tear production), <u>rhinorrhea</u> (runny nose), pupillary dilation, <u>piloerection</u> (hair standing on end), sweating, diarrhea, yawning, fever, or insomnia. Withdrawal symptoms in individuals who use short-acting opioids such as heroin may begin as early as 6 hours after the last use. Among intravenous opioid users, as many as 90% test positive for a hepatitis infection, and as many as 60% in some areas are reported to have HIV.

When an opioid-related disorder is suspected, an opioid antagonist such as naloxone may be administered to verify that the symptoms are indeed caused by an opioid and not another substance, general medical condition, or mental disorder. The administration of 0.4 to 2.0 mg of naloxone is also indicated in cases in which opioid intoxication has caused loss of consciousness and respiratory drive. Naloxone can cause the intoxicated individual to rapidly awaken from a state of substance-induced euphoria, which may lead to violent behavior. It is commonly suggested that naloxone be given in small, slow doses only to the point at which the patient's respiratory status improves but the patient is not completely awakened. However, in some cases of intoxication with synthetic opioids, such as fentanyl, the amount of naloxone required to reverse the effects has been recorded to be as high as 40 mg.

Phencyclidine-Related Disorders

Phencyclidine (PCP) and similarly acting compounds such as ketamine or cyclohexamine were originally developed as dissociative anesthetics. PCP is commonly called "angel dust" or simply "dust." Nystagmus, tachycardia, hypertension, muscle rigidity, incoordination, slurred speech, and heightened sensitivity to sounds may be present in individuals with PCP intoxication. Other less common effects of PCP may range from fever to <u>rhabdomyolysis</u> (the breaking down of skeletal muscle tissue) with renal impairment. Rhabdomyolysis is diagnosed by a laboratory test that identifies myoglobin in the bloodstream.

Dissociation of the mind-body connection allows intoxicated individuals to endure extreme pain and exhibit feats of superhuman strength. Violent outbursts are possible in an individual with PCP or ketamine intoxication. In some cases, individuals will do physical harm to themselves and not feel any pain or distress. Because of this, they will continue to be resistant or combative, further injuring themselves or others. Controlling or restraining patients can be very difficult and dangerous. This task should not be handled without the assistance of law enforcement personnel, who may have to secure the individual with handcuffs. Although no antagonist that reverses the effects of these drugs is available, a benzodiazepine (Valium® or Ativan®) or haloperidol (Haldol®) may be administered for sedation, treatment, and transportation.

Sedative-, Hypnotic-, or Anxiolytic-Related Disorders

CNS depressants include barbiturates, benzodiazepines, and similarly acting substances. Often these substances are used as anti-anxiety, anticonvulsant, and sleep medications. An individual with sedative, hypnotic, or anxiolytic intoxication may present with signs similar to alcohol intoxication, including slurred speech, incoordination, unsteady gait, nystagmus, attention or memory impairment, and stupor or coma. An overdose of medications in this category can be life threatening and may lead to a decrease in mental status and respiratory drive, so the patient's airway should be constantly monitored for patency. In some cases, death can occur. Short-acting benzodiazepines mixed with alcohol create special problems because of their chemical interactions.

Sedative, hypnotic, or anxiolytic withdrawal may be accompanied by hand tremor, insomnia, hallucinations, anxiety, depression, diaphoresis, abdominal cramping, or convulsions. In case of barbiturate withdrawal, treatment should initially revolve around preventing convulsions and cardiovascular collapse. The administration of flumazenil (a benzodiazepine antagonist) via a slow intravenous push (0.2 mg/min) may be considered in cases of benzodiazepine (eg, diazepam) overdose. In case of barbiturate (eg, phenobarbital) overdose, administration of 1–2 mEq of sodium bicarbonate may be considered. The sodium bicarbonate will keep the barbiturate in its ionized form and will promote its excretion in the urine.

Prehospital Management

A good physical examination is imperative in the management of individuals with a substance-related disorder. Individuals may deny some symptoms because of the illicit status of certain substances, and other symptoms may be masked by the use of more than one substance. With some substances, such as amphetamines, the range of symptoms is very wide. In those cases, obtaining a detailed history may be the best method of discovering which substance caused the disorder.

The treatment for any substance-related disorder in the prehospital setting is fairly straightforward and mainly supportive. Using the SAFER-R model will provide you with a guide for these complicated patients.

The emergency responder must ensure that a patent airway exists and that breathing is adequate. Individuals who use depressants such as alcohol, opioids, sedatives, hypnotics, or anxiolytics have an increased risk of respiratory compromise and need to be closely monitored. All patients should be given a high concentration of oxygen, and individuals in severe substance-induced stupor or coma might require an advanced airway in order to prevent aspiration. An exception is made for opioid intoxication, when the administration of an opioid antagonist such as naloxone could restore the patient's consciousness and respiratory drive without the use of an advanced airway.

Vascular access should be obtained in case of hypotension caused by stimulant use or substance-related injury. Certain symptoms of substance-related disorders can be alleviated, counteracted, or prevented by the use of medication available in the prehospital environment. Electrocardiography, pulse oximetry, and capnometry should be applied to all patients showing signs of drug use. Normal saline or lactated Ringer's can be given as a fluid challenge according to local protocol or at a rate of 20 mL/kg, providing the patient is not presenting with pulmonary edema. Transportation to an appropriate facility and conveying the detailed history obtained on the scene to the receiving hospital staff will ensure proper definitive care.

SAFER-R for Field Intervention

Stabilize: Present yourself in a professional manner, knowing that patients with substance-related disorders are often in denial or embarrassed by their condition. Be empathetic and supportive.

Acknowledge: Acknowledge that you are there to help and recognize that patients may feel out of control of the current situation. Advise them that you will do your best to allow them to make appropriate choices regarding their care.

Facilitate: Recognize that substance-related disorders affect not only the patient, but family members as well. Facilitate the transfer of information from the patient and family to medical direction when possible.

Encourage: Constant reassurance is important for the substance-related disorder patient because of poor self-esteem, denial, and overall condition. Recognize that patients are often very self-conscious about their situation and ensure them that you will do your best to protect their privacy.

Recovery: Be sure to discuss and reinforce your plan for getting patients to the hospital and that you are there to take care of their needs and that they are in good hands.

Referral: Suggest to family members that they seek out community resources or search the Internet for local and national information to help their loved one.

Final Thoughts

This chapter has presented to you a variety of different drug-related conditions on an individual basis, including specific clinical symptoms of each substance. The reality of some of our patients is that they may also experience polysubstance abuse, defined as taking more than one chemical at a time. In these particular situations, the patient may present with a confusing mixture of symptoms and may also be in a severe crisis state both medically and psychologically.

As an EMS provider, it is extremely important for you to recognize that patients presenting with signs of depression or psychosis may have a potentially life-threatening medical condition as well. Your ability to be a good detective and to rely on your experience during your assessment will be very valuable tools for you when dealing with patients suffering from substance-related disorders. As always, be safe and be thorough.

Selected References

American Psychiatric Association: *Diagnostic and Statistical Manual of Mental Disorders, Fourth Edition, Text Revision (DSM-IV-TR)*. Washington, DC, American Psychiatric Association, 2000.

BehaveNet.com. Available at: http://www.behavenet.com/. Accessed April 1, 2007.

National Institute on Drug Abuse. Drugs of abuse information. Available at: http://www.drugabuse.gov/drugpages.html. Accessed July 20, 2008.

Pollack AH, Elling B, Smith M (eds): *Nancy Caroline's Emergency Care in the Streets*, ed 6. Sudbury, MA, Jones & Bartlett Publishers, 2008.

Prep Kit

Ready for Review

- Substance-related disorders can be very complex. However, by understanding the four key concepts of substance dependence, substance abuse, substance intoxication, and substance withdrawal, you can perform a thorough evaluation and devise an appropriate treatment plan.

- Substance abuse and dependence have similar definitions. To abuse a chemical, one needs to use the substance despite the impairment or distress caused during or shortly after the use of the drug. Dependence moves toward a more chronic condition and implies that the individual uses the substance despite actual physiologic changes and negative life events.

- Intoxication is a condition commonly seen in the prehospital environment. Technically speaking, intoxication means that one is under the influence of a drug. In most cases, this state is recognizable because patients show signs of physiologic change in the central nervous, cardiovascular, or respiratory system.

- Reducing or discontinuing a drug can result in substance withdrawal. The majority of people only experience unpleasant symptoms when withdrawing from a drug. These symptoms include nausea, vomiting, headache, muscle tremors, and cravings. However, in the case of alcohol and barbiturates, patients can experience severe CNS symptoms that can result in seizures or death.

- Many patients seen in the prehospital arena have very confusing presentations. Do not become a caregiver who puts on blinders when assisting an individual who appears to be intoxicated. Often, illnesses such as diabetes, hypoxia, stroke, or depression can mimic a substance-related disorder.

Vital Vocabulary

abuse Abuse occurs when an individual continues the use of a substance despite significant impairment or distress caused during or shortly after the use of the substance.

anhedonia The inability to experience pleasure.

anxiolytic Classification of a group of medications given to reduce anxiety.

bradycardia Slow heart rate.

craving A strong drive to use a substance, often seen as a common sign of substance dependence.

dependence When an individual continues to use a substance despite adverse physiological changes and negative life events.

diplopia Double vision.

hallucination False perceptions that relate to any of the five senses.

hypnotic A class of drug that induces sleep.

illusion A false interpretation of an external sensory stimulus, commonly auditory or visual in nature.

intoxication Being under the influence of a drug, possibly causing a loss of senses.

labile mood Unstable, unsteady, not fixed; denotes free and uncontrolled moods or behaviors expressing emotions.

lacrimation Increased tear production.

nystagmus Rapidly oscillating eye movement.

piloerection When one's hair stands on end; commonly called goose bumps.

polysubstance abuse Abuse of more than one substance.

psychomotor agitation Excessive motor activity, such as pacing or wringing of the hands; often seen as unintentional and purposeless and commonly caused by inner tension.

psychomotor retardation An abnormal slowing of movement, physical reaction, or speech that is directly related to brain activity.

rhabdomyolysis A condition in which skeletal muscle cells break down, releasing myoglobin, which carries oxygen in the muscle, along with enzymes and electrolytes from inside the muscle cells. Two major risks with this condition are the continuing breakdown of the muscle, and, because myoglobin is toxic to the kidneys, renal failure.

rhinorrhea Nasal discharge; a runny nose.

septal erosion Wearing away of the wall of the nasal septum, commonly seen as the result of repeated inhalation of drugs such as cocaine or inhalants.

sympathomimetic Substances that mimic epinephrine (adrenalin) or norepinephrine.

tachycardia Fast heart rate.

tolerance When a higher amount of substance is required in order to produce the effect previously induced by a lower dose of substance.

toxidrome A group of clinical signs that suggest a specific type of overdose or poisoning.

vein sclerosis A scarring, hardening, or thickening of the venous tissue secondary to repeated needle injections; commonly seen in intravenous drug users.

withdrawal A series of symptoms experienced by the individual when the substance is no longer taken.

Assessment in Action

Answer key is located in the back of the book.

1. You arrive on the scene of a patient who reportedly has been drinking alcohol for much of the evening. He is cooperative but appears confused and has difficulty walking. Additionally, when you evaluate his eyes, they uncontrollably move back and forth. This classic sign of alcohol intoxication is called:

   A. lacrimation.
   B. piloerection.
   C. normal eye movement.
   D. nystagmus.

2. You are dispatched to a local club where you find a 20-year-old college student sitting in the corner of the dance floor where he collapsed. He is now awake but confused. Several of his friends are there but also appear under the influence of some substance so they are not very helpful. They are pouring water over him, saying that he is very hot and needs to cool down. One patron tells you that he was seen earlier sucking on a baby pacifier and seemed to be dancing by himself. You suspect which of the following?

   A. Stimulant use, such as methamphetamine
   B. Hallucinogen use, such as ecstasy
   C. Opioid use, such as heroin
   D. Sedative use, such as sleeping pills

3. From the following choices, select the statement that is FALSE.

   A. Crack cocaine is smoked and has a quick onset but also has a quick half-life, requiring users to smoke it more often for the effect.
   B. A person who uses more than one drug to obtain a high is known as a polysubstance abuser.
   C. A person who continues to use a substance despite adverse physiological changes and negative life events has a dependence problem.
   D. Because caffeine is a legal chemical commonly found in coffee, tea, and chocolate, one does not have to worry about it having physiological effects on the patient.

4. You are called to a local halfway house for recovering addicts. Upon arrival, you are led to a patient who is having a grand mal seizure. Which of the following conditions BEST describes the seizure activity?

   A. Substance withdrawal
   B. Substance abuse
   C. Substance dependence
   D. Substance intoxication

5. From the following choices, select the statement that is TRUE.

   A. Drugs taken by intravenous or intranasal routes will have a higher chance of creating dependency.
   B. Drugs with a slow onset tend to create dependency and addiction quickly.
   C. Weight loss or diet pills are commonly classified as anxiolytics.
   D. Alcohol is considered a stimulant because it is known for making you feel good when you drink it.

Chapter 13

Psychosis and Schizophrenia

Background

The psychiatrist Thomas S. Szasz said, "If you talk to God, you are praying; if God talks to you, you have schizophrenia." It is common for the prehospital provider to care for a person who appears to be detached from their environment. When you arrive on the scene, a patient may be talking to himself in a language that does not exist or she may be witnessing an event that is not actually happening. He or she might even report hearing voices inside of his or her head. These behaviors may lead a provider to suspect that the person may be suffering from hypoglycemia, substance abuse, or a serious head injury.

Another possibility is that the patient is experiencing delusions and hallucinations associated with a type of psychosis or schizophrenia. <u>Delusions</u> are false beliefs that significantly hinder a person's ability to function. An example of a delusion would be a server at a fast-food restaurant believing that he is the CEO of the company for which he works. <u>Hallucinations</u> are false perceptions that relate to any of the five senses, such as seeing or talking to significant individuals from history. It is common for patients to claim that they have special powers that allow them to see and talk with spiritual leaders, past presidents, or people who have been dead for many years.

Individuals experiencing delusions and hallucinations are said to be experiencing <u>psychosis</u> or to be psychotic. Psychosis is a persistent, often chronic mental disorder that involves disturbances in content of thought, form of thought, perception, <u>affect</u>, sense of self, motivation, behavior, and interpersonal functioning. Thinking may be disconnected and illogical and may include delusions or hallucinations. Peculiar or disorganized behaviors may be associated with social withdrawal and disinterest. In general, the person appears out of touch with reality. The severity of the psychosis determines how much of a person's life the delusions and hallucinations may control.

The *DSM-IV-TR* identifies eight distinct schizophrenic and psychotic disorders.

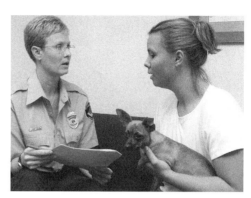

Figure 13-1 General questioning provides you with an opportunity to begin the trust-building process.

- Schizophrenia
- Schizophreniform disorder
- Schizoaffective disorder
- Delusional disorder
- Brief psychotic disorder
- Shared psychotic disorder
- Psychotic disorder due to a general medical condition
- Substance-induced psychotic disorder

Despite these distinctions, schizophrenia and psychosis are imperfect categories, and patients may not fit neatly into any one description.

Assessment

The assessment of the patient with a psychotic disorder can be difficult and challenging. Those with psychotic disorders often are out of touch with reality, and many are delusional or experiencing hallucinations, leading them to believe that they are not safe. As is the case with any patient, the safety of the EMS provider should be considered above all else. When treating a patient with any form of psychosis, proper composure and distance are necessary until the scene is deemed secure.

Previous experience with a specific individual can help you to establish rapport and expedite the assessment and transport component of the call for that person (**Figure 13-1**). This is of particular importance with individuals experiencing <u>paranoia</u> who have previous experience with EMS providers with whom trust has already been established. Reminding familiar patients of how things have been done on past occasions will provide structure for both evaluating and treating the patient.a

Using the standard SAMPLE and OPQRST format for questioning will help the emergency responder to gather pertinent psychological and medical history on the patient. General questioning also provides you with an opportunity to begin the trust-building process.

SAMPLE History

Signs and symptoms: Symptomatology will vary depending on the disorder, and can range from **catatonia** to hyperactivity. Patients may complain that aliens or the government is spying on them. In some cases, feelings of special religious connections may be present.

Allergies: Allergies are common in some patients as they attempt new medications.

Medications: Various antipsychotic medications, called neuroleptics, are common; however, patients tend to be non-compliant because of disturbing side effects. Common side effects include drowsiness, dizziness, weight gain, decrease in sexual interest, and complications with menstrual periods.

Past medical history: Medical conditions are usually not directly connected to any of the psychotic disorders except for a psychotic disorder due to a general medical condition. The EMS provider should gather a thorough medical history to document the patient's disorder. Remember that many of the symptoms will mimic other CNS disorders, such as tumors or temporal lobe epilepsy.

Last oral intake: It is common for patients experiencing psychotic episodes to skip meals, resulting in dehydration and malnourishment.

Events leading up to today's event: In many cases, it is not the patient who calls for EMS but a neighbor or bystander who reports an individual who is acting strangely.

OPQRST

Onset: When did the symptoms begin? Does the patient have a history of schizophrenia or other psychotic disorder? Is this something new that would lead you to suspect a medical condition?

Provocation: What happened today to trigger EMS or the police being called? Patients with severe active schizophrenia may be standing out in the yard wearing aluminum foil, screaming that the aliens are coming. However, many other patients may be quiet or muted and withdrawn in their apartments.

Quality: How severe is the presentation? Is it to a point that the psychological syndrome is causing physical symptoms or distress? Has the condition impeded the daily function of the individual?

Radiation: Does the patient's behavior affect family, friends, colleagues, or neighbors?

Severity: On a scale of 0 to 10, how severe is the distress today for the patient? For the first-time patient, this may be a difficult question to answer. For patients with a history of psychotic events, you can question them about how this day compares to previous episodes.

Time: How long has the current condition been occurring? Has the condition worsened over time? It may be necessary to obtain this type of information from others because the patient may be unable to answer these questions appropriately.

The SEA-3 mental status exam will complete the information-gathering process. It can help determine the type of psychosis the person is experiencing by focusing strictly on the components important to the psychological aspect of these complicated patients.

Psychosis and Schizophrenia
Schizophrenia

Schizophrenia is a disorder that involves disturbances in content and form of thought, perception, affect, sense of self, motivation, behavior, and interpersonal functioning. It is one of the most commonly discussed mental disorders and often seen on television. Approximately one person in 100 develops schizophrenia. Schizophrenia presents equally as often in males and females; however, males tend to experience their first episode in their late teens or early 20s while women usually report their first episodes in the late 20s and early 30s. The onset in most cases is gradual, so many individuals and their families may not be aware of the illness for several months or years.

The symptoms present in these individuals will often hamper the individual's functional and personal life. Symptoms are classified as positive and negative. Positive symptoms encompass delusions, hallucinations, and disorganized speech and behaviors. Negative symptoms include affective flattening, alogia, avolition, and anhedonia. Affective flattening means decreased emotions, facial expression, and responsiveness to the surrounding environment. Alogia is speechlessness. Avolition is the unwillingness to respond or act, and anhedonia is the inability to experience pleasure. In some cases, the severity of symptoms is so dramatic that the EMS provider will need to depend upon family and friends to determine the history. The cause of schizophrenia is unknown, but seems to be a combination of genetic and environmental factors during prenatal and childhood development. Imbalance of the neurotransmitters dopamine and serotonin is present in schizophrenia.

The onset symptomatology often differs greatly between the sexes. Men will present with more negative symptoms, such as a flat affect or social withdrawal, while women will present with more positive symptoms, such as paranoid delusions and hallucinations.

A schizophrenic patient does not develop the debilitating symptoms of schizophrenia in a single day. Instead, signs and symptoms come and go through phases. There are three phases of schizophrenia: prodromal, active, and residual. The prodromal phase is the initial phase in which the individual begins to withdraw from society. Interpersonal and workplace relationships begin to deteriorate. A marked decline in productivity is evident in this stage. The individual experiences thought and perception disturbances, such as visual hallucinations, hearing voices (often it will be two

In the Field

A *positive symptom* is the addition of something that the patient does not normally have, such as delusions or hallucinations. A *negative symptom* is the subtraction of a normal function, such as the ability to experience pleasure.

SEA-3 Mental Status Exam

Speech: A disorganized speech pattern is common in cases involving psychosis. Sentences may lack structure and flow or be filled with words that are completely unrecognizable. Catatonic patients may not speak at all or have **echolalia**, a senseless repetition of words or phrases. Paranoid patients may limit speech because emergency personnel may be seen as part of a conspiracy. Speech may also appear normal, with rational content, distinguishable words, and appropriate flow. With delusional patients, the speech pattern may be clear, but what is being said may not make sense given the circumstances.

Emotion: The emotional pattern of a person with psychosis is the most distinguishable and dynamic aspect of these illnesses. Emotions can range from completely flat to very active. The emotions of someone experiencing substance-induced or brief psychotic disorder can change drastically over a short period of time. The emotional status of a person with delusional disorder can vary with the type of delusion.

Appearance: Many schizophrenic and psychotic patients have been pushed out of society because of their illness and difficulties with social and professional relationships, resulting in homelessness. Patients may appear disheveled and unkempt and may not have bathed or had anything substantial to eat in days or weeks. Patients may be dressed in clothing inappropriate for the season or with strange things attached to what they are wearing. This may be due to the illness or to protect items from being stolen by others. In another instance, the house where a delusional patient lives could be filled with countless pictures of a particular celebrity or the windows may be covered with aluminum foil to stop the spies from looking into the residence. Because these are unusual findings, be sure to document what you see at the scene.

Alertness: The level of alertness varies. Some patients are alert and oriented, while others are completely out of touch with reality. It is important to remember that, with few exceptions, patients suffering from psychosis are not normally sedate because of the mental condition. Lack of alertness may be the sign of a medication interaction, accidental overdose, or attempted suicide.

Activity: Activity level will also vary. Patients in catatonia will be stoic and nearly stone-like, while active paranoid schizophrenics may feel intimidated or threatened by emergency workers' presence and become defensive. In some situations, patients may need to be either physically or chemically restrained for transportation to the emergency department.

voices talking about the person), and incoherent muttering. The prodromal phase always precedes the active phase.

In the **active phase**, the person experiences a variety of symptoms that persist until the phase is over. This is by far the worst stage of schizophrenia, because the person is completely detached from reality and the surrounding environment. Members of society withdraw themselves from the person because of abnormal or unnatural behaviors, which increases the person's isolation. The individual believes and lives in a confabulated or made-up world, and often experiences increased mental pain and suffering.

The **residual phase** marks the end of the active phase. Individuals may be listless, have trouble concentrating, and be withdrawn. Many of the symptoms present in the prodromal phase are also present in the residual phase. The person experiences schizophrenia in a transient manner as symptoms come and go.

A strong understanding of these phases will enhance the emergency responder's ability to recognize the most appropriate ways to interact with schizophrenic patients.

Types of Schizophrenia

The *DSM-IV-TR* classifies schizophrenia into five different subtypes, each of which has specific criteria for a diagnosis. Catatonic and paranoid types are more easily diagnosed, while the prognosis of disorganized, undifferentiated, and residual types is not clearly understood.

Catatonic Type Schizophrenia

Individuals who manifest peculiar and bizarre psychomotor disturbances fall into the <u>catatonic type</u>. The *DSM-IV-TR* defines catatonic type schizophrenia as one that is "marked by marked psychomotor disturbances that may involve motor immobility, excessive motor activity, extreme negativism, mutism, peculiarities of voluntary movement, echolalia, or <u>echopraxia</u>." Echolalia is an involuntary parrot-like repetition of a word or phrase that has just been spoken by another individual. Echopraxia is the repetitive imitation of movements of others.

Patients are often hyperactively mobile and move around in a purposeless manner, pacing, walking in circles, making loud noises, or throwing their arms into the air. These activities tend to have no motivating cause. Another name for this activity is *catatonic excitement*. The emergency responder must watch and monitor hyperactive catatonic patients because they may be a danger to themselves, others, and the provider. You should make every effort to talk with the person and get him or her to cooperate with you. However, in some incidents, the patient may have to be restrained or handcuffed by police if transport is required.

Conversely, some catatonic schizophrenics may not possess any hyperactive symptoms at all. Instead they may appear rigid and immobile, as though they were statues. Even when trying to fix their posture, they will fall back into pose, and all effort to maintain or correct the situation is futile. Catatonic individuals tend to shut themselves off from the outside world and keep to themselves.

Disorganized Type Schizophrenia

<u>Disorganized type</u> is considered to be the most severe and debilitating form of schizophrenia. The components for the disorganized type include disorganized speech, thought, and actions, along with extremely bizarre behavior. Patients demonstrate the loss of emotional expression and present with an inappropriate, blank, or flat affect. Individuals have no problems talking, but their speech is odd and bizarre, as are their actions. In the long-term, unusual actions may affect the individual's ability to provide self-care. Hallucinations and delusions may also be present.

Paranoid Type Schizophrenia

<u>Paranoid type</u> schizophrenia is classified by the presence of delusions and hallucinations in the form of visions or voices, often aimed against a government figure or agency. Individuals suffering from paranoid type schizophrenia do not have any disorganized speech or behavior. Their delusions and hallucinations mainly affect their lives as they become increasingly suspicious of friends and family and become untrusting and isolated. They often complain of being followed, watched, or spied on by aliens or government officials.

Paranoid patients hear either a single voice commenting on their lives or two voices talking about the individual. Aggression and combativeness are rare unless the patient feels trapped. The interviewer needs to demonstrate patience and diplomacy in dealing with such patients to assure them that they are safe. Provide constant reassurance that you are there to help them and, when possible, allow the patient to make choices. For example, allowing patients to walk to an ambulance or police car for transport provides them with an opportunity for control while still accomplishing the mission of getting them to a hospital for evaluation (**Figure 13-2**).

Undifferentiated Type Schizophrenia

Individuals who show complex signs and symptoms of schizophrenia but do not meet the criteria for the aforementioned types are diagnosed as having <u>undifferentiated type</u> schizophrenia. They may show delusional symptoms at times and disorganized symptoms at other times, often talking to themselves in an incomprehensible language. These individuals need to be treated and handled according to the state of mind demonstrated at the time of assessment.

Residual Type Schizophrenia

Residual type schizophrenia is a diagnosis used to refer to patients who have recovered from prominent symptoms such as delusions, hallucinations, or disorganized behavior but still show some mild evidence of the continuing disease process, such as a flat affect or poverty of speech. Patients may act and function normally in life when they are free of symptoms, but relapses are possible and delusions and hallucinations may return.

Schizophreniform and Schizoaffective Disorders

Schizophreniform and schizoaffective disorders are related to schizophrenia. In the case of schizophreniform disorder, the individual shows the same psychotic symptoms attributed to schizophrenia but lacks the required duration. Symptoms typically last between 1 to 6 months and may not cause social and occupational deterioration or dysfunction. For instance, a person who tried to raise money for a charity may inaccurately believe that he or she has earned a lot of money to donate. He or she writes a check for $10 million. When the charity supervi-

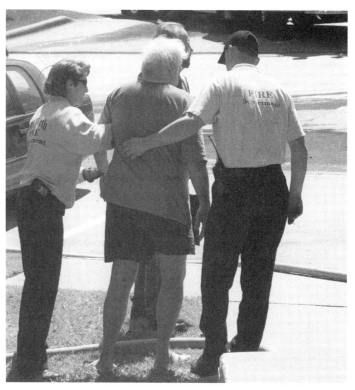

Figure 13-2 Allowing patients to walk to an ambulance or police car for transport provides them with an opportunity for control.

sor questions the check, the person believes the charity is conspiring to prevent him or her from doing what is right. While this example is not a life-threatening emergency, you may be called to evaluate this individual by a neighbor who is concerned for his or her welfare. These types of wellness checks are common for prehospital providers and should be conducted in the presence of law enforcement personnel. Depending on the assessment, you may be instrumental in providing safe and efficient transport to the emergency department for further evaluation.

What is termed schizoaffective disorder is actually a combination of two disorders: the active phase of schizophrenia and severe mood disorder, which must be either preceded or followed by at least 2 weeks of delusions or hallucinations (without prominent mood symptoms). The mood disorder can be a major depressive episode, a manic episode, or a mixed episode. Unlike most mental disorders, schizoaffective disorder can last for many months or even years.

Delusional Disorders

An individual with a delusional disorder has a firm belief based on something that is not true. The patient may try to convince emergency care personnel that his or her delusion is real. While it is human nature to agree with individuals experiencing delusions out of kindness, this is not the correct thing to do. It is best to say that you appreciate what the patient is telling you, but that you are not aware of the subject of his or her delusion. For example, if an individual tells you that his or her neighbor has planted listening devices in the patient's apartment and is spying on the patient, do not agree with the patient. Ask the patient to show you why he or she believes this and tell the patient that you will record it in your report. Surprisingly, if you agree with some patients, they will quickly point out to you that they know they have psychosis and that you are lying to them; at this point, you have lost your credibility.

There are five different types of delusional disorders that all share the same psychotic symptom: an organized system of non-bizarre false beliefs.

Erotomanic type is a delusion that a celebrity or other famous person is madly in love with the individual experiencing the delusion. An example would be a male patient who believes that a particular rock star is madly in love with him. Whenever he watches her video on television and she sings a particular song, he believes the star is singing that song just for him. These individuals commonly make the news as the result of stalking and harassment.

Grandiose type is diagnosed when a person believes that he or she is of extreme importance. Often the individual believes that he or she is more powerful or more talented than other people. In some cases these delusions can be of a religious nature. For example, the individual might believe that he or she has a special relationship with a powerful spiritual leader such as the Pope or Dalai Lama.

Jealous type occurs when the delusional person believes his or her sexual or romantic partner is being unfaithful even though there is no evidence to support the claim. The weekly washing of bed linens might be misinterpreted by the delusional person as an attempt to hide the spouse's infidelity. The jealous-type patient may go as far as planting evidence to prove his or her theory.

A person suffering from *persecutory type* delusions believes he or she is always being harassed or oppressed. Often patients feel that they are being cheated, conspired against, or obstructed in their attempt to reach long-term goals. Unfortunately, as the delusion continues, these individuals spend tremendous time and money pursuing their battles in courts and through various governmental agencies.

Somatic type delusions are diagnosed when a person believes that something is wrong with his or her health or some body function. Individuals suffering from this delusion may believe that some bodily process is not working and believe their bodies are emitting a foul smell. The patient might also believe that he or she has an organ that is not working properly or that she has been diagnosed with a terrible disease, such as AIDS, and is dying. It is important to note that this is not the same as hypochondria, which is a chronic concern about one's health that is usually associated with anxiety or depression.

Brief Psychotic Disorder

Brief psychotic disorder occurs after a person has experienced an extremely traumatic or stressful event. Psychotic symptoms such as hallucinations, delusions, or disorganized speech and behavior appear, but last for a short period of time. A person who experiences a brief psychotic disorder shows symptoms for less than one month and does not meet the criteria for schizophrenia. Symptoms of brief psychotic disorder tend to have a rapid onset, but eventually subside as the patient is further removed from the stressor or event.

Typical events that can trigger this disorder include divorce, death of a loved one, or a sudden change in environment, such as a student leaving home for college for the first time. These cases are highly unusual; however, you should manage the patient as you would any other psychotic event. Respectful and compassionate care and a thorough history and physical evaluation will provide you with the information needed to determine your treatment plan based on your local protocols.

Shared Psychotic Disorder

There are times when psychotic symptoms appear to become contagious and start affecting other people. In shared psychotic disorder, one person presents with active delusions. When that person has a close relationship with another person, the delusions carry over and the once-sane individual begins to share the same delusions. The French term *folie a deux,* meaning a folly of two, is used to describe two people sharing the same delusion.

It is difficult for people with shared psychotic disorder to receive help, because each individual supports and confirms the other's delusions. When the relationship ends, it is common for the person who was once nonpsychotic to return to normal functioning.

Shared psychotic disorder can also affect groups of people in the form of radical cults. In this case, the leader shares his delusion with his followers, who quickly become swept into believing whatever the leader preaches. An example of a large shared psychotic disorder includes the Branch Davidian cult, led by David Koresh, in 1993. Over 75 adults and children died in a standoff with the federal government. Those who survived the siege have been able to return to society after being separated from their leader.

Psychotic Disorder Due to a General Medical Condition

Psychotic disorder due to a general medical condition also presents with hallucinations and delusions; however, the psychotic symptoms are directly linked physiological effects of some medical condition and not better described by another mental disorder.

In addition to the presence of substantial behavioral symptomatology, the patient's history, physical examination results, and laboratory findings are taken into consideration in making this diagnosis. Causes of this form of psychotic disorder include temporal lobe epilepsy, brain tumors, cerebrovascular disease, multiple sclerosis, migraine headaches, electrolyte imbalance, and a variety of endocrine conditions. As an emergency responder, you would treat the patient based upon the symptoms presented until the actual cause has been diagnosed.

Substance-Induced Psychotic Disorder

Prehosptial providers respond to various emergencies related to drug use and abuse. Substance-induced psychosis is the development of psychotic symptoms such as prominent hallucinations or delusions that are the direct physiological effects of drug abuse, prescribed medication, or toxic exposure. Substance induced psychotic disorder occurs when a user begins to show psychotic signs and symptoms within a month of intoxication or withdrawal from the drug. In order for a person to be diagnosed with this disorder, the person must present with two or more active-phase criteria, which include delusions, hallucinations, disorganized speech, extremely disorganized or catatonic behavior, or negative signs and symptoms.

The patient may only show one of these characteristics and still be diagnosed with substance-induced psychotic disorder if the delusions are bizarre, the hallucinations consist of a voice that is always commenting on the patient's behavior, or the patient hears two or more voices conversing with each other.

The emergency responder must take an accurate and thorough history from the patient or friends and family members. If the patient started acting abnormally before taking the drugs or has

SAFER-R Field Intervention

Stabilize: Create a calm environment by presenting yourself with a professional demeanor. Offer words of support that will make the patient and family feel safe. If the patient is agitated or distrustful, maintain a sufficient distance to ensure your safety.

Acknowledge: Assess and recognize the current situation by gathering information. Make an effort to explain to the patient why you are there. Acknowledge triggers that may cause agitation or anger.

Facilitate: Understand the situation by determining if cognitive processes are intact or disturbed. Begin thinking about what type of help the patient and family need. Be honest with the patient at all times. Lying about seeing or hearing what the patient does will only cause more distrust.

Encourage: Continue to build rapport with the patient and family by attempting to reorient the patient and move him or her toward transportation and definitive care. Explain the consequences should the patient decide not to go to the hospital with you.

Recovery: Reinforce treatment and transportation plans with the patient. If you have seen this patient before, use that knowledge to your benefit. Talk with the patient about the differences you observe in his or her behavior.

Referral: Assist the family by suggesting community contacts such as local mental health agencies sponsored by city, county, or state social services. If the police decide not to write an emergency petition, suggest that the family might contact the court system for assistance.

been acting strange for more than a month, it is possible that another form of psychosis may be present such as schizoaffective disorder, mood disorder, bipolar or major depressive disorder, or schizophrenia.

Prehospital Management

The prehospital management of psychotic patients can be confusing. Generally speaking, patients sick enough to require a call to the local EMS provider probably should be transported to a hospital for psychiatric evaluation. Because many schizophrenic patients are excluded from society as a result of their illness, it is possible that they have not had the opportunity to be seen by a psychologist or psychiatrist for treatment for many months or years, if ever.

State laws protect individuals from being taken from their homes against their will unless a licensed mental health professional, police officer, or court representative orders the transport. EMS alone cannot take a patient for evaluation if the patient states that he or she does not wish to go, even if you feel that the person is extremely sick or at risk of dying.

A detailed assessment can result in the writing of an emergency petition (EP) or emergency protective order by one of the above individuals. In most states, this requires that the person (1) is demonstrating the symptoms of a mental disorder and (2) appears to be of danger to himself, herself, or others. Once the EP is written, EMS may transport the patient against the patient's will.

As stated earlier, the safety of the emergency responders takes first priority. While sizing up the scene, emergency personnel must determine if additional resources will be needed to effectively and safely treat the psychotic patient. When making the initial contact with the psychotic patient, it is important to maintain a calm environment. The SAFER-R model is an effective tool for preparing to manage your patient.

Extra effort to convince the patient that he or she needs to be transported to the hospital for evaluation may be needed. If time permits, work at the patient's pace when transitioning to the ambulance. An ambulance can be a foreign and threatening environment to psychotic patients. It is important to take great care in introducing the patient to that environment and, whenever possible, to transport the patient without lights and sirens. Patients with paranoid schizophrenia or persecutory delusions may believe that the ambulance will kidnap them and transport them to a dangerous place. Stress that the ambulance is safe and the personnel in the back of it are there to help, not hurt, the patient. If necessary, additional resources such as police or the fire department can aid in the safe transportation of the psychotic patient.

In some unfortunate situations, physical restraints are necessary to transport the patient to the emergency department. This can be both physically and psychologically traumatizing to the patient, family members, and EMS providers. There should be a plan addressing this possibility. Commercial devices are made for the purpose of providing safe and secure restraint of the potentially violent patient.

Pharmacological Considerations

An alternative to physical restraints is chemical restraint. Many EMS providers have now implemented a chemical restraint protocol, generally using an antipsychotic medication such as haloperidol (Haldol®). Prehospital providers should follow local protocols in the administration of this medication.

Long-term treatment for schizophrenia and psychosis includes antipsychotic medications, psychotherapy sessions, or a combination of both. If the cause of the disorder is genetic or biological in nature, patients are prescribed antipsychotic or neuroleptic medications. If the cause is attributed to the environment, then a psycho-behavioral approach is adopted. When the origin is unknown, a combination therapy is used.

Commonly prescribed neuroleptic medications include risperidone (Risperdal®), olanzapine (Zyprexa®), quetiapine (Seroquel®), and ziprasidone (Geodon®). In some cases, patients may be on a combination of these medications.

It is important to note that many patients tend to go on and off of these medications for various reasons. First, these medications are very expensive and many patients are unable to hold a job that provides good insurance. Second, once patients start feeling better, they stop taking the medication and lapse back into an active form of the disorder. Also, many antipsychotic drugs have prominent and unpleasant side effects, including repetitive, involuntary, purposeless movements of the lips, face, legs, or torso; sexual dysfunction; tachycardia; significant weight gain; liver toxicity; and hypotension.

Final Thoughts

Individuals suffering from psychosis and schizophrenia are very complex patients with severe mental illness. Physical and psychological symptoms vary greatly from patient to patient, which makes the job of the prehospital provider extremely difficult. The SAMPLE and OPQRST histories combined with the SEA-3 mental status exam will provide you with a good picture of your patient.

Safe and careful intervention can result in effective treatment and will deliver very sick patients to the help they need. From the moment you arrive on the scene until the patient is transferred over to hospital staff, the emergency responders must be aware of safety for both the patient and their team.

Selected References

AllPsych Online. Available at: http://allpsych.com. Accessed July 20, 2008.

American Psychiatric Association. *Diagnostic and Statistical Manual of Mental Disorders, Fourth Edition, Text Revision (DSM-IV-TR)*. Washington, DC, American Psychiatric Association, 2000.

Bledsoe BE, Clayden DE: *Brady's Prehospital Emergency Pharmacology*, ed 6. Upper Saddle River, NJ, Pearson Education, 2005.

Centre for Addiction and Mental Health: About mental health and addictions. Available at: http://www.camh.net/About_Addiction_Mental_Health/index.html. Accessed July 20, 2008.

Frances A, First MB, Pincus HA: *DSM-IV Guidebook*. Washington, DC, American Psychiatric Press, 1995.

Getzfeld AR: *Essentials of Abnormal Psychology*. Hoboken, NJ, John Wiley & Sons, 2006.

Halgin RP, Whitbourne SK: *Abnormal Psychology: Clinical Perspectives on Psychological Disorders,* ed 4 updated. New York, NY, McGraw Hill, 2005.

Mosby's Medical, Nursing, and Allied Health Dictionary, ed 4. St Louis, MO, Elsevier, 1994.

PsychNet-UK. Disorder information sheet. Available at: http://www.psychnet-uk.com/dsm_iv. Accessed July 20, 2008.

Prep Kit

Ready for Review

- Patients with psychosis and schizophrenia often present as odd, peculiar, and even frightening in some cases. Emergency responders must realize that the disease process is something beyond patients' control and patients need compassionate and competent care.

- Delusions, hallucinations, and disorganized thought are the prominent symptoms that patients present. It is important that you acknowledge what is told to you; however, do not lie to the patient by agreeing with what you know to be false.

- The addition of something that the patient does not normally have, such as delusions or hallucinations, is known as a positive symptom. A negative symptom is the subtraction of a normal function, such as the inability to experience pleasure.

- The patient may experience three phases of schizophrenia: prodromal, active, and residual. The prodromal phase is the initial phase in which symptoms begin and the patient starts to experience deterioration of lifestyle because of the onset of delusions or hallucinations. The active phase is the worst phase, because the individual becomes isolated as a result of the severity of the symptoms. The residual phase occurs at the end of the active phase, when symptoms are now controlled and may only be mildly present.

- Schizophrenia is divided into five subtypes: catatonic, paranoid, disorganized, undifferentiated, and residual.

- Catatonic type schizophrenia presents with peculiar psychomotor disturbances ranging from hyperactive behavior to motor retardation and muscular stiffness.

- Disorganized type schizophrenia is the most severe and debilitating form of the disease, in that individuals develop extremely bizarre behaviors, including disorganized speech, thought, and actions.

- Paranoid type schizophrenia is classified by the presence of delusions and hallucinations either through voice or vision.

- Undifferentiated and residual type schizophrenias present with general symptoms but do not meet the special criteria set forth by the *DSM-IV-TR* for a diagnosis of catatonic, disorganized, or paranoid types. These two types are recognized for patients with mild symptoms or those who have not met the time requirements of the disease for an official diagnosis.

- There are five types of delusional disorders: erotomanic, grandiose, jealous, persecutory, and somatic. These disorders present with a patient's false beliefs about himself or herself and others, such as extreme beauty or greatness or that others are pursuing, in love with, or harassing the patient.

- Medical conditions such as diabetes, cardiovascular blockages, or tumors can sometimes mimic psychosis or schizophrenia. Be sure to complete a thorough history and physical on all patients who present with the signs of altered mentation that have been presented in this chapter.

- Psychotic events can occur without an actual diagnosis of schizophrenia. The exposure to severe stress, life change, pregnancy, death, and substances can cause the brain to react and develop psychotic-like symptoms.

- Neuroleptic or antipsychotic drugs have prominent and unpleasant side effects that can cause patients to stop taking the medication. Side effects include repetitive, involuntary, purposeless movements often of the lips, face, legs, or torso; sexual dysfunction; tachycardia; and hypotension, to mention a few.

Vital Vocabulary

active phase The second phase of schizophrenia. During this phase, the person is completely detached from reality and the surrounding environment, often resulting in isolation. The individual believes and lives in a confabulated or made-up world and commonly experiences increased mental pain and suffering.

affect The observable emotion or feeling, tone, and mood attached to a thought; one's emotional presentation to the evaluator.

affective flattening Exhibiting decreased emotions, facial expression, and responsiveness to one's surrounding environment.

alogia The inability to speak because of a medical or psychological reason.

anhedonia The inability to experience pleasure.

avolition An unwillingness to respond or act.

brief psychotic disorder A condition lasting less than one month in which an individual presents with a sudden onset of the symptoms of psychosis such as delusions, hallucinations, or gross disorganization as the result of a stressful or traumatic event.

catatonia A state of psychologically induced immobility with muscular rigidity; can be interrupted with agitation.

catatonic type schizophrenia A type of schizophrenia with marked psychomotor disturbances that may involve motor immobility, excessive motor activity, extreme negativism, mutism, peculiarities of voluntary movement, echolalia, or echopraxia.

delusion False beliefs that significantly hinder a person's ability to function.

delusional disorder A condition in which the individual has a firm belief based on something that is not true. Delusional disorders are classified according to the prominent delusional theme as erotomanic, grandiose, jealous, persecutory, or somatic.

disorganized type schizophrenia Considered to be the most severe and debilitating form of schizophrenia, with a presentation that includes disorganized speech, thought, and actions, along with extremely bizarre behavior.

echolalia An involuntary parrot-like repetition of a word or phrase that another individual has just spoken.

echopraxia The repetitive imitation of movements of others.

hallucination False perceptions that relate to any of the five senses.

paranoia A psychological condition exemplified by extreme suspiciousness, usually focused on one central theme. It often includes delusions of grandeur or persecution.

paranoid type schizophrenia A type of schizophrenia distinguished by the presence of delusions and hallucinations in the form of visions or voices often aimed against a governmental figure or agency.

prodromal phase The initial phase of schizophrenia in which the individual begins to withdraw from society, interpersonal and work place relationships begin to deteriorate, and productivity declines markedly. The individual may also experience thought and perception disturbances such as visual hallucinations, hearing voices (usually two voices talking about the person), and incoherent muttering.

psychosis Mental disorder with the presence of delusions or hallucinations.

psychotic disorder due to a general medical condition The presentation of psychotic symptoms such as hallucinations and delusions that are directly linked to the physiological effects of some medical condition and not better described by another mental disorder.

residual phase The third phase of schizophrenia that marks the end of the active phase. Individuals may be listless, have trouble concentrating, and be withdrawn, as well as experience thought and perception disturbances like those present in the initial prodromal phase.

residual type schizophrenia A type of schizophrenia in which patients who have recovered from prominent symptoms such as delusions, hallucinations, or disorganized behavior still show some mild evidence of the continuing disease process, such as a flat affect or poverty of speech.

schizoaffective disorder A condition that is actually a combination of two disorders: the active phase of schizophrenia and severe mood disorder, which must be either preceded or followed by at least two weeks of delusions or hallucinations (without prominent mood symptoms). The mood disorder can be a major depressive, manic, or mixed episode.

Prep Kit | continued

schizophrenia A persistent, often chronic disorder that involves disturbances in content of thought, form of thought, perception, affect, sense of self, motivation, behavior, and interpersonal functioning. Thinking may be disconnected and illogical, and present with delusions or hallucinations. Peculiar behaviors may be associated with social withdrawal and disinterest.

schizophreniform disorder A condition in which the individual shows the same psychotic symptoms attributed to schizophrenia, but lacks the required duration. Symptoms typically last between 1 and 6 months and may not precipitate social and occupational deterioration or dysfunction.

shared psychotic disorder A condition, commonly called folie a deux, in which an otherwise mentally healthy individual develops delusions while in a close relationship with someone who has an actual psychotic disorder.

substance-induced psychotic disorder The development of psychotic symptoms such as prominent hallucinations or delusions that are judged to be due to the direct physiological effects of a substance such as drug abuse, prescribed medication, or toxic exposure.

undifferentiated type schizophrenia A category of schizophrenia in which individuals show very complex signs and symptoms of the disease but do not meet specific *DSM-IV-TR* criteria to be diagnosed as paranoid, disorganized, or catatonic type.

Assessment in Action

Answer key is located in the back of the book.

1. There are five types of schizophrenia. The most common type is:

    A. catatonic.
    B. paranoid.
    C. disorganized.
    D. undifferentiated.

2. The French term *folie a deux,* meaning a folly of two, is characteristic of which type of disorder?

    A. Brief psychotic disorder
    B. Erotomanic type delusional disorder
    C. Schizoaffective disorder
    D. Shared psychotic disorder

3. The inability to experience pleasure best defines:

    A. avolition.
    B. anhedonia.
    C. alogia.
    D. prodromal.

4. You are dispatched to evaluate a 67-year-old male who is standing in the middle of the local fast-food restaurant. He appears disheveled and unkempt. The manager tells you that he is a local homeless man who "has something wrong with him because he thinks he is God." When you enter the restaurant, he is standing on a table telling the customers that he is God and has the power to strike them dead whenever he wishes to do so. His belief of his power is an example of a(n):

    A. dementia.
    B. hallucination.
    C. delusion.
    D. catatonia.

5. From the following list, select the psychotic disorder that also includes a mood disorder.

    A. Schizophreniform disorder
    B. Schizoaffective disorder
    C. Persecutory type delusional disorder
    D. Paranoid type schizophrenia

Chapter 14

Mood Episodes and Disorders

How many times have your heard someone say "he's in a bad mood today" or "she's always in a good mood?" To truly understand these statements, we need to understand exactly what mood is. <u>Mood</u> is a pervasive and sustained emotion that influences a person's perception of the world. It is something that changes constantly and may be prolonged or last for only a short period of time. Mood is the way a person feels inside and is generally characterized by a positive or negative emotion.

Short, significant, disruptive mood changes are classified as <u>episodes</u>. An episode is a time-limited period during which a person experiences specific, intense symptoms of a disorder. The *DSM-IV-TR* classifies an episode as a time period of at least 2 weeks during which an individual may experience fluctuations in mood, from extreme elation to severe sadness, or a combination of the two. Episodes may be the result of brain chemistry changes or changes in one's environment, such as winning a huge prize or experiencing the death of a loved one.

<u>Mood disorders</u> have identical symptoms, but are measured in longer periods of time. These disorders are mental conditions in which the normal functioning of mood is altered (**Figure 14-1**). Individuals with mood disorders experience mental changes that can last a few hours, several months, or, in some cases, years.

Mood disorders are also commonly called <u>affective disorders</u> because they are characterized by a prevalent change in mood that affects one's

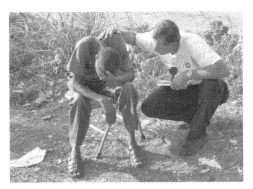

Figure 14-1 Individuals suffering from mood disorders may experience extreme mood fluctuations.

thoughts, emotions, and behaviors. In some cases, the individual will exhibit overwhelming feelings of anguish, also known as **dysphoria**, while other patients will present with **euphoria**, or a sense of exaggerated well-being. Emotional changes for these individuals are far more extreme than normal day-to-day fluctuations in mood. Mood alterations are distorted, inappropriate to the circumstances, and can happen at any time.

Many prehospital providers believe that mood disorders are "adult" disorders; however, since the 1980s, mental health professionals have recognized the signs and symptoms of mood changes in children and adolescents. The emergency responder cannot discount the possibility of a mood disorder in children and adolescents and must look for other acting-out behaviors.

In the prehospital environment, where situations are often unpredictable, it can be very difficult to distinguish what is appropriate and inappropriate behavior. Paying close attention to the interview and assessment of the patient will allow the provider to determine if the situation is medical or psychological in nature.

Background

Although the medical community clearly understands many physical diseases, progress on understanding diseases of the mind, especially mood disorders, has been slower. Conventional wisdom might lead us to suspect that mental disorders are caused strictly by chemical changes in the brain. That is not the case. The diagnosis of a mood disorder is a very complex process and various etiologic and contributing factors must be taken into consideration, including psychological, social, and biological factors.

Conditions discussed in this chapter will be divided into four categories. They are:

- **Mood episodes:** major depressive episode, manic episode, mixed episode, and hypomanic episode
- **Depressive disorders:** major depressive disorder and dysthymia
- **Bipolar disorders:** bipolar I disorder, bipolar II disorder, and **cyclothymia**
- **Other mood disorders:** mood disorders resulting from general medical conditions or substance abuse

Assessment

Prehospital assessment of any patient with psychiatric symptoms is a very difficult and complex process. When responding to a call dispatched as a behavioral emergency, the provider must remember that this scene may not be predictable. You should have a higher index of suspicion on a behavioral emergency call, request additional resources if necessary, and never enter the scene before it is cleared. A provider is of no help to anyone if the provider becomes a patient. The emergency provider should obtain information quickly and adapt to a rapidly changing scene.

As with all patients in the prehospital environment, the provider must form a general impression of the patient, assess the airway, breathing, and circulation; and identify any life-threatening issues. Additionally, the provider should perform a mental status examination to evaluate whether the patient's speech, thought patterns, or memory has been affected. Remember that when dealing with patients with a mood disorder, the provider's most important skill is the ability to be a good listener and historian.

Prehospital professionals must establish rapport with the patient and gather a detailed SAMPLE history. Gather accurate information about the patient's symptoms, such as when they started, how long they have been present, and whether the patient has experienced them before. Be aware that patients with mood disorders will demonstrate a wide range of presentations, from mania or excitement to extreme sadness and depression. It is important to determine if the patient has a known diagnosis of mood or other mental disorder. The provider should ask patients to disclose any treatment they may have received in the past for their condition.

Because mood disorders can be so psychologically devastating, it is important to find out if the patient has the desire to commit suicide, has a plan to do so, or has attempted suicide in the past. The provider should ask the patient how he or she currently feels and if he or she has any desire to harm himself or herself. Patients generally will be honest and willing to share their plans with you; some may even experience relief that someone has asked. Always remember that a person who is truly suicidal and suspects that you will stop the attempt must also be considered homicidal, and extra precautions should be taken.

SEA-3 Mental Status Exam for Mood Disorders

Speech: Speech patterns in patients with depression generally will be very quiet, soft-spoken, or possibly even muted. It takes energy to speak, and patients may tell you that they simply do not have that energy. The manic patient will be speaking boisterously with a rush of ideas that may be difficult to follow. Speech may appear pressured, as though there is a need to be talking at all times.

Emotion: Depressed patients will demonstrate various degrees of sadness, from simply being somber to openly weeping. Patients commonly will report that their crying is uncontrollable and may not be able to tell you why they are crying. Other patients may not even realize that they are depressed, but their actions will indicate otherwise. Elevated mood is easily recognizable after a few minutes of interviewing. Manic patients feel very good about themselves and have an inflated sense of self-esteem or grandiosity. The elation may be described as euphoric and might be confused with the symptoms of a person who is taking some form of amphetamine or other stimulant.

Appearance: Appearance varies according to the degree of depression. In cases of mild depression, there may be no obvious changes. If subtle changes are present, they may be easy to miss; you might only see that the patient recently has grown a beard because "he doesn't feel like shaving." On the severe end of the spectrum, patients may lose the motivation to care for themselves to the point of creating severe medical problems. Failure to bathe, severe weight loss or gain, going without sleep, or wearing the same clothes repeatedly is common. Manic patients generally will be dressed normally and take care of themselves relatively well. However, because of extreme changes in sleep habits, visual signs of fatigue may be present even though the individual may deny feeling tired.

Alertness: Under normal circumstances, patients with depression are alert and oriented unless there is a problem with medication regulation. Many of the drugs used to treat this category of mental illness have severe side effects that include lethargy and drowsiness. Manic patients are extremely alert but are easily distracted. As a result of their mania, patients are often unable to maintain a focus on one topic and may appear confused.

Activity: Some of the most important information for assessment is obtained in the activity component of the interview. It is common for patients to describe activities that would demonstrate low energy levels or motivation. Poor eating and sleeping habits, failure to complete tasks, calling in sick to work, and sitting around the house feeling sad and depressed are common. In some cases, the patient will acknowledge having intrusive suicidal thoughts and wanting the mental anguish to go away. A person experiencing a manic episode often demonstrates constant motion; however, you must evaluate the effects of that activity. Is the patient doing things that are harmful to himself or herself, such as not sleeping or failing to eat?

Prehospital personnel should also ask questions to evaluate other excessive behaviors such as gambling, unrestrained buying, sexual indiscretions, or foolish business investments. Questions such as: "What do you do in your free time?" "Do you have any hobbies?" "Are you dating anyone?" or "What type of work do you do?" may provide useful information.

OPQRST for Mood Episodes and Disorders

Onset: When did symptoms begin? Were they gradual or sudden? Symptoms are usually gradual in onset; however, mania tends to come on, or at least become recognizable, more acutely.

Provoking factors: Any of a variety of factors can bring on either depression or mania. Some examples are sensitivity to stress, response to negative events, personal feelings of failure, feelings of inadequacy, termination from a job, marital infidelity, death of a loved one, genetic predisposition, hormonal changes, or injury to the brain.

Quality: What is the person's quality of life? A person can generally maintain a functional life if he or she has mild depression or hypomania; however, severe cases of mania, depression, and bipolar disorder can be debilitating.

Radiation: Mood and bipolar disorders can radiate out and affect peers, friends, and family members, resulting in stressed relationships.

Severity: How severe is the presentation? Mood and bipolar disorders vary according to the type of disorder and degree of mania. Individuals can remain functional and able to perform daily activities or be completely debilitated, requiring professional assistance such as day programs or a residential home.

Time: How long has the patient been experiencing symptoms? Episodes can be brief, lasting only a few hours or days; however, severe disorders can be chronic and episodes can occur intermittently for a lifetime.

A valuable tool in assessing a patient with a mood disorder is the SEA-3 evaluation. Using this tool, the provider evaluates the speech, emotion, appearance, alertness, and activity of the patient. The SEA-3 evaluation tool will provide you with the structure needed to assess whether the person is quiet with a flat **affect**, depressed, or manic. You should inquire about the person's ability to eat and sleep and care for himself or herself to form an impression of the patient's presentation. Is he quiet and muted or energetic and talkative? How is she dressed? Is the patient wearing appropriate clothing or is the patient unbathed and wearing multiple layers of clothing inappropriate for the weather? Once the provider begins talking to the patient, the provider should assess the speech for tone, character of voice, and ability to respond appropriately to questioning. This can supply clues about the patient's current mood and alertness and whether the patient is oriented to person, place, and time.

The interviewer also should observe the patient's activity level and body language. Patients with severe **depression** may present with sluggish movements, lack of interest, and concentration difficulties, whereas patients experiencing a manic episode may present with a highly engaging and creative outlook, the inability to focus or concentrate, and an inability to commit to thoughts, actions, or feelings.

SAMPLE History for Mood Episodes and Disorders

Signs and symptoms: An individual experiencing depression presents with an overall feeling of sadness, lack of energy, poor eating and sleep habits, and a sense of hopelessness, helplessness, and haplessness. Persons with mania will demonstrate signs that represent an abnormally persistent elevated or high mood.

Allergies: Although allergic reactions to antidepressants are rare, side effects such as dry mouth, loss of sexual drive, nausea, headache, nervousness, insomnia, and agitation are common.

Medications: Medication regimens vary with each patient and with the philosophy of each physician who prescribes the drug. Most patients with the disorders discussed in this chapter will be taking a minimum of one mood regulator, and it is common for patients to be on a multi-drug regimen (**Figure 14-2**). A list of common medications is shown in **Table 14-1**.

Past medical history: Unless this is the first presentation of a mood disorder, most patients will present with a significant mental health history. Prehospital personnel should take a complete history with emphasis on patterns of behavior, previous clinical diagnoses, and past hospitalizations.

Last oral intake: Every effort should be made to determine the patient's compliance to the prescribed medication regimen.

Events leading up to today's event: If depression is the presenting sign, the emergency responder may find a person who is feeling sad, hopeless, hapless, and helpless. It is common for EMS to be activated following a suicide attempt. If the patient is manic, friends or family may note that the patient exhibits strange behavior or hyperactivity or fails to care for himself or herself.

Mood Episodes

The American Psychiatric Association recognizes four types of <u>mood episodes</u>: major depressive, manic, mixed, and hypomanic. *Depression* is a feeling of being sad or having other significant symptoms such as lack of energy, changes in eating or sleeping habits, lack of self-worth, and dejection.

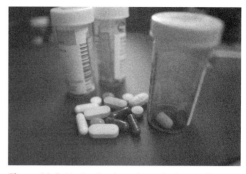

Figure 14-2 Medication is an important part of treatment regimens for mood disorders.

Major depressive episodes, also known as <u>unipolar mood disorder</u>, are characterized by depression only, rather than episodes of depression and mania (elation) as in bipolar mood disorders. Unipolar disorders are five times more common than bipolar disorders, and are diagnosed two to three times as frequently in women as in men. The onset of symptoms usually occurs in younger or middle-aged individuals.

To be diagnosed with major depressive disorder, one must, in addition to experiencing a depressed mood every day and loss of interest or pleasure, exhibit three or more of the following signs and symptoms over a 2-week period: increased or decreased appetite with significant weight change, changes to sleeping habits including insomnia or hypersomnia, psychomotor agitation or retardation, fatigue or malaise, feeling worthless or experiencing excessive or inappropriate guilt, decreased ability to think or concentrate, inability to make decisions, and recurrent thoughts of death, suicidal ideation, or suicide plan or attempt.

<u>Mania</u> means that the patient presents with an abnormally persistent elevated or high mood. Mania has two forms: manic episodes and <u>hypomanic</u> episodes. The *DSM-IV-TR* criteria for these two forms are very similar; however, there is one major difference that is easy for the prehospital provider to evaluate. Can the patient still go to work? Are friendships stressed? Has the patient's high feeling led to multiple problems? If the answer is yes, and if the condition has restricted the patient's daily routine, the patient is likely experiencing a manic episode. Hypomania presents with the same symptoms, but to a lesser extent, allowing the patient to be functional in his or her daily routines.

Although ADHD and mania may present with similar symptoms, they are not the same and should not be confused. The manic or hypomanic patient will present with three or more of the following: inflated self-esteem or grandiosity, insomnia or feeling rested with only a few hours of sleep, extreme talkativeness, flight of ideas or thoughts, distraction, increased goal-directed activities, or excessive involvement in pleasurable activities that have a high potential for extreme consequences.

Mixed episodes occur when the patient experiences both manic episodes and major depressive episodes nearly every day over a period of time, lasting at least one week. During the mixed episodes, <u>rapid cycling</u> or alternating moods occur. Moods may include sadness, irritability, and euphoria, accompanied by the symptoms discussed above. These individuals present with agitation, insomnia, appetite changes, psychotic features, and suicidal thoughts. Social and occupational impairment is common when patients are experiencing an acute mixed episode.

Prehospital personnel are usually activated by concerned or stressed friends and family members. Unless the depressive episode is so severe that suicidal ideation or attempt is imminent, patients are not generally classified as emergent, but may be in need of care and transport to an emergency facility for evaluation.

Depressive Disorders

Depressive disorders are divided into two specific disorders: <u>major depressive disorder</u> and <u>dysthymia</u>. Distinguishing between the two is difficult; they can coexist, and many mental health professionals consider them to be two aspects of the same disorder.

Table 14-1 Common Antimanic and Antidepressant Medications

Antimanic Medications

Brand name	Generic name
Cibalith-S	lithium citrate
Depakote	valproic acid, divalproex sodium
Eskalith	lithium carbonate
Lamictal	lamotrigine
Lithane	lithium carbonate
Lithobid	lithium carbonate
Neurontin	gabapentin
Tegretol	carbamazepine
Topamax	topiramate

Antidepressant Medications

Brand name	Generic name
Adapin	doxepin
Anafranil	clomipramine
Asendin	amoxapine
Aventyl	nortriptyline
Celexa	citalopram
Desyrel	trazodone
Effexor	venlafaxine
Elavil	amitriptyline
Lexapro	escitalopram
Ludiomil	maprotiline
Luvox	fluvoxamine
Marplan	isocarboxazid
Nardil	phenelzine
Norpramin	desipramine
Pamelor	nortriptyline
Parnate	tranylcypromine
Paxil	paroxetine
Pertofrane	desipramine
Prozac	fluoxetine
Remeron	mirtazapine
Serzone	nefazodone
Sinequan	doxepin
Surmontil	trimipramine
Tofranil	imipramine
Vivactil	protriptyline
Wellbutrin	bupropion
Zoloft	sertraline

In order to be diagnosed with major depressive disorder, an individual must have undergone one or more depressive episodes without experiencing mania or the feeling of elation. Dysthymia is defined as a chronic mild condition present for many years leading to a depressed mood for at least a consecutive 2-year time period. The *DSM-IV-TR* criteria for this disorder require two or more of the following symptoms: poor appetite or overeating; sleep disturbance, including either insomnia or hypersomnia; diminished energy or fatigue; low self-esteem; poor concentration or decision-making difficulty; and feelings of hopelessness.

Major depressive disorders and dysthymia may be triggered by psychological, cognitive, social, or biological factors, or some combination. An individual's sensitivity to stress, response to negative events in his or her life, personal feelings of failure, belief that he or she is inadequate, termination from a job, genetic predisposition, hormonal changes, or injury to the brain may all serve as catalysts for the development of a major depressive disorder. Other catalysts include marital infidelity and the death of a loved one.

Bipolar Disorders

The American Psychiatric Association recognizes three bipolar disorders: bipolar I, bipolar II, and cyclothymia.

The *DSM-IV-TR* defines bipolar I disorder as a condition in which a person has been "clinically diagnosed with having one or more manic episodes with the possibility of having one or more major depressive episodes." Research has shown that more than 90% of patients who experience one manic episode go on to have subsequent episodes and, if untreated, have an average of 8 to 10 episodes per year. These individuals have most likely already experienced one or more major depressive episodes.

The average age of onset for bipolar I disorder is 21 years old, and it is equally prevalent in men and women. The presence of bipolar I disorder usually results in damaged relationships, poor job and school performance, and suicidal ideation. Completed suicide occurs in individuals with bipolar I disorder at a rate of 10% to 15%. Patients may present with symptoms for 2 weeks or for 4 or 5 months. Bipolar I disorder can be severely debilitating and can prevent the individual from leading a productive normal life.

The *DSM-IV-TR* defines bipolar II disorder as a condition that is characterized by "one or more major depressive episodes, and at least one hypomanic episode." Hypomania is a mild degree of mania characterized by optimism, excitability, energetic productive behavior, marked hyperactivity and talkativeness, heightened sexual interest, quick anger and irritability, and decreased need for sleep. A hypomanic state may be observed just before a full-blown manic episode and feel appropriate to the person experiencing it.

These episodes may sometimes be associated with good functioning and enhanced productivity; however, persons exhibiting signs and symptoms of hypomania have an increased chance of reverting to mania or depression. Typically, patients will have several major depressive episodes in addition to hypomania prior to their first manic episode, leading to a shift in diagnosis from bipolar II to bipolar I disorder.

Individuals suffering from a cyclothymic disorder also experience rapid fluctuations in mood, ranging from elation to depression. However, even though these mood shifts may be dramatic and recurrent, they are not as intense as those seen with bipolar I and II disorder. The *DSM-IV-TR* classifies cyclothymic disorder as the presence of numerous hypomanic episodes in addition to minor depressive episodes that do not meet the criteria for major depressive episodes. In this disorder, a patient's mood may change within hours, weeks, or months, and changes are unrelated to life events. In some cases, cyclothymia may appear as just a characteristic of an individual's personality; however, it interferes with normal day-to-day functioning, classifying it as a mood disorder.

Cyclothymia is a chronic condition that must last a minimum of 2 years in adults and a minimum of 1 year in children and adolescents to be diagnosed. This disorder affects less than 1% of the population, and individuals suffering from it may act appropriately in work and social situations even when not receiving treatment, but they typically do not function at full capacity. Unfortunately, because the signs and symptoms for cyclothymic disorder are mild, individuals experiencing these symptoms will not usually seek medical treatment.

An increase in stressful life events, such as a schedule disruption due to lack of sleep, changes in job situations or personal relationships, changes in menstrual cycles, and changes in work shifts, has been noted to stimulate these disorders. Additionally, goal-attainment events may precipitate manic or depressive episodes. Individuals feel a sense of achievement after attaining specific goals, including job promotions, acceptance into specific groups, organizations, or schools, or beginning a new relationship. These events can lead to a period during which excess activity culminates in a spiral of positive or negative emotion, developing into a manic or depressive episode.

Evidence has shown that individuals who have first-degree biological relatives with mood disorders will tend to have an earlier age of onset if they develop the disorder; therefore, genetics may play a role in bipolar disorder. Ongoing research is attempting to identify specific areas of the brain and changes in various neurotransmitters, such as serotonin, norepinephrine, and dopamine, that may cause these disorders.

Other Mood Disorders: Mood Disorders Due to General Medical Conditions or Substance Abuse

Approaching any patient with a suspected behavioral emergency should always make the prehospital provider suspicious of any underlying conditions that may contribute to the patient's behavior. For example, medical conditions such as multiple sclerosis, stroke, brain lesions, and hypothyroidism are disease processes that may present as a mood disorder.

During your assessment, it is imperative to take both a good psychological and medical history. Every effort should be made to investigate and document the onset of symptoms, identify what

Table 14-2 Common Side Effects of Antimanic and Antidepressant Medications

- Loss of sexual drive
- Headache
- Nausea
- Nervousness
- Insomnia
- Agitation and feeling jittery
- Dizziness
- Drowsiness
- Weight gain
- Hand twitching or tremors

SAFER-R for Mood Episodes and Disorders

Stabilize: Ensure that life-threatening problems have been corrected. If the patient is experiencing a mood disorder, attempt to calm and support the patient. Assure the person that help has arrived and that you are willing to listen to his or her problems.

Acknowledge: Acknowledge why you are on scene. If the patient initiated the call, thank the person for calling you and ask why he or she called. If a family, friend, or someone else called, be honest and identify why you are there and why others are concerned.

Facilitate: Attempt to understand the patient's feelings. Patients with either mania or depression may not recognize that their symptoms are creating a problem for themselves or others. If the person has attempted suicide, move the patient to a neutral location such as the back of the ambulance and provide medical care as soon as possible. Reassure the person again that he or she is safe.

Encourage: If the patient does not wish to seek immediate help, encourage him or her to accept your offer of assistance. In most cases, your patience and perseverance will get the patient to agree to be transported. Explain to the patient your concerns and the consequences of his or her decision. If necessary, offer to make phone calls to family or friends who may be supportive in the treatment and recovery process.

Recovery: By being empathetic and understanding, you can begin the recovery process while the patient is in your care. Constant reinforcement of why you are there and how you care about the outcome will provide a simple but powerful message. Realize that severely depressed patients often feel that you do not care and that they have no reason to live.

Referral: Upon arriving at the emergency department, make sure that your story is heard by the receiving nurse, physician, and possibly social worker. Both patients and families need advocates and referrals for long-term mental health care.

has made the symptoms worse, and determine whether the symptoms have lessened or disappeared. Additionally, assess whether there is anything about the current mood presentation that does not seem to fit the normal criteria, such as an onset of symptoms at an unusual age or the absence of a family history of the disorder.

Intoxication with alcohol or illicit substances, medication abuse, or exposure to specific toxins may lead to signs and symptoms related to a mood disorder. The intake of alcohol, depressants, or tranquilizers can easily mimic depression, just as amphetamines or cocaine can cause hyperactivity that would mimic mania. However, it is important that the emergency provider does not dismiss the possibility of a mood disorder simply because intoxication is present. Individuals with mood disorders are more likely to develop substance abuse problems as a coping mechanism for their illness. Intoxicants such as alcohol, cocaine, heroin, tranquilizers, and pain pills are often used to combat the disorders and the side effects of various medications (**Table 14-2**). It can be difficult to tell if the psychological emergency is a result of a mental illness, medical condition, or substance abuse, or some combination of these. Performing a comprehensive history and physical examination will allow the prehospital provider to speculate about the origin of the emergency and to provide appropriate care.

Prehospital Management

Mood disorders can be particularly challenging to manage in the prehospital environment. EMS providers are familiar with "load-and-go" situations that are common in prehospital emergencies. Unless the patient has attempted suicide, there will probably be no reason to rush this patient to the hospital using red lights and sirens. If the patient is suffering from suicidal and/or homicidal ideation, the scene must be secured by police before any emergency responder attempts to provide care for the patient.

If you have reason to believe that a patient is suffering from a mood disorder, the SAFER-R model will be the most appropriate way to provide support to your patient in the field environment. This method will prove to be the most professional and effective means to encourage patients with mood disorders to seek further medical help.

Much of your time on the scene with the patient affected by a mood disorder should be dedicated to assessment and planning for safe transport to the emergency department. Patients suffering from a mood disorder may not be aware of the severity or even the existence of their symptoms. Once the patient is placed in a safe zone, emergency responders should respectfully begin to take a SAMPLE history, being sure to ask about feelings of guilt and hopelessness, sleeping habits, eating habits, perceptual disturbances, and homicidal or suicidal ideation. Be sure to note if the patient is demonstrating impaired judgment, seems withdrawn from friends and family, is unable to distinguish right from wrong, is seeking dangerous activities, is experiencing heightened sexual awareness, or is unable to commit to thoughts or feelings.

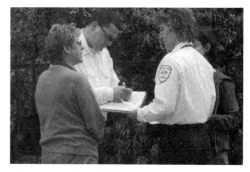

Figure 14-3 If possible, interview friends and family of the patient.

In addition to the patient, be aware that family and friends will need your support and compassion. EMS is often activated by family members and friends who can no longer deal with the day-to-day stress of caring for a loved one with a severe mood disorder. Patients with mania will be up for most of the night, disturbing the sleep of others in the home. On other occasions, family members live in fear that severe depression will lead to suicide (**Figure 14-3**).

Your transport to the hospital could mean that their loved one will be committed to a facility for ongoing psychiatric care. Every effort should be made to provide compassionate care for the patient as well as empathy to those family and friends who are also intimately involved. Your calm, professional, and knowledgeable approach will provide reinforcement that the patient is in good hands. Additionally, your organization might wish to develop a special brochure listing local and national support groups to give to family members in these situations.

Pharmacologic Considerations

When caring for a patient with a mood disorder, it is particularly important to pay attention to the medications that have been prescribed for the patient. It is common for patients to be on multiple medications, many of which have serious side effects, especially antidepressants or mood stabilizers (Figure 4-2). Table 14-1 provides a comprehensive list of common mood stabilizers and antidepressants.

In the prehospital environment, an EMS provider seldom administers any medication to the patients discussed in this chapter. Medications given for any of the mood disorders take days or weeks to have a therapeutic effect.

Final Thoughts

Depressive mood disorders can present with a vast array of symptoms, including loss of energy, change in sleep habits, loss or gain in weight, irritability, and poor judgment—just to mention a few. Those with mania present at the opposite end of the continuum, showing signs of hyperactivity, lack of sleep, and poor attention span. Without a thorough and proper interview, prehospital personnel might easily mistake some of these symptoms for a medical condition such as a brain tumor, drug intoxication, or stroke.

For a person who is severely depressed, getting out of bed or answering your questions may truly be difficult to accomplish. Likewise, a patient

In the Field

The National Alliance on Mental Illness (NAMI) is an excellent referral source for families of patients with mental illness. Their web site is www.nami.org.

experiencing a manic episode will have difficulty focusing on the task at hand or on your questions. In the absence of a life-threatening emergency such as a suicide attempt, the key to treating the patient with a mood disorder is care, understanding, and patience.

Selected References

American Psychiatric Association: *Diagnostic and Statistical Manual of Mental Disorders, Fourth Edition, Text Revision (DSM-IV-TR)*. Washington, DC, American Psychiatric Press, 2000.

Bledsoe BE, Porter RS, Cherry RA: *Essentials of Paramedic Care,* ed 2. New Jersey, Prentice Hall, 2007.

Dryden-Edwards R, Lee D: Depression. Available at: http://www.medicinenet.com/depression/article.htm. Accessed September 10, 2008.

Grohol JM: Depression treatment: (2006). Available at: http://psychcentral.com/disorders/sx22t.htm. Accessed March 7, 2007.

Halgin RP, Whitbourne SK: *Abnormal Psychology: Clinical Perspectives on Psychological Disorders,* ed 4. Boston, MA, McGraw Hill, 2005.

Mental disorders (n.d.). Available at: http://psyweb.com/Mdisord/jsp/mental.jsp. Accessed March 3, 2007.

Myers T (ed): *Mosby's Dictionary of Medicine, Nursing and Health Professions.* St Louis, MO, Elsevier, 2006.

National Institute of Mental Health: Depression. Available at: http://www.nimh.nih.gov/publicat/depression.cfm#ptdep2. Accessed March 7, 2007.

National Institute of Mental Health: Medications. Available at: http://www.nimh.nih.gov/health/publications/medications/complete-publication.shtml. Accessed July 14, 2008.

Oltmanns T, Emery R: *Abnormal Psychology,* Upper Saddle River, NJ, Pearson Prentice Hall, 2004.

Psychologynet.org. Available at: http://www.psychologynet.org/dsm.html. Accessed March 7, 2007.

Seidel HM, Ball JW, Dains JE, Benedict GW: *Mosby's Guide to Physical Examination,* ed 6. Canada, Elsevier, 2006.

Wikipedia: Bipolar disorder. Available at: http://en.wikipedia.org/wiki/Bipolar_disorder. Accessed March 3, 2007.

Wikipedia: Major depressive disorder. Available at: http://en.wikipedia.org/wiki/Clinical_depression. Accessed June 6, 2008.

Prep Kit

Ready for Review

- A mood disorder is a category of mental health disorder that is represented by a disturbance in mood, such as extreme sadness, apathy, euphoria, or irritability.
- Types of mood disorder discussed in this chapter include mood episodes, depressive disorders, bipolar disorders, and mood disorders caused by medical conditions or substance abuse.
- A person's mood is a subjective symptom of how the patient feels inside.
- An episode is an event or presentation that is time limited, lasting usually less than two weeks.
- Rapid cycling is the occurrence of four or more episodes of depression and/or mania within a 12-month period.
- Medical conditions such as multiple sclerosis, stroke, brain lesions, and hypothyroidism can mimic and present with symptomatology like that of a mood disorder. Likewise, intoxication from alcohol or another substance can present like that of either depression or mania.
- It is rare that a patient with a mood disorder will require a red light and siren response to the hospital. The one exception might be that of a serious suicide attempt. In most situations, the patient will need calm, empathetic, and supportive care during transport.

Vital Vocabulary

affect The observable emotion or feeling, tone, and mood attached to a thought; one's emotional presentation to the evaluator.

affective disorder See mood disorder.

bipolar disorder A major mental disorder characterized by episodes of mania, depression, or mixed mood.

cyclothymia (or cyclothymic disorder) A disorder of mood wherein the essential feature is a chronic mood disturbance of at least 2 years' duration, involving numerous periods of mild depression and hypomania.

depression A syndrome in which a depressed mood is accompanied by several other symptoms, such as fatigue, loss of energy, difficulty in sleeping, and changes in appetite.

dysphoria A disorder of affect characterized by depression and anguish.

dysthymia (or dysthymic disorder) A chronic mild depressive condition that has been present for greater than two years, in which the patient exhibits at least two of the following six symptoms: poor appetite or overeating, insomnia or hypersomnia, low energy or fatigue, low self-esteem, poor concentration or difficulty making decisions, and feelings of hopelessness.

episode A time-limited period during which specific, intense symptoms of a disorder are evident.

euphoria An exaggerated or abnormal sense of physical and emotional well-being that is usually not based on reality or truth and is inappropriate for the situation and disproportionate to its cause.

hypomania An episode of increased energy that is not sufficiently severe to qualify as a full-blown manic episode.

major depressive disorder Also known as major depression or unipolar depression; a disorder characterized by a pervasive low mood, loss of interest in a person's usual activities, and diminished ability to experience pleasure.

mania A disturbance in mood characterized by such symptoms as elation, inflated self-esteem, hyperactivity, and accelerated speaking and thinking; an exaggerated feeling of physical and emotional well-being.

mood The pervasive feeling, tone, and internal emotional state of a person; how one feels.

mood disorder Disorders in which a disturbance in mood is the predominant feature, such as depression, mania, or hypomania.

mood episode The presentation of a mood disturbance such as depression or mania that appears for a short period of time, lasting only days or a few weeks.

Prep Kit | continued

rapid cycling Changing from one mood to the other and back again at short intervals, sometimes several times a day and even several times an hour, commonly between depression and elation.

unipolar mood disorder A type of mood disorder in which the person only experiences episodes of depression.

Assessment in Action

Answer key is located in the back of the book.

1. Time-limited periods in which one exhibits signs and symptoms of a disorder are called _____.

   A. disorders
   B. situations
   C. syndromes
   D. episodes

2. A chronic condition that has been present for many years and has mild depression as its key aspect is _____.

   A. cyclothymia
   B. dysthymia
   C. euphoria
   D. hypomania

3. A mood describes subjectively what the patient tells you about his or her feelings, whereas affect is your objective evaluation as to how the patient appears.

   A. True
   B. False

4. Upon arriving at the scene of a call for an unresponsive patient, you find a 36-year-old male sitting in his living room chair sleeping. He is arousable but sleepy. You must rule out all of the following possible field diagnoses except _____.

   A. alcohol or substance abuse
   B. antidepressant medication overdose
   C. severe depression
   D. All are possible causes of drowsiness

5. The psychiatric condition that presents with both depression and hypomania is _____.

   A. bipolar I disorder
   B. major depressive disorder
   C. bipolar II disorder
   D. dysthymia

Chapter 15

Anxiety Disorders

Anxiety is a feeling that is familiar to nearly everyone. It is a natural response to unfamiliar or high-stress situations and is no stranger to those working in the prehospital setting. Most prehospital providers experience anxiety at some point during their training or careers (eg, when responding to the scene of a mass casualty or a cardiac arrest call or when going through the smoke house during their first fire fighter course). The anxiety can be heard in a jittery voice, seen in shaky hands, and felt in the adrenaline rush while en route to the scene of the next big call. In some instances, anxiety can become so overwhelming that an individual will develop an anxiety disorder.

This chapter will focus on the recognition and treatment of patients experiencing anxiety disorders and will discuss how to best manage these patients in the prehospital environment. Conditions discussed in this chapter are:

- Panic attack
- Panic disorder (with and without agoraphobia)
- Social phobia (social anxiety disorder)
- Specific phobias
- Obsessive-compulsive disorder

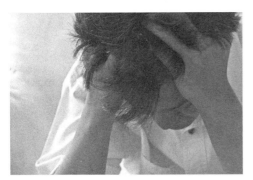

Figure 15-1 Anxiety disorders affect 18% of the population in the United States.

- Acute stress disorder
- Post-traumatic stress disorder (PTSD)
- Generalized anxiety disorder

Background

Anxiety is the sense of fear, apprehension, or worry that something terrible is going to happen in the near or distant future. Anxiety disorders are mental health conditions; they hinder the ability of an individual to function in daily life and are marked by chronic symptoms of anxiety. Anxiety disorders affect approximately 40 million people, or about 18% of the population in the United States in any given year (**Figure 15-1**). The economics of the disease are staggering; patients suffering from anxiety disorders consume $42 billion in mental health services or almost one third of the $148 billion mental health bill in the United States alone.

It is important to remember that the disorders discussed in this chapter can often cause such intense anxiety as to be physically and emotionally distressing or debilitating to the individual. Anxiety disorders frequently occur in tandem with other mental and physical illness. The stress caused can be so great as to overwhelm an individual's normal coping mechanisms and may present with physical symptoms similar to many other illnesses such as chest pain, shortness of breath, sweating, and muscle tremors. These classic conditions will require a thorough assessment by the emergency responder. The behavior of some individuals may be odd or perplexing to you, especially because most patients present with anxiety that appears irrational or unwarranted. Respect and patience will go a long way in helping the individual cope with or recover from feelings of anxiety.

Assessment of Patients With Anxiety Disorders

The assessment of a patient suffering from an anxiety disorder will differ very little from your typical, routine medical assessment. With the exception of panic disorder and panic attacks, most of these disorders will never be your primary focus as an EMS provider in the field. The important difference between other patients and those suffering from anxiety disorders is the integral, often damaging effects that trauma or illness can play in the development of their conditions. Many patients with severe anxiety disorders such as PTSD can become very isolated and prisoners in their own world. Because you are their first point of contact with the medical profession, it is absolutely necessary for you to display empathy and compassion when dealing with complaints.

It is important to remember when assessing patients with an anxiety disorder that their condition may be the result of a previous traumatizing stimulus. Their lives are often preoccupied by intense, irrational worrying, which may center around illness, trauma, and sudden death. If this is the case, their initial stimulus may lead to physical symptoms indicative of extreme fear.

Assessment of these patients should first focus on ruling out other life-threatening physical ailments. This is especially true for patients who call 911 with other, nonpsychiatric chief complaints. For many such patients, you may only identify the existence of an anxiety disorder when inquiring about past medical history. Often, the stigma of being seen as crazy may cause individuals to hide or deny the presence of a disorder. Past experience may tell these patients to avoid telling health care providers for fear that their complaint will be taken less seriously or passed off as simple anxiety. This is extremely common among individuals who suffer from sudden chest pain as well as a history of panic disorder. For example, women are prone to suffer from atypical-presentation myocardial infarction, and their symptoms often differ from the typical complaint of chest pain found among men. They may present with trouble breathing, heart palpitations, abdominal pain, and other physical symptoms that are identical to a panic attack. If the patient has an anxiety disorder, it may be difficult for the patient as well as the emergency services provider to determine immediately whether the symptoms represent a myocardial infarction or a panic attack.

Interview the patient utilizing the SAMPLE and OPQRST inventories to assess the nature of the complaint quickly. Always perform a brief physical exam if the patient complains of physical pains or discomfort before forming your differential diagnosis. Remember the symptoms of panic attacks can mimic or accompany those experienced by patients suffering from many cardiac abnormalities. The EMS provider should maintain a high index of suspicion during the assessment.

A rapid mental status examination must always be performed on patients suffering from anxiety disorders. The SEA-3 mental status exam is the fastest and easiest way to make a quick determination of the patient's state of mind while simultaneously looking for signs and symptoms indicative of anxiety or other mental disorders. Many of these findings are found through simple observation and conversation, rendering them less intrusive and embarrassing to patients who may be self-conscious about their disorder.

SAMPLE History for Anxiety Disorders

Signs and symptoms: Patients may be experiencing hyperventilation, dyspnea, chest pain, palpitation, signs of anxiety, or other stress-like symptoms.

Allergies: Allergies are common in some patients as they attempt new medications, especially for depression.

Medications: Antianxiety medications (anxiolytics) are very common; many patients are taking some type of anti-depressant medication.

Past medical history: Patients may have a history of calling EMS because of anxiety symptoms such as difficulty breathing. If the patient is alone, obtaining a history may be difficult because the patient may only be able to provide one- or two-word responses.

Last oral intake: This is dependent upon the diagnosis of the patient; most will report a regular diet and intake.

Events leading up to today's event: This may be one of the most important pieces of information gathered. What happened that caused the patient to present to EMS today? Often you will *not* be called to the scene for an anxiety disorder but for some other true medical or trauma situation.

Anxiety Disorders

Panic Attack and Panic Disorder

The *DSM-IV-TR* defines a panic attack as "a discrete period in which there is the sudden onset of intense apprehension, fearfulness, or terror, often associated with feelings of impending doom." During the panic attack, patients will present with a variety of other medical signs and symptoms that can easily confuse the emergency responder during a sometimes chaotic situation. It is common to have patients complain of shortness of breath, chest pain, and cardiac palpitations, which could easily result in the patient being treated for a myocardial infarction instead of panic. Likewise, individuals experiencing panic attacks can present with rapid respirations and be misdiagnosed as having <u>hyperventilation syndrome</u>.

Panic attacks are divided into three subgroups. Attacks that occur suddenly and without warning are called <u>unexpected (uncued) panic attacks</u>. These often occur in the absence of a

OPQRST for Anxiety Disorders

Onset: When did the symptoms begin? Does the patient have a history of an acute or chronic anxiety disorder?

Provocation: What happened today to trigger the attack? Has the patient done anything or taken any medications to calm himself or herself? Beware of patients who self-medicate and then call EMS because they may worsen in your care quickly and without notice.

Quality: How severe is the presentation? Is it to a point that the psychological syndrome is causing physical symptoms, such as chest pain or hyperventilation?

Radiation: How has the disorder affected the client, family, and peers? Do panic attacks and phobias restrict the patient from leaving home? Has handwashing or other obsessive rituals limited the patient's activity?

Severity: On a scale of 0 to 10, how severe is the distress today for the patient? For the first-time patient, this may be a difficult question to answer. For patients with chronic anxiety disorders, you can question the person about how today's anxiety compares to previous episodes.

Time: When did today's episode begin? Has there been more than one episode? If so, how long did it last?

SEA-3 Mental Status Exam for Anxiety Disorders

Speech: Patients suffering from anxiety disorder generally will be capable of speaking, although the rate, quality, amplitude, and flow may be vastly different depending on the individual and the disorder. There is no set pattern of speech that is indicative of any one disorder, although abnormalities should be noted. Accelerated speech may be present. The individual may describe the need to just "get out their thoughts."

Emotion: Emotion will remain relatively constant in most individuals suffering from anxiety disorders unless the individual is also suffering from a comorbid mood disorder. Depression is common among individuals with anxiety disorder and will greatly affect the mood of the patient. Be sure to note any manic or depressive episodes and the regularity with which they occur. Fear and anxiety are common among those suffering from any one of the anxiety disorders.

Appearance: The appearance of a patient suffering from anxiety disorder may range from appropriate to very disheveled and dirty. This will be entirely dependent on the severity and nature of the disorder. In many cases, individuals suffering from severe forms of an anxiety disorder may become so preoccupied with their feelings of anxiety or obsession that they completely ignore their appearance and personal hygiene.

Alertness: Nearly all patients suffering from anxiety disorder will be alert to person, place, and time (or event) and generally retain all of their cognitive functions. Patients are generally of average to above-average intelligence. For the most part, individuals with anxiety disorders should be fairly good historians, although patients with PTSD may experience significant emotional pain in trying to recount specifics of their symptoms. Patients will generally exhibit good impulse control but poor judgment when it comes to how best to manage their crisis.

Activity: The level of activity can be a significant clue for the prehospital provider and suggest an anxiety disorder, especially those disorders that may involve avoidant behavior. Question the individual about daily activities, including how often he or she leaves the home for work and pleasure. Decreased social activities may indicate social phobia, whereas avoidance of public places may indicate agoraphobia.

known situational cue or trigger. Attacks that occur in response to known, established triggers are called situational bound (or cued) panic attacks. If the attack occurs occasionally, but not every time the patient is exposed to the trigger, the attack is said to be a situationally predisposed panic attack.

Panic disorder is a condition in which an individual experiences panic attacks, or periods of time marked by intense fear, opposition, and physical discomfort. The patient may report uncontrollable terror and feel as if he or she is dying or losing control of the surroundings. The individual will experience a variety of symptoms, including heart palpitations, tachycardia, sweating, trembling or shaking, sensations of shortness of breath, chest pain, nausea, abdominal pain, feelings of being dizzy or lightheaded, paresthesia (numbness or tingling) in the extremities, and hyperventilation. The patient may also exhibit akathisia, or the feeling of having to constantly move or leave. Individuals diagnosed with panic disorder have recurrent panic attacks that are accompanied by fear or apprehension of having additional attacks. Patients experiencing these symptoms will require much patience and reassurance by the emergency responder, along with a thorough assessment (**Figure 15-2**). It is important to provide them with a comfortable, safe environment as you evaluate their needs. Panic attacks can mimic serious medical conditions such as heart attack or pulmonary embolism, so never assume that the above symptoms are purely psychologically based.

Patients may also fear the consequences of such an episode. Approximately 6 million Americans (about 2%) suffer from panic disorder in the United States, and 15% of the population will suffer an attack at some time during their lifetime. While relatively uncommon within the general population, the prevalence among those individuals suffering from other medical ailments is high. Of particular concern to the EMS provider is the relative commonality of panic attacks in patients suffering from chest pain. Up to 60% of all patients treated for symptoms of chest pain experience panic disorder. This is understandable given the stressful, often terrifying, experience that accompanies many medical emergencies.

Occasionally an individual with panic disorder may develop agoraphobia. Agoraphobia is the intense fear of being trapped, stranded, or embarrassed in a situation without help if a panic attack were to occur. The disorder commonly develops after repeat panic attacks, as the person attempts to curb exposure to the situation or event that generally causes an attack. People with agoraphobia tend to condition themselves to avoid the place where they may feel predisposed to suffering from an attack. This form of panic disorder is perhaps the most debilitating, often causing individuals to stay at home all the time or avoid social situations completely.

Panic disorder most commonly develops in younger patients, especially those in their 20s, but is seen among patients of all ages. It is indiscriminate to ethnic, social, and racial status, although it is twice as likely to be diagnosed in women. There is some evidence to suggest that the disorder has a familial or genetic property. Biological relatives of those who suffer from panic disorder are eight times as likely to experience the condition during their lifetime.

Social Phobia (Social Anxiety Disorder)

Like agoraphobia, social phobia, also known as social anxiety disorder, is characterized by a rather extreme, often irrational fear of being in public places. However, unlike agoraphobia, social phobia tends to appear in very specific situations and is a response to the belief that the individual will be victim to sudden public embarrassment. For example, a person may be so afraid of speaking in front of other people that he or she will avoid entirely any situation that may necessitate such speaking. This can become

> ## In the Field
>
> ### Signs and Symptoms of Panic Attacks
> - Palpitations, pounding heart, or accelerated heart rate
> - Sweating
> - Trembling or shaking
> - Sensations of shortness of breath or smothering
> - Feelings of choking
> - Chest pain or discomfort
> - Nausea or abdominal distress
> - Feeling dizzy, unsteady, lightheaded, or faint
> - Derealization (feelings of unreality) or depersonalization (being detached from oneself)
> - Fear of losing control or going crazy
> - Fear of dying
> - Paresthesia (numbing or tingling sensations)
> - Chills or hot flushes
> - Sense of impending doom

so crippling that it may hinder job performance or social life. In the adult patient, you will find that he or she is aware that the fears are irrational; this awareness adds to the person's experience of great internal emotional distress. The emergency responder may receive a call to check on the welfare of someone when he or she has not left the home or apartment for many days. Upon arriving, you might find an individual who presents with not only anxiety or fear, but also the signs of depression in serious scenarios. As with all patients with an anxiety disorder, extreme compassion and understanding will be paramount to the successful assessment and transport of individuals suffering from social phobias.

On the other hand, children have an underdeveloped sense of appropriate fears and behaviors and often cannot pick and choose their environmental situations as easily as adults. This may lead them to exhibit other signs of social phobia such as tantrums or general antisocial behavior.

Empathy and respect will be your best tools when treating patients with a diagnosis or symptoms of social phobia. Likewise, it will be important for emergency personnel to recognize this disorder, especially in those patients who have fallen ill or been injured in public areas. Protecting a patient's modesty, such as covering the person or protecting the person's identity from onlookers, will be just as important as treating the physical illnesses. Failure to do so could lead to crippling anxiety that may manifest into physical signs of abnormal stress or full-blown panic attacks. The appearance of such signs and symptoms may complicate your treatment of the underlying physical disorder and cause greater harm to the patient.

Specific Phobias

Almost everyone can identify one thing about which they are absolutely terrified. You might be afraid of spiders, snakes, heights, or any one of a thousand different things. You may feel some discomfort

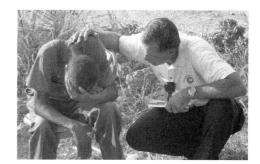

Figure 15-2 Patients experiencing panic attacks require patience from the responder.

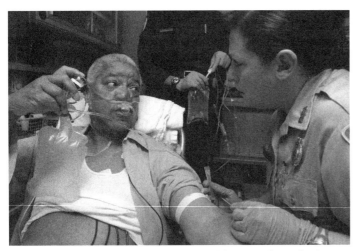
Figure 15-3 The inside of your ambulance may trigger a panic reaction in a patient who suffers from claustrophobia.

when you are exposed to these objects or situations and try to avoid them if possible. The mild anxiety that you experience is called an <u>aversion</u>. An aversion occurs when a person experiences a normal response of discomfort or dislike to a particular object or situation. When these aversions become disproportionate to the level of threat posed by these objects, situations, or activities, causing severe discomfort and anxiety, they become <u>specific phobias</u>. As is true with all phobias, absolute avoidance and social disruption almost always follow the feelings of severe anxiety.

Specific phobias are the most common form of anxiety disorder. It is estimated that some 19 million people in the United States suffer from specific phobias, making it the most prevalent of the anxiety disorders. It is the most common mental illness in women and the second most common in men. Theories abound as to exactly why human beings suffer from phobias, but it is likely that they have been evolutionarily adapted in response to common elements within our environment that could cause harm. There is evidence of a familial or genetic component to the disorder. For instance, it is advantageous for human beings to avoid falling from great heights. You would not be practicing EMS if all of your ancestors had haphazardly walked off cliffs. In response, some people develop irrational fears of heights known as <u>acrophobia</u>. It is important to remember that although many people you know may experience acrophobia, it is only classified as a specific phobia when it becomes a hindrance to the person's daily quality of life. For example, a flight paramedic would be at a significant disadvantage if he or she suffered from acrophobia that was so severe that he or she might have to change jobs. It is easy to see how phobias, be they specific or social, can cause significant turmoil in an individual's life.

Phobias will most likely be of little concern to the prehospital provider in the field, although there are some specific phobias of which you should be aware. <u>Claustrophobia</u> is the fear of being in small or confined spaces. Your ambulance is the perfect place for a patient to experience a sudden panic attack while en route to the hospital. Although unavoidable, it is important to recognize and reassure the patient (**Figure 15-3**). Stay by the patient's side and provide assistance should the attack become severe.

<u>Mysophobia</u>, sometimes simply called <u>germophobia</u>, is the irrational fear of harmful pathogens such as viruses or bacteria. Utilizing a proper aseptic technique and providing reassurance will go a long way with these patients. <u>Trypanophobia</u> is the fear of medical procedures or medical injections. Obviously, this is a phobia that will be difficult for emergency responders to deal with, because many lifesaving procedures involve the use of needles or other fairly invasive medical devices. Patients will

In the Field

Tips for Calming the Claustrophobic Patient

- Never leave the patient's side or sight unless you tell the person specifically of your location.

- If in an emergency vehicle, do not use lights and sirens unless the patient's condition is life threatening.

- Ensure that there is good ventilation or a cool breeze blowing near the patient.

- Provide constant reassurance.

- Have the patient close his or her eyes and encourage the patient to visualize being in a place that feels safe, such as an open field. You can ask the patient what type of place feels safe and help the patient with this step.

- Allow the patient to walk to the ambulance if possible, instead of being strapped to a stretcher.

generally voice their concern prior to the initiation of IV therapy or any other procedure uncomfortable to them. You must reassure the patient that the procedure is needed to treat the ailment properly and that refusing such care may be detrimental to the patient's health. It is important to note that phobias are generally a result of a fear of pain, suffering, or death. Being honest with the patient and identifying the dangers associated with a refusal may help the patient overcome these irrational beliefs; however, do not threaten the patient with dire consequences.

Obsessive-Compulsive Disorder

Obsessive-compulsive disorder (OCD) came to widespread public attention in 1997's movie *As Good as It Gets,* starring Jack Nicholson as an author suffering from severe OCD. The movie portrays one man's interactions with the world around him, while simultaneously dealing with his internal struggle to acknowledge and deal with one of the most debilitating anxiety disorders. Although the movie serves as good comedy, the life of an individual suffering from severe, clinical OCD is anything but fun.

In order to understand OCD, you must first understand the two unique, but integral, components necessary for the diagnosis of the disorder. There is both an obsessive and a compulsive component to the disorder; the patient must exhibit symptoms of at least one in order to fully meet the criteria. The *DSM-IV-TR* defines obsessions as "persistent ideas, thoughts, impulses, or images that are experienced as intrusive and inappropriate and that cause marked anxiety or distress" and compulsions as "repetitive behaviors, either observable or mental, that are intended to reduce the anxiety engendered by obsessions."

People with OCD suffer from recurrent intrusive, often unavoidable, thoughts that cannot be forgotten or dismissed. These thoughts generally are characterized by intense worrying about some idea or action and can take on the form of intense, often vivid images of a terrible event happening. Such thoughts may include a plane crashing, catching a disease, or a close family member dying tragically. In order to suppress these images and thoughts, individuals suffering from OCD develop abnormal rituals and patterns in an effort to suppress the thoughts. These rituals define the compulsive nature of the disorder. Obsessions generally fall into one of four categories: (1) checking-related obsessions, (2) obsessions rooted in the need for symmetry and order, (3) obsessions related to cleanliness or hypochondrias, or (4) hoarding-like behaviors.

You may not see the obsessive components of the disorder unless the patient expressly mentions them to you; instead, you will most likely see signs of compulsions. For instance, as you prepare a 30-year-old male patient for transport, he may enter the kitchen and do a rather routine check to see if every appliance is turned off. Although checking the toaster may seem reasonable at first, you may notice that he does this many times. This repetitive behavior is fairly common among people with OCD and is an effort by the individual to suppress some horrible, intrusive

In the Field

Helping Patients With a Fear of Medical Procedures

- Ask the patient to explain to you why he or she is afraid. Knowing the history will help you to avoid situations that might increase the patient's anxiety.
- Elicit the patient's help when you need to perform a medical procedure. For example, allowing the patient to hold onto a dressing that you will use during an injection or IV attempt will offer the patient an opportunity for control and will provide some distraction.
- Be patient! Rushing a patient with any type of anxiety disorder will only escalate the situation and increase the chances that the patient will refuse needed medical care.
- Do not use red lights and sirens unless absolutely necessary because emergency signals often cause patients to secrete adrenaline and increase the "fight-or-flight" responses; these responses are already activated during a panic attack.
- Assure the patient that he or she is in a safe environment and that you are using safe, clean techniques for all of your procedures.
- Ask the patient how much he or she wants to know about his or her condition or the procedures that you will be performing. Information provides another source of control for the patient and will often serve to calm patients.

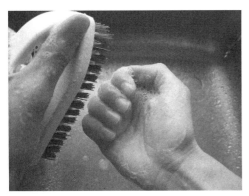

Figure 15-4 Every effort should be made to accommodate a patient suffering from OCD in the prehospital setting.

thought. As a result, extra patience on your part will be needed in order to prepare the patient for transport to the hospital. While you may have been called for an emergency of a different etiology, the need to check the lights or the stove will occupy the patient's mind and outweigh his or her current medical condition. Every effort should be made to accommodate the patient before initiating transport to the hospital if time permits (**Figure 15-4**).

OCD will be one of the most perplexing disorders you will see in your career. Unlike many of the other anxiety disorders that can be rationalized through fears or past exposure, OCD is one of the oddest and most often misunderstood of the mental disorders. All in all, some 2.2 million Americans suffer from full-blown, debilitating OCD. This is important to note, because although the disease has become such a cliché in describing obsessive behavior in society, OCD is a disease only when it significantly interferes with the individual's daily quality of life. The obsessive nature of your partner to recheck the supplies in the ambulance is simply good practice, not OCD.

Acute Stress Disorder

Traumatic experiences are not new to EMS personnel. Prehospital providers have been at the scene of every major disaster of the last half century in some capacity. We have served in times of environmental disaster as well as extreme acts of violence and terrorism both at home and abroad. These experiences have led to a deep understanding of traumatic stress and its effects on the psychological health in both provider and patient populations.

A **traumatic experience** is any event that has disastrous consequences for the person involved, both psychologically and physically. The pain and emotional trauma that result can often be so debilitating as to cause the development of **acute stress disorder**, or the appearance of signs and symptoms consistent with extreme fear and anxiety that have detrimental effects on an individual's quality of life. Patients suffering from acute stress disorder may develop symptoms that last anywhere from 2 to 28 days after the event has occurred. Symptoms usually consist of extreme fear and anxiety. These symptoms may result in the patient reliving the experience and manifest themselves as visions, sometimes known as **flashbacks**, which can cause retraumatization. More common is the development of extreme anxiety that sometimes leads to **panic attacks** or other physical symptoms. The individual also may experience dissociative symptoms, such as numbness and detachment from the environment or reality. Symptoms can vary in those suffering from acute stress disorder, ranging from severe episodic flashbacks to anxiety and overwhelming emotional stress.

Regardless of the symptoms exhibited, all sufferers of acute stress disorder have one thing in common: they all have been exposed to some experience or event that brings about disastrous

In the Field

Common Obsessions or Compulsions Seen in Patients With OCD

- Multiple handwashings, to a point that the skin might begin to break down
- Counting items or steps to accomplish a task
- Locking and relocking doors
- Brushing one's hair or teeth repeatedly
- Checking repeatedly to see if appliances are unplugged or turned off
- Frequent thoughts of violence and harming loved ones
- Intrusive thoughts of sexual misconduct
- Having things orderly and symmetrical

consequences to their health and state of mind. These experiences can be relatively personal events, such as rape or witnessing a murder, or global events, such as disease and war. The prehospital provider must be aware that the severity and traumatic nature of an event is dependent upon the individual. For example, you may handle the death of a child much differently than your partner. An event becomes a crisis for an individual when the person's unique psychological coping mechanisms fail. There are no set criteria for when and where this may occur, and it differs significantly from one person to the next. You must always be prepared to look for the signs and symptoms of acute stress disorder following any traumatic event.

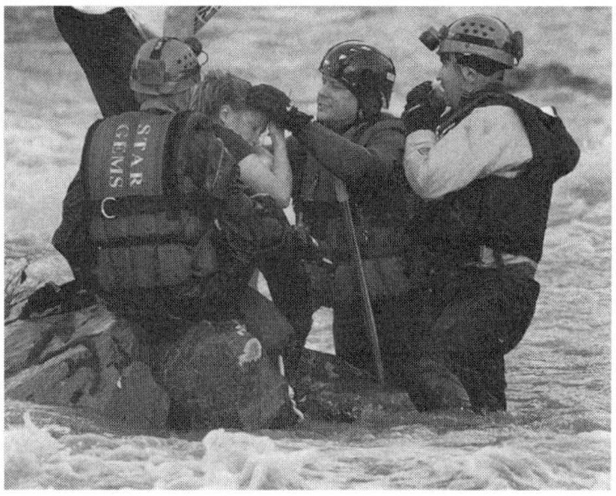

Figure 15-5 PTSD develops in patients who have experienced traumatic events.

Post-Traumatic Stress Disorder

Post-traumatic stress disorder (PTSD) is not a new disorder, even though it first appeared in the *DSM-IV-TR* only in 1980. Decades of American wars, most notably Vietnam, have produced generations of young Americans who returned stateside with a variety of symptoms indicating severe emotional and psychological trauma. Descriptors such as shell shock, combat stress, combat fatigue, and soldier's heart were used to describe this disorder in the decades before it was labeled as PTSD. Today we know that PTSD is one of the most severe and debilitating of all mental disorders. It is especially worrisome because it develops easily in individuals who have experienced severe traumatization. War produces its fair share of psychological victims. Estimates put the incidence of PTSD in Vietnam War veterans at anywhere from 25% to 70% of those who saw high concentrations of intense fighting, and there are indications that many veterans of the war in Iraq and Afghanistan are experiencing PTSD as well. Soldiers are not the only people who experience the disorder; environmental disasters such as Hurricane Katrina leave many victims suffering from the effects of PTSD, and people who have experienced assault, domestic or sexual violence, or rape may experience PTSD as well (**Figure 15-5**).

PTSD has many of the hallmark presentations of acute stress disorder. The difference is the chronic, unrelenting nature of PTSD. Individuals diagnosed with PTSD must suffer from symptoms of stress and anxiety for more than one month after a traumatic event. Often these patients present with symptoms for months or years if untreated and can spiral into extreme levels of despair and psychosis. Like acute stress disorder, patients suffering from PTSD have experienced some traumatic event for which they have been unable to compensate psychologically. They present with four types of unique, but equally important, symptoms. The patient will present with signs of **intrusion** and subsequent **avoidance**. The patient will experience intrusive, recurrent thoughts, dreams, or flashbacks that cannot be blocked or forgotten and thus will attempt to avoid situations that stimulate or trigger such thoughts. PTSD also includes symptoms such as **hyperarousal** and **numbing**. Hyperarousal is a condition of unusual and intense nervousness due to persistent stimulation of the autonomic nervous system. The patient will exhibit loss of interest in daily activities and suffer from otherwise unexplainable irritability and sleep loss. Numbing is an insensitivity that results in the individual feeling detached from reality. Individuals will often present with a relatively flat affect.

PTSD can be found in almost any individual as long as the individual has experienced some form of significant traumatic event. Statistically, it occurs in about 10% of the population. Prehospital providers working in disaster areas, such as those affected by hurricanes, tornadoes, or floods, must be constantly alert for the signs and symptoms of PTSD in both patients and providers. Likewise, EMS providers who work in systems with high call volumes, excessive violence, or trauma watch for signs of acute or chronic stress. In most cases, individuals and providers with the symptoms listed above should be referred to the agency's employee assistance program or to a private counselor for evaluation. It is common for fire, police, and EMS personnel to deny having any problems, so extra understanding and compassion may be needed as you try to assist them.

Generalized Anxiety Disorder

Generalized anxiety disorder (GAD) is a disorder marked by severe, often nonspecific anxiety that plagues an individual throughout most of his or her daily activities. Unlike the other anxiety disorders, GAD does not generally result from a specific stimulus. Individuals suffering from the disorder report an all-encompassing, unrelenting feeling of anxiety all of the time and may experience both physical and psychological symptoms similar to those of other anxiety disorders. Individuals with this disorder may report worrying about a specific aspect of their lives, say their finances, but when asked will report several other unrealistic and irrational worries. In some ways, GAD serves as a catchall for individuals who do not meet the criteria for any other anxiety disorder, but whose lives are adversely affected on a routine basis by overwhelming anxiety.

GAD is far more prevalent in women. Two thirds of the general population suffering from the disorder are women. GAD sufferers have a high comorbidity with other psychological problems, especially depressive disorders. It also happens to be one of the least studied and least understood of the anxiety disorders. Treatment is usually long-term and may last throughout the patient's lifetime. Individuals suffering from GAD will prove to be complex patients to work with in the field, mostly because there is no specific stimulus the emergency responder will be able to identify. This will significantly decrease avenues for which to provide assistance. Unlike the patient suffering from panic disorder or a phobia, there is no "safe place" for a GAD sufferer. Reassurance and understanding will be your best bet for handling these patients. Make every effort to help the person understand your actions and what your treatment plan is going to encompass. A calm and professional presentation is the best way to support your patient.

Management and Intervention

Treatment of patients suffering from anxiety disorders will almost always consist of supportive care. As a prehospital emergency provider you are not prepared to diagnose and treat these types of medical ailments; however, you can make a significant difference in the person's quality of life and self-image by showing empathy and respect in the field. For many patients, especially those who experience a sudden panic attack, you will be the first medical professional to witness and treat their disorder. At this stage, trust is the most important aspect of the provider-patient relationship. Like all mental illnesses, a thorough understanding will go a long way in accomplishing this task. Recognizing these disorders as severe, debilitating diseases is the first step. The second is to implement interventions quickly that will facilitate these patients getting the help they need as defined by their specific condition.

Most of the anxiety disorders will present with relatively harmless, albeit unusual symptoms.

In the Field

Tips for Establishing Rapport and Building Trust With Your Patient

- Exhibit professionalism at all times.
- Always be honest; getting caught in a lie will ruin your credibility and increase the patient's anxiety.
- Get at the patient's level and speak "with" the patient, not "at" the patient.
- Make good eye contact.
- Allow the patient to maintain as much control of the situation as possible.
- Follow through with the patient from start to finish. Don't downgrade patients or pass them off to other providers.
- No surprises! Tell patients exactly what you are doing and why you are doing it.

Panic disorder and panic attacks are an exception to this rule. Occasionally an individual suffering from a panic attack may suffer from a condition known as hyperventilation syndrome, or rapid breathing. Remember that panic attacks manifest themselves as many physical signs and symptoms. As an individual begins to experience extreme fear and panic, he or she may begin to hyperventilate. As this occurs, a series of physiologic changes will occur within the body that primarily affect blood pH. Rapid accelerated breathing causes the body to lose carbon dioxide, which in turn makes the blood extremely alkaline. This shift in blood pH leads to muscle cramping and tingling, or paresthesia, in the fingers and hands. If this becomes severe, the patient may pass out and the rate of respiration will return to normal. These feelings can often exacerbate the patient's belief that her or she is going to die and lead to extreme, terrifying fear. Hyperventilation is usually self-limiting and not life threatening. Coax the patient to consciously slow the rate and depth of breathing by using the 7-11 counting technique.

If the patient's anxiety and feelings of fear are relatively controlled, you can take a series of steps to ensure that the patient receives the proper care. Again, it is important to recognize the embarrassment that a patient may experience along with his or her mental illness. If you have reason to believe that a patient is suffering from an anxiety disorder, the SAFER-R model will be the most appropriate way to provide support to your patient in the field environment and will prove to be the most professional and effective means to encourage patients with anxiety disorders to seek further medical help.

Pharmacologic Considerations

In severe instances of some anxiety disorders, especially panic attacks, prehospital providers may have to resort to pharmacologic intervention in order to provide a safe environment for the patient. Anxiolytics such as Valium®, Versed®, or Ativan® may be warranted to control the patient's fear and anxiety. Anxiolytics should only be given as directed by your local protocol. Patients requiring long-term treatment will utilize a variety of pharmacologic methods and psychotherapy. Common prescription drug regimens include anxiolytics and selective serotonin reuptake inhibitors (SSRIs).

In the Field

Controlling Hyperventilation—7-11 Technique

The emergency responder can use several techniques to help a patient with hyperventilation syndrome to regain control of his or her breathing. Patients can try to slow their respirations by breathing in slowly for 7 seconds and breathing out for 11 seconds.

SAFER-R for Anxiety Disorders

Stabilize: Ensure that other life-threatening problems have been corrected. If the patient is experiencing a panic attack, attempt to calm the patient. Assure the person that help has arrived and that you are willing to listen to the problem.

Acknowledge: Acknowledge that there is a problem. If a critical, traumatic, or triggering event has occurred, acknowledge that the person's behavior is a reaction to the event, regardless of the perceived severity. Make an effort to understand the trigger. If the attack has no identifiable trigger, be empathetic to the patient's condition and recognize that an anxiety disorder may be present.

Facilitate: Attempt to understand the patient's feelings. Remember that the anxiety and fear common among anxiety disorders can be terrifying. If you suspect a trigger, quickly move the patient to a neutral location such as the back of the ambulance. Assure the patient that he or she is safe and ask what the patient would like you to do.

Encourage: If the patient does not wish to seek immediate help, encourage the person to so before the next attack occurs. Anxiety disorders can become more debilitating if left untreated. Explain your concerns to the patient, along with the consequences of the patient's decision. If necessary, offer to make phone calls to family or friends who may be supportive in the treatment and recovery process.

Recovery: If this is a patient that you see frequently, look for signs of recovery. Have the symptoms progressively increased or decreased? Has the patient's quality of life changed for the better or worse?

Referral: If signs of recovery are absent, consider referring the patient for further treatment. Provide the patient with information on local social and psychiatric services. It is important to realize when to transfer the patient to a more specialized health care professional. The emergency department social worker can be a good referral source for the patient.

Final Thoughts

As with all patients experiencing mental disorders, safety is *always* your primary concern. Most individuals with anxiety disorders can be managed easily in the field environment. However, if you feel endangered at any time, request police assistance immediately.

The role of the prehospital provider is to help stabilize the patient so he or she can be transported to definitive care. Unlike patients with respiratory or diabetic conditions, an ampule or syringe of medication will not correct long-term problems for patients suffering from anxiety disorders. Many of the anxiety disorders such as OCD or PTSD will require years of counseling to correct the condition. Professional and compassionate care is the first line of attack for these conditions.

Selected References

American Psychiatric Association: *Diagnostic and Statistical Manual of Mental Disorders, Fourth Edition, Text Revision (DSM-IV-TR)*. Washington, DC, American Psychiatric Association, 2000.

Anxiety Disorder Association of America (n.d.): Statistics and facts about anxiety disorders. Available at: http://www.adaa.org/AboutADAA/PressRoom/Stats&Facts.asp. Accessed March 10, 2007.

Bringager CB, Dammen T, Friss S: Nonfearful panic disorder in chest pain patients. *Psychosomatics*, 2004;45:69–79.

Chamberlain SR, Blackwell AD, Fineberg NA, Robbins TW, Sahakian BJ: The neuropsychology of obsessive compulsive disorder: the importance of failures, cognitive and behavioural inhibition as candidate encephenotypic markers. *Neurosci Biobehav Rev*, 2005;29:399–419.

Halgin HP, Whitbourne SK: *Abnormal Psychology: Clinical Perspectives on Psychological Disorders*, ed 5. New York, NY, McGraw-Hill, 2007.

McPhee ST, Papadakis MA, Tierney LM Jr: *Current Medical Diagnosis and Treatment*, ed 46. New York, NY, McGraw-Hill, 2007.

National Institutes of Mental Health: Anxiety disorders. Available at: http://www.nimh.nih.gov/publicat/anxiety.cfm. Accessed March 10, 2007.

Prep Kit

Ready for Review

- Anxiety is the sense of fear, apprehension, or worry about something terrible happening in the near or distant future.
- Everyone experiences some type of anxiety at some point in life. The conditions discussed in this chapter are anxiety conditions that have the ability to become overwhelming and to debilitate the patient.
- Individuals with anxiety or panic disorders will present with a variety of symptoms that will mimic other medical conditions. Heart palpitations, sweating, trembling, shortness of breath, chest pain, and nausea are all classic presentations for many illnesses. A thorough assessment and history is necessary to provide the appropriate care to your patient.
- Stress disorders can be either acute or chronic. In most cases, they result in some form of psychological intrusion, including flashbacks or visions of an event or situation, that causes anxiety.

Vital Vocabulary

acrophobia Irrational fear of heights.

acute stress disorder An anxiety disorder that develops after a traumatic event, with symptoms such as depersonalization, numbing, dissociative amnesia, intense anxiety, hypervigilance, and impairment of everyday functioning that last for less than one month after a stressor.

agoraphobia The intense fear of being trapped, stranded, or embarrassed in a situation without help if a panic attack were to occur; also the fear of open spaces.

akathisia A feeling of restlessness, having to constantly move or leave.

anxiety The sense of fear, apprehension, or worrying about something terrible happening in the near or distant future.

anxiety disorder A class of mental health disorders characterized by irrational fear and intense anxiety that leads to significant detriment to an individual's quality of life.

aversion Normal response of discomfort or dislike to a particular object or situation.

avoidance A type of intrusive symptom commonly seen in PTSD in which the traumatic event is so distressing that the individual attempts to avoid contact with those things or people that may trigger memories of the event.

claustrophobia The fear of being in small or confined spaces.

compulsion Repetitive behaviors, either observable or mental, that are intended to reduce the anxiety engendered by obsessions.

flashback A symptom commonly seen in PTSD in which the individual re-experiences or relives a traumatic event as though he or she were actually there.

generalized anxiety disorder (GAD) An anxiety disorder characterized by anxiety that is not associated with a particular object, situation, or event but seems to be a constant feature of a person's day-to-day existence.

germophobia See mysophobia.

hyperarousal A condition of unusual and intense nervousness due to persistent stimulation of the autonomic nervous system; commonly seen as a sign of PTSD.

hyperventilation syndrome An episodic disorder wherein the individual breathes faster than normal.

intrusion A condition caused by traumatic events where unpleasant thoughts or memories cannot be ignored or supressed.

mysophobia The irrational fear of harmful pathogens such as viruses and bacteria.

numbing Insensitivity to outside stimulation.

obsession Intrusive, recurrent, unwanted ideas, thoughts, or impulses that are difficult to dismiss, despite their disturbing nature.

obsessive-compulsive disorder (OCD) An anxiety disorder characterized by recurrent obsessions or compulsions that are inordinately

Prep Kit | continued

time-consuming or that cause significant distress or impairment.

panic attacks Periods of time marked by intense fear, opposition, and physical discomfort in which an individual feels helpless or as if he or she is about to lose control or even die.

panic disorder An anxiety disorder in which an individual has recurrent panic attacks or has apprehension about the possibility of future attacks.

post traumatic stress disorder (PTSD) An anxiety disorder in which the individual experiences several distressing symptoms for more than a month following a traumatic event, such as re-experiencing the traumatic event, avoiding reminders of the trauma, numbing of general responsiveness, and increasing arousal.

situational bound (cued) panic attack A form of panic attack that occurs immediately following the exposure to, or anticipation of, some event, trigger, or situational stimulus.

situationally predisposed panic attack A form of panic attack that is similar to situationally bound panic attacks but does not occur every time the individual is exposed to a trigger.

social phobia Anxiety disorder characterized by an irrational and constant fear of being scrutinized by one's peers or strangers, causing the individual to feel extreme embarrassment in social situations.

specific phobia An irrational and unabating fear of a particular object, activity, or situation.

trypanophobia The fear of medical procedures or medical injections.

traumatic experience Any event that has disastrous psychological and/or physical consequences for the person involved; it may include witnessing others' distress.

unexpected (uncued) panic attack A form of panic attack that occurs suddenly and without warning and is not associated with an internal or external situational trigger.

Assessment in Action

Answer key is located in the back of the book.

The "Assessment in Action" for this chapter is based on the following case scenario.

Bobby, a 36-year-old construction worker, has developed anxiety-like symptoms while at work. These symptoms have been bothering Bobby for about a year. He cannot explain what brings on these feelings, but when he recognizes that he is feeling them he has to immediately stop whatever he is doing. Bobby is unable to put a finger on exactly how he is feeling. The only symptom he is sure of having is a feeling like his heart skips a beat.

On a summer day Bobby was in his neighbor's yard helping with some housework. While walking toward a shaded area he suddenly developed an intense fear accompanied by physical discomfort. Bobby's neighbor decided to call 911 after he saw Bobby slouched in a nearby chair.

After your arrival, Bobby states that he felt fearful but couldn't say exactly what he was scared of. He described a feeling of high anxiety followed by heart palpitations, sweating, shaking, nausea, vomiting, and crushing chest pain. You decide that this patient may need a cardiac workup. You immediately take a 12-lead electrocardiograph to rule out a myocardial infarction. Further investigation, including a proper cardiac workup, reveals no indication of myocardial infarction.

1. Based on the presentation of symptoms, you suspect which of the following conditions?

   A. Social phobia
   B. Post traumatic stress disorder
   C. Panic attack with agoraphobia
   D. Panic disorder

2. In this case, the emergency responder might initially want to diagnose the patient as experiencing general anxiety disorder (GAD), even though that is not the situation here. Which of the following statements is false?

   A. GAD is pervasive throughout most of the day.
   B. GAD does not result from a specific stimulus.
   C. GAD is often a catchall diagnosis when the patient fails to meet other criteria.
   D. GAD presents as a fear of being trapped should an attack occur.

3. Which signs or symptoms would not suggest that a cardiac evaluation was appropriate?

   A. The skipping of his heartbeat
   B. The fear that occurred when walking toward his house
   C. Nausea and vomiting
   D. Crushing chest pain

4. Given the presentation, you would anticipate future calls to this residence for possible suicide attempts.

   A. True
   B. False

5. The best treatment for Bobby would be

   _____.

   A. sedation with an antianxiety medication
   B. calm, compassionate care
   C. supportive care such as rebreathing or oxygen at low flow until you determine the cause of Bobby's condition
   D. b and c are both correct

Chapter 16

Dissociative Disorders

The concept of <u>dissociation</u> can be very difficult to understand. Simply put, it means to cease associating with someone or something, or to separate. In the context of mental illness, it refers to people whose memory processes may be impaired. Emergency responders will interact with patients who dissociate for various reasons on a regular basis. Patients suffering from dissociative disorders often present with amnesia or different personalities that will challenge your interviewing techniques and ability to obtain a thorough history.

Background

The *DSM-IV-TR* defines a dissociative disorder as a "disruption in the usually integrated functions of consciousness, memory, identity, or perception of the environment." Dissociative disorders are typically linked to trauma, especially childhood trauma and abuse. Other traumatic events that trigger dissociative episodes include war, high stress, kidnapping, torture, natural disaster, invasive medical procedures, and financial problems.

The *DSM-IV-TR* identifies five distinct categories of dissociative disorders. Conditions that will be discussed in this chapter are:

- Dissociative amnesia
- Dissociative fugue
- Dissociative identity disorder

- Depersonalization disorder
- Dissociative disorder not otherwise specified (NOS)

Dissociative disorder is a broad diagnosis that encompasses one of the five disorders previously listed. Additionally, dissociative disorders have five characteristics in common:

- Dissociative episodes have sudden onset and termination.
- Episodes are often triggered by stressors.
- Severe gaps in memory (except in depersonalization disorder) may occur.
- The patient may experience difficulty functioning or a feeling of distress.
- The condition may be idiopathic, meaning that the disorder is not caused by drug use, an underlying medical condition, or another psychological disorder.

> ## SAMPLE History for Dissociative Disorders
>
> **Signs and symptoms:** Confusion and disorientation are common. Patients may confabulate or make up a story to fill in gaps in memory.
>
> **Allergies:** Allergies can exist for any medication, many of which will cause confusion.
>
> **Medications:** Some patients with dissociative disorders take amobarbital, a barbiturate, to relieve anxiety and help with insomnia. This will be particularly important if you administer any other medications.
>
> **Past medical history:** Medical history will vary. This may be the first reported episode, or there may be documentation of previous occurrences. Document any psychological trauma that is reported.
>
> **Last oral intake:** May be unobtainable, depending upon the patient's level of dissociation.
>
> **Events leading up to today's event:** Assess to determine if EMS was called for an acute or chronic condition. Prior events are usually a stressful or traumatic situation. The patient may or may not be able to recall the event. The provider should include where the patient was found.

Assessment

As with all prehospital environments, the safety of the prehospital providers is essential. In order to assess the patient successfully, keep in mind that scene control and the reduction of stimuli are the best ways of handling a patient with a dissociative disorder. Another key for managing patients with dissociative disorders is to remember that these are true psychological conditions. The person may dissociate into multiple personalities, exhibit amnesia, or not know where he or she is or how he or she arrived at the present location.

As we will discuss later, you will see that patients with dissociative identity disorder (DID), formerly known as multiple personality disorder, may have some psychotic and/or violent personalities that may require restraint and/or additional resources. In most cases, a patient with DID will not become violent unless he or she feels threatened, so a calm, safe environment is paramount. This can usually be accomplished by maintaining a nonthreatening distance, remaining professional, and minimizing stimulation (**Figure 16-1**). Some patients, particularly those with a condition known as dissociative fugue, are prone to outbursts of violence, so extra human resources or the administration of physical or chemical restraints may be necessary.

As always, assessment tools such as the SAMPLE and OPQRST history will provide you with useful information. The SEA-3 mental status examination is also a great way to document the EMS provider's findings.

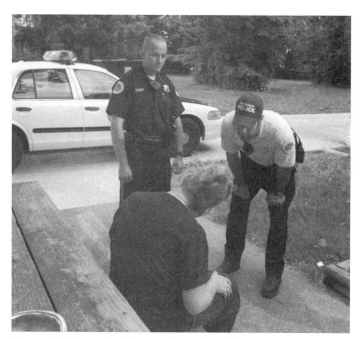

Figure 16-1 It is important to maintain a nonthreatening distance when assisting patients with dissociative disorders.

OPQRST for Dissociative Disorders

Onset: When did the symptoms begin? The onset of the dissociative episode is usually sudden.

Provocation: Provoking factors in a dissociative episode are external stimuli. Examples of external factors that can worsen the episode are lights, noises, and many people in confined spaces.

Quality: How pervasive or significant are the patient's feelings and emotions at the time of assessment?

Radiation: Is the state of confusion experienced by the patient radiating out to family members, neighbors, or others? Has it affected important components of the patient's life such as employment, or simply the patient's ability to live alone?

Severity: Have the patient rate his or her current psychological distress with a 1-to-10 scale. In most cases of dissociative disorders, the family and friends of the patient are more distressed than the patient about the loss of memory and/or the state of dissociation.

Time: The timeline of the episode is important. How much time is unaccounted for? How long has the patient been feeling this way?

SEA-3 for Dissociative Disorders

Speech: The amplitude, quality, flow, and organization of speech may change with dissociative identity disorder as the patient changes among identities.

Emotion: The full spectrum ranges from inappropriate emotion for the time and place to depression, anger, hostility, confusion, apprehension, anxiety, fear, and absence of emotion.

Appearance: The patient may have an unusual facial expression and may look confused or dazed because of the dissociation.

Alertness: The patient may still have intellectual function and cognitive thought, although memory and orientation to person, place, and time may be distorted or absent.

Activity: The patient may exhibit anything from normal behavior to possible outbursts of violence, varying with the type of dissociative disorder.

Dissociative Amnesia

Dissociative amnesia is a condition in which the individual has lost some component of his or her memory. This disorder is usually triggered by an extremely stressful or traumatic event (**Figure 16-2**). The event is so traumatic that it causes the patient to be unable to recall personal information. There are several types of memory disturbances that have been labeled as dissociative amnesias, specifically (1) selective amnesia, (2) generalized amnesia, (3) localized amnesia, (4) continuous amnesia, and (5) systematized amnesia.

The patient presenting with selective amnesia can recall the traumatic event, but cannot recall the parts of that event that he or she found disturbing. For example, the patient remembers being in a ferry crash, but the patient cannot remember witnessing the death of a friend.

In the case of generalized amnesia, the patient cannot recall any personal information. The patient retains all learned behaviors, habits, tastes, and skills, but the patient cannot recall who he or she is. The patient would still be able to ride a bike, write, read, and any and all other learned behaviors but would be unable to give a correct name, address, or any other personal identifying information. Despite the frequency with which dissociative amnesia appears in soap operas, it is very rare for a patient to be unable to recall all personally identifying information.

With continuous amnesia, the patient cannot recall anything following an incident. This is another rare form of dissociative amnesia. The patient remembers all information he or she had learned prior to the incident but has become unable to learn new information. The patient has difficulty functioning because of the inability to learn new information, which causes impairment with school, work, and social life. The patient may be able to continue working at the current job because he or she already learned how to perform the required skills prior to the incident, but the person could not change positions or move up in the workforce because of the inability to learn new skills.

Localized amnesia, the most common type of dissociative amnesia, occurs when the patient cannot recall the specific time period in which the stressful or traumatic event occurred. The patient has no recollection of the traumatic event. An example of localized amnesia is a survivor of a mass-casualty incident who cannot recall the time period surrounding the incident. The patient may have localized amnesia of the event for anywhere from hours to years. In some cases, this form of amnesia can be permanent.

Systematized amnesia is when the patient cannot recall all information about one aspect of life such as work, family, or personal relationships, as if the one aspect never existed in the patient's mind. An example would be a patient who has no recollection of her ex-boyfriend as the result of a very emotional breakup. She would not recall the person, that they dated, or any event that occurred while with that person. Systematized amnesia is a rarely seen form of dissociative amnesia.

Dissociative Fugue

<u>Dissociative fugue</u> occurs when an individual suddenly and unexpectedly leaves a location and is unable to recall past personal information. Because of the inability to recall personal information, the patient may become confused about his or her identity or assume a new identity. In order to function despite the loss of personal information, the individual may not think about the past or may <u>confabulate</u> or make up events to replace the lost memories.

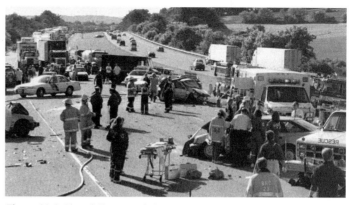

Figure 16-2 Dissociative amnesia is usually triggered by an extremely stressful or traumatic event.

Dissociative fugue often follows a stressful event, such as a natural disaster in which the person is fleeing for his or her life. The person quickly leaves home and is unable to recall any past personal information.

It is very unlikely that the prehospital provider would be dispatched for a patient "diagnosed" with this disorder. Instead, you would probably be sent to evaluate a person who is experiencing altered mental status. This form of amnesia may initially present with symptoms that would seem to indicate that the patient is under the influence of a substance, is diabetic, or is suffering from a brain lesion. However, by performing a good history and physical examination, you will in most cases come up with a perfectly healthy individual who simply cannot remember how he or she ended up where you found the person. It should be noted that patients diagnosed as having or showing signs of dissociative fugue may be prone to outbursts of violence, so extra precautions should be taken for your safety, including involving law enforcement or keeping a safe distance when necessary.

Dissociative Identity Disorder

<u>Dissociative identity disorder (DID)</u>, formerly called *multiple personality disorder,* is diagnosed when a patient has two or more personalities. The creation of additional personalities may occur for various reasons. Multiple personalities may serve as an outlet for patients to express their true feelings or as a coping mechanism in stressful situations. Only one personality reacts with the environment at a time; however, the separate personalities may be either aware or unaware that the other personalities exist. The patient may deny knowledge of a second personality but report hearing voices. The change between personalities is sudden and often triggered by a stressful event. In most cases, the separate personality is aware of the lost time while the other personality was in control and may be extremely distressed because of it.

The types of personalities vary among patients. They may include a dominant personality, a subordinate personality, personalities of varying age, including children, personalities of the opposite gender, and/or a "protector" personality. Some of the personalities may be psychotic and/or violent. The protector personality typically takes over when the patient feels threatened. Patients with dissociative identity disorders often have a wide array of other conditions that have an unknown cause or are idiopathic in nature and linked to the disorder. The conditions include amnesia, depression, suicidal ideation, anxiety, panic attacks, and episodes of depersonalization. The patient may have varying medical conditions and even different vital signs for each personality, all of which are completely real.

It is extremely important that the prehospital provider does not attempt to provoke or contact the various personalities. This is an extremely complex condition that is sometimes unpredictable even in controlled environments. For example, a patient may have been repeatedly sexually and physically abused as a child, and, as a result of intense abuse and emotional pain, the patient's mind attempts to protect itself from further harm. In doing so, it develops various personalities that may talk to each other to try to prevent further injury. If the patient feels threatened, the defensive personality may come forward and confront you. This could include assaulting you as you are taking a blood pressure, securing the patient to the stretcher, or starting an intravenous line.

Depersonalization Disorder

Depersonalization disorder is characterized by a feeling of detachment from oneself in the form of derealization episodes. A derealization episode is characterized by a feeling that the outside world is unreal or strange. The patient is aware that the derealization episode is not real. It often presents as a distorted view of objects' shape and size. The patient may also have the sense that other people are robotic or lifeless in nature. Derealization episodes often occur in the late teens and early 20s and are triggered by a stressor. They often start and end quickly, so they may not impair everyday function.

Patients often report that they sometimes detach from themselves or their body, even to a point that they feel that they are floating or living in a dream or movie. An individual may even tell an emergency responder that he or she feels as if he or she is going crazy. In order to manage these patients, simple reassurance and compassionate care will suffice until you arrive at an emergency department for evaluation.

Dissociative Disorder Not Otherwise Specified (NOS)

The *DSM-IV-TR* uses very detailed criteria when outlining a diagnosis of a mental disorder, such as age of onset or length of symptoms. Nevertheless, there are cases that have some of the characteristics of a disorder but do not meet all of the criteria for a definitive diagnosis. Dissociative disorder not otherwise specified (NOS) is diagnosed when a patient does not meet the full criteria for the other dissociative disorders but demonstrates some of the characteristics of derealization. Examples include brainwashing, Ganser's syndrome, and dissociative trance disorder.

An individual who has been subjected to prolonged periods of intense coercive mental persuasion is commonly said to be brainwashed. Brainwashing is a process that, after time, will actually alter the mental pathways and the way a person thinks. Brainwashed patients are often seen following prolonged capture in prison camps, after spending time in religious cults, or when placed in situations demanding severe thought reform.

Ganser's syndrome is an unusual condition in which the patient gives answers that appear deliberately false. With this condition, the patient is incapable of giving a correct or appropriate answer to the question asked. For example, if you were to ask the patient the color of the sky, the patient might respond that it is red, even though it is a clear and sunny day outside and the sky is obviously blue. Patients with Ganser's syndrome have a form of dissociation that only pertains to answering questions.

Dissociative trance disorder is not common in the United States. Dissociative trance is often associated with spiritual beliefs in which the individual sharpens awareness of the immediate surroundings and engages in stereotyped behaviors or movements. The person takes on a new identity that is often attributed to divine intervention followed by amnesia of the event. One similar event in the United States is a vision quest, a cultural practice of Native Americans. In some Native American cultures, teenage boys participate in a vision quest as a rite to manhood. The vision quest requires the participant go into a form of dissociative trance; however, the person remembers the event. Because the activity is intentional and the person does not have amnesia after the event, a vision quest is not classified as a dissociative trance disorder.

Prehospital Management

Patients with dissociative disorders may require the provider to use a different approach to medical assessment. Because the person may see and hear things as unreal or strange, stimuli may be exaggerated and cause more anxiety and stress. Providing a calm, safe, and uncrowded assessment area for the patient should reduce anxiety, stress, and fear (**Figure 16-3**).

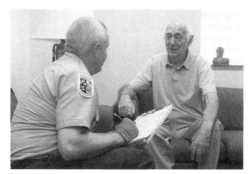

Figure 16-3 Providing a calm, safe environment is essential when interviewing patients suffering from dissociative disorders.

Because dissociative disorders are characterized by a distorted view of objects and individuals, it is vital that the providers identify themselves as health care professionals who are there to help. Explanation prior to and during any medical assessment is critical; patients with dissociative disorders are stressed, anxious, and fearful, and they may misunderstand the provider's intent. The patient may take the provider's intentions as hostile, causing the patient to become violent toward the provider. The SAFER-R model is a good tool for managing the dissociative patient.

Acknowledge that a stressful event has occurred and that the patient is having a normal response to an abnormal event. The provider should understand that this is an abnormal event and express concern and a willingness to help the patient.

Simply talking with the patient and finding out what would make the current episode better or worse for the patient can be extremely helpful. The patient and provider may decide to limit stimuli, remove the patient from the stressful environment, and/or seek psychiatric assistance. Including the patient when building a plan helps to calm the patient and gives him or her a sense of control.

In most cases, you should be able to get a patient who has been diagnosed with a dissociative disorder refocused within 15 to 30 minutes. Because these are rarely emergencies, you can make attempts at simply reorienting the patient to person, place, and time. Often the initial step is to get the patient to recognize that he or she is having some type of disruption in the function of consciousness, memory, identity, or perception of the environment. Once the patient has recognized that he or she is experiencing a dissociative episode and is safe, you can move toward transporting the patient to the emergency department. If the patient fails to reorient after a few minutes, simply explain that you need to take him or her to a medical facility for evaluation.

In rare cases, some patients will require physical restraints. Avoid physical restraints whenever possible; documentation has shown that many patients have suffered broken bones and injured muscles while trying to get untied from ambulance stretchers.

Pharmacologic Interventions

Rarely will the prehospital provider need to medicate a patient in order to accomplish transportation to the emergency

SAFER-R Field Intervention for Dissociative Disorders

Stabilize: Create a calm environment by presenting yourself with a professional demeanor. Offer words of support that will make the patient and family feel safe.

Acknowledge: Assess and recognize the current situation by gathering information.

Facilitate: Understand the situation by determining if cognitive processes are intact or disturbed. Begin thinking about what type of help the patient and family need.

Encourage: Continue to build rapport with the patient and family by attempting to reorient the patient and move him or her toward transportation and definitive care.

Recovery: Reinforce the treatment and transportation plan with the patient.

Referral: Assist the family by suggesting community contacts such as local mental health agencies sponsored by city, county, or state social services.

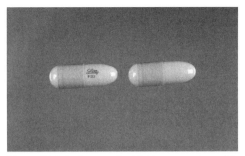

Figure 16-4 Sodium amobarbital is commonly used to treat dissociative disorders in the outpatient setting.

department. However, if the patient becomes violent, chemical restraint using some form of tranquilizer, such as diazepam (Valium®), or an antipsychotic, such as haloperidol (Haldol®), may be administered according to local protocol.

One prescription medication is of particular importance to the prehospital provider. Sodium amobarbital (Amytal®) is commonly administered for the treatment of dissociative disorders (**Figure 16-4**). Amobarbital is classified as a sedative-hypnotic with analgesic properties. It is the drug of choice for the treatment of dissociative disorders, because it releases the patient's inhibitions while calming the patient enough to allow for the recollection of the traumatic event. Because of the actions of the medication, patients may appear groggy or sleepy during transport.

Patients with dissociative disorders are prone to suicidal ideation, so an overdose of sodium amobarbital is possible and must be considered during your evaluation. Symptoms of overdose of sodium amobarbital include severe confusion and drowsiness, decreased or loss of reflexes, fever, irritability, poor judgment, shortness of breath, bradycardia, slurred speech, trouble sleeping, extrapyramidal eye movements, and severe weakness. Additionally, there is a long list of drugs that may interact with sodium amobarbital. If you identify any of the medications in **Table 16-1**, you may wish to consult with your local poison control center to see if the patient's presentation is related to a drug interaction.

Table 16-1 Medications That Interact With Amobarbital Intoxication and Withdrawal

- Alcohol
- Antiarrhythmics
- Antidepressants
- Antiepileptics
- Antihistamines
- Antihypertensives
- Benzodiazepines
- Caffeine
- Chloramphenicol
- Chlorpromazine
- Cyclophosphamide
- Cyclosporin
- Digitoxin
- Doxorubicin
- Doxycycline
- Methoxyflurane
- Metronidazole
- Narcotic analgesics
- Quinine
- Steroids
- Theophylline

Final Thoughts

Dissociative episodes are almost always triggered by a stressful or traumatic event, so removing the patient from that environment to a calm and nonthreatening environment is the best course of action for the emergency medical service provider. The request for extra manpower may be necessary with dissociative patients of a more violent nature to ensure the safety of the provider. Proper documentation of patients experiencing a dissociative episode is important, because emergency medical service providers are often the first to evaluate the patient. All physical assessment and environmental findings should be included in the report, as this is helpful to the receiving facility as well as a first step in the patient's treatment.

Selected References

American Psychiatric Association: *Diagnostic and Statistical Manual of Mental Disorders, Fourth Edition, Text Revision (DSM-IV-TR)*. Washington, DC, American Psychiatric Press, 2000.

Comer JR: *Fundamentals of Abnormal Psychology*, ed 3. New York, NY, Worth Publishers, 2002.

Morrison J: *DSM-IV Made Easy*. New York, NY, The Guilford Press, 1995.

Mosby's Medical, Nursing, and Allied Health Dictionary, ed 4. St Louis, MO, Elsevier, 1994.

Nevid S, Jeffrey R, Spencer A, Greene B: *Abnormal Psychology in a Changing World*, ed 4. New Jersey, Prentice Hall, 2000.

Prep Kit

Ready for Review

- Dissociative disorders are a disruption in the usually integrated functions of consciousness, memory, identity, and perception of the environment.
- Although these disorders may be unusual and difficult to understand, they are not life threatening to the patient.
- There are five types of dissociative amnesia discussed in this chapter: selective, generalized, localized, continuous, and systematized. Many of these involve either psychological or physical trauma.
- The feeling of detachment from oneself is known as depersonalization.
- Because patients with dissociative disorders may be confused at times, you should exhibit patience as you interview and attempt to reorient them to their current location and situation.

Vital Vocabulary

confabulation The fabrication of events or experiences to fill in gaps in memory.

continuous amnesia A form of dissociative amnesia in which the individual cannot recall anything following a traumatic incident and becomes unable to learn new information, often resulting in impairment in the person's school, work or social life.

depersonalization disorder Condition characterized by a persistent or recurrent feeling of being detached from one's mental processes or body that is accompanied by intact reality testing.

derealization A feeling that the outside world is unreal or strange.

dissociate To cease associating with or to separate.

dissociative amnesia Condition characterized by an inability to recall important personal information, usually of a traumatic or stressful nature, that is too extensive to be explained by ordinary forgetfulness.

dissociative disorder not otherwise specified (NOS) Condition in which the predominant feature is a dissociative symptom, but does not meet the criteria for any specific dissociative disorder.

dissociative fugue Condition characterized by sudden, unexpected travel away from home or one's customary place of work, accompanied by an inability to recall one's past and confusion about personal identity or the assumption of a new identity.

dissociative identity disorder (DID) Condition characterized by the presence of two or more distinct identities or personality states that recurrently take control of the individual's behavior, accompanied by an inability to recall important personal information; the condition is too extensive to be explained by ordinary forgetfulness. It is a disorder characterized by identity fragmentation rather than a proliferation of separate personalities.

dissociative trance disorder A rarely seen condition where a person enters a trance-like state for the purpose of sharpening one's awareness to their immediate surroundings, often taking on a new identity during the trance; commonly seen in religious or spiritual ceremonies.

Ganser's syndrome An unusual condition in which the patient gives answers that appear deliberately false.

generalized amnesia A form of dissociative amnesia in which the individual cannot remember any personal information such as name or address or other personal identifying information.

idiopathic Arising from an unknown cause.

localized amnesia A common form of dissociative amnesia in which the individual cannot recall the specific time period in which a stressful or traumatic event occurred.

selective amnesia A form of dissociative amnesia in which the individual can recall a traumatic event, but is unable to remember specific parts of the trauma that are particularly disturbing.

Prep Kit | continued

systematized amnesia A form of dissociative amnesia in which the individual cannot recall all of the information about one specific aspect of their life such as work, family, or personal relationships.

Assessment in Action

Answer key is located in the back of the book.

1. Dissociative disorders have five characteristics that are common among them. From the following list, select the one does NOT belong to this group of disorders.

   A. They usually present with sudden onset and termination.
   B. The cause is generally unknown or idiopathic.
   C. Episodes are triggered by stressful events in the person's life.
   D. Individuals will experience syncopal episodes and become unresponsive for 15 to 30 minutes.

2. While interviewing a patient who is alert and oriented, you ask the patient to add 2 and 2. He responds with the answer 5. Given a medical history of dissociative disorder, you suspect which of the following?

   A. Ganser's syndrome
   B. Dissociative identity disorder
   C. Depersonalization
   D. Dissociative fugue

3. From the following list, select the one patient who may be prone to violent outbursts.

   A. Dissociative identity disorder
   B. Depersonalization disorder
   C. Systematized amnesia
   D. Dissociative fugue

4. There are various types of amnesia. From the following list, select the one that is most common and is diagnosed when the patient cannot recall the specific time period in which the stressful or traumatic event occurred.

   A. Continuous
   B. Localized
   C. Selective
   D. Generalized

5. Many patients who have lapses in memory will make up events or fill in the gaps with stories about events that never occurred. This process is known as _____.

   A. perseveration
   B. illusion
   C. confabulation
   D. delusion

Chapter 17

Eating Disorders

The American Psychiatric Association recognizes <u>eating</u> <u>disorders</u> as diagnosable mental illnesses that present with possible life-threatening medical consequences. Research has shown that more than 90% of those experiencing eating disorders have been young women between the ages of 12 and 25 years. However, in recent years, that percentage has shifted to include older women and more men and boys. A study of Division I National Collegiate Athletic Association athletes reported that more than one third of females were at risk of <u>anorexia nervosa</u>, a condition in which the individual refuses to maintain a healthy body weight (**Figure 17-1**). Male athletes who participate in sports that focus on diet, appearance, or size and weight requirements, such as wrestling, are also at high risk for eating disorders.

Statistically, anorexia nervosa has one of the highest death rates of any of the mental disorders. Most individuals with eating disorders make every effort to keep their body weight below a minimal normal level through excessive exercise, control of food intake, and other means. It is common for individuals with eating disorders to limit food intake to the point of starvation, engage in <u>bingeing</u> and <u>purging</u>, induce vomiting, or use <u>laxatives</u> to lose weight.

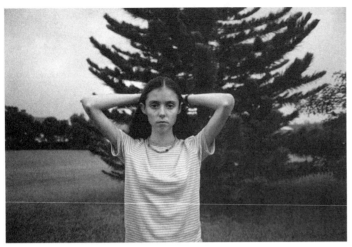

Figure 17-1 Eating disorders have possibly life-threatening medical consequences.

Background

Eating disorders are sometimes difficult for the prehospital provider to understand. The medical community itself did not widely recognize eating disorders until 1980, following the death of pop singer Karen Carpenter at the age of 30 years old. Though more prevalent in the late 20th century, some eating disorders, particularly anorexia nervosa, were described more than 300 years ago, when cultural pressures were very different than today.

Organizations and researchers often find it difficult to report statistics surrounding eating disorders accurately, because many people remain either hidden or difficult to diagnose. It is suspected that actual numbers are significantly higher, especially among males. Several national organizations such as Anorexia Nervosa and Related Eating Disorders, Inc., American Anorexia/Bulimia Association, Inc., and National Depressive and Manic-Depressive Association collect data and compile statistics on eating disorders. They report that overall in the United States approximately 8 million people suffer from some form of eating disorder, and females make up 90% to 95% of those experiencing anorexia. About 30% to 50% of anorectics (ie, people with anorexia) also exhibit signs of bulimia nervosa or bulimia. Estimates show that 2% to 5% of anorectics will commit suicide, and 10% to 15% will die from the disease. Males are 10% to 15% of the population suffering from bulimia. Often these men are athletes who need to meet weight requirements, such as wrestlers and jockeys.

This chapter discusses three common eating disorders:

- anorexia nervosa
- bulimia nervosa
- binge-eating disorder

What Causes an Eating Disorder?

To understand the cause of an eating disorder, one must first understand the individual. Many people with an eating disorder also experience other conditions such as depression, anxiety, or substance abuse. The National Eating Disorder Association outlines four factors that contribute to the development of eating disorders: psychological, interpersonal, social, and biological.

The *psychological factor* is related to how the patient views himself or herself in the world. It is common for individuals to have feelings of low self-esteem and inadequacy. Patients report that they lack control in their lives and suffer from feelings of loneliness, depression, anxiety, or anger. Patients believe that controlling food intake is one way to regain or reclaim control, and many patients tie feelings of self-worth to their ability to maintain this control.

Many patients with eating disorders will have long histories of troubled family and personal relationships. These *interpersonal factors* may result in the individual feeling that he or she cannot talk or express his or her true feelings about situations with peers and loved ones. Women who have been physically or sexually abused particularly fall into this category. Others in this category include those with a history of being teased or tormented about their size or weight.

The *social factor* has been the focus of news reports in recent years, following the deaths of several professional models. Although some fashion designers and modeling agencies now require a minimum body mass index for models there continues to be great pressure on models to be extremely thin. This affects both the models themselves and women in general, as society expects women to conform to this unhealthy body shape.

Biological factors may also contribute to the development of eating disorders. Although it is known that eating disorders run in some families, it is not always possible to identify why this occurs. In recent years, scientists have identified specific neurotransmitters, such as norepinephrine and serotonin, that may control hunger, appetite, and digestion. These neurotransmitters often are out of balance in the individual with an eating disorder. Scientists have also identified significant genetic markers that are linked to eating disorders, especially among monozygotic twins.

Assessment

Family members will often initiate the emergency call in cases involving eating disorders, because patients tend to deny that the condition exists. Many patients with eating disorders experience a comorbid depression. The loss of control over their eating and their habits will often lead to severe distress between the patient and their family members and friends. Isolation is a common trait seen in these individuals.

Gathering information can be difficult, because patients suffering from eating disorders are typically very reluctant to discuss their habits and disease, many will deny the existence of any disorder. To conduct a full assessment, you will need to ask additional questions specific to eating disorders.

Anorexia Nervosa

The primary characteristics of anorexia nervosa are self-starvation and extreme weight loss; some patients may also exercise excessively (several hours each day) as well as or instead of starving themselves. While the great majority of patients are female, males can also be anorectic. Anorexia nervosa should not be confused with the general medical term **anorexia**, which simply means a loss of appetite. When most medical providers use the term anorexia, they are implying anorexia nervosa, so be sure to clarify. For example, many patients with cancer undergoing chemotherapy lose their appetite, and the symptom would be reported as anorexia. In that case, the loss of appetite is due to the medication regimen, not self-image.

SEA-3 Assessment for Eating Disorders

Speech: The speech patterns of patients with an eating disorder are usually clear and concise.

Emotion: Patients with eating disorders will have varied emotions. They may be angry that help has been called or crying because their situation has reached a point at which medical attention is necessary. Some patients will demonstrate signs of depression or anxiety.

Appearance: Anorectics tend to be thin and malnourished, bulimics often are of normal size, and binge eaters range from normal weight to morbidly obese.

Alertness: In most cases, patients are alert and oriented unless they are in crisis because of electrolyte, respiratory, or cardiac emergency. Evaluate the patient for shortness of breath, chest pain, irregular heart rate, or changes in the 12-lead electrocardiogram if available.

Activity: Activity levels will vary from those addicted to exercise to those who are so thin or obese that they cannot move from their bed.

SAMPLE History for Eating Disorders

Signs and symptoms: These vary by condition; however, expect fluctuations in weight along with symptomatology specific to the disorder.

Allergies: There are no specific allergies associated with eating disorders; however, allergies can exist for any medication.

Medications: It is common for patients with eating disorders to take medications for depression or anxiety. Also, many anorectics and bulimics will take medications such as laxatives or diuretics to help them lose weight.

Past medical history: Eating disorders tend to be long-term or life-long disease processes. Expect histories to focus on eating patterns, along with possible electrolyte, cardiac, and respiratory disorders. Anorectics may also present with **amenorrhea** or the absence of menstrual cycles.

Last oral intake: Extra effort may be needed to determine the *actual* last oral intake because the patient is likely to attempt to hide his or her disorder. When questioning the patient, be sure to have him or her clarify exactly what was consumed.

Events leading up to today's event: Assess to determine if emergency responders were called for an acute or chronic condition and who called for your assistance. Often family members will call for help because patients tend to deny that the condition exists. In cases in which families have been dealing with a loved one's condition for an extended time, family members often will need emotional support.

OPQRST for Eating Disorders

Onset: Nearly all eating disorders are chronic. Focus on the time frame surrounding the acute onset of the event that triggered the call.

Provocation: What changed that resulted in EMS being called? In many cases, family members make the decision to call out of concern for the patient's well-being.

Quality: How significant is the patient's presentation? Is he or she alert and cooperative or in respiratory or cardiac distress?

Radiation: Is the eating disorder experienced by the patient now radiating out to family members, neighbors, or others? Has it affected important components of the patient's life such as employment or simply the ability to live alone?

Severity: Have the patient rate his or her current psychological distress with a 1-to-10 scale. In most cases of eating disorders, the family and friends of patients are more distressed than the patient.

Time: The timeline of the disorder is important. Be sure to document how long the patient has had the condition as well as any significant changes in pattern, lifestyle, eating habits, or weight changes.

In the Field

Sample Questions When Assessing a Patient With an Eating Disorder

- How many meals do you eat each day? How many did you eat yesterday?
- What do you eat at each meal? What did you eat yesterday?
- How much of each food did you eat?
- Do you avoid some foods or skip meals?
- Do you count calories?
- Do you use laxatives? If so, how often and how many?
- What is your normal exercise routine?
- Do you ever hide food and eat it when no one is around to see you?
- Have you been on diets before? What happened when you dieted?
- Did you ever eat until you vomited?
- Do you ever make yourself vomit, such as by sticking your fingers into the back of your throat?
- Do you ever feel out of control when eating?

Anorexia nervosa is often a true medical emergency and is potentially life threatening. The individual will so limit food and nutrition intake that the body begins to attack itself. As a result, the body metabolically slows itself down to conserve energy (**Figure 17-2**). The end results are serious medical side effects such as bradycardia, hypotension, muscle loss, dehydration, kidney failure, electrolyte imbalances, cardiac irregularities (dysrhythmias), dry and brittle bones, fatigue, fainting, and hair loss. In severe cases of anorexia, patients will grow very fine hair over their body when they fail to have enough fat to keep them warm. This fine hair is called <u>lanugo</u> and is also seen on a fetus still in the uterus and on infants for a short period after birth.

The *DSM-IV-TR* further classifies anorexia nervosa into restricting and binge-eating/purging types. Restricting type is exactly as the name implies: The individual severely limits the amount of food consumed without any type of bingeing or purging behaviors. Binge-eating/purging occurs when the individual will eat food but then regularly purge through self-induced vomiting or misuse of laxatives, diuretics, or enemas. In some cases, bingeing can result in a person eating an abnormally large amount of food during a specific time period or meal.

It is common for many anorectics to be living at home with parents, because this disease often affects young adults. Use parents and family members at the scene as a resource for information during an emergency. Interpersonal relationships often suffer during anorexic episodes because of isolation and an unwillingness to go out to restaurants or socialize. During your assessment, ask specifically about eating habits. Determine whether the patient eats three meals per day, avoids most foods or meals, eats only small amounts of food, or strictly counts calories.

Bulimia Nervosa

The anorectic patient is typically extremely thin and fragile. However, the patient with bulimia nervosa is usually of normal weight. Bulimia involves the repeated process of binge eating, followed by the purging of consumed food to avoid gaining weight. It is common for <u>bulimics</u> to routinely and secretly have uncontrolled or binge-eating sessions and then self-induce vomiting, misuse laxatives and diuretics (fluid pills), and exercise excessively (**Figure 17-3**).

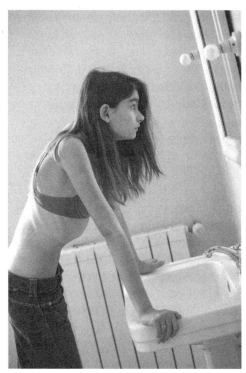

Figure 17-2 In severe cases of anorexia, the body metabolically slows itself down to conserve energy.

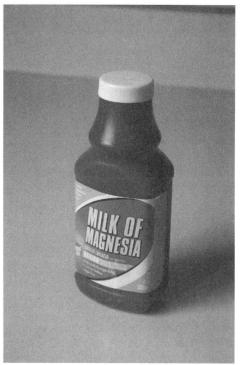

Figure 17-3 Patients suffering from bulimia nervosa may use laxatives or diuretics to control their weight.

Bulimia nervosa generally begins in adolescence or early adulthood. Studies show that the cause often is depression, boredom, or difficulty dealing with anger issues. Because it is a disease associated with normal weight, the problem can be difficult to identify because individuals are able to hide or explain away any signs or suspicions.

Bulimia nervosa can be an extremely dangerous and potentially life-threatening disease. The recurrent binge-and-purge cycles can result in severe damage to the esophagus and digestive system. In the upper gastrointestinal (GI) tract and esophagus, repeated vomiting will allow gastric acids to eat away at the linings of the digestive system. In worst-case situations, the esophagus can bleed or rupture because of frequent vomiting, resulting in a hemorrhagic emergency. Stomach acid eats away the enamel of the teeth, causing tooth decay and bleeding from the gums. Chronic laxative use will cause irregular bowel movements and constipation in the lower GI tract. Laboratory studies identify the presence of potentially severe electrolyte imbalances. As a result, dysrhythmias, heart and kidney failure, swollen salivary glands, and dehydration are common.

In the Field

Medical Problems Associated With Anorexia Nervosa

- Bradycardia
- Hypotension
- Vomiting
- Light-headedness
- Increased bowel movements or diarrhea
- Increased urination
- Heart failure
- Electrolyte imbalance
- Brain damage
- Brittle hair and nails
- Yellow-colored dry skin, with a covering of soft hair called lanugo
- Mild anemia
- Swollen joints
- Reduced muscle mass
- Brittle bones due to calcium loss (severe cases)

(*Source:* National Mental Health Information Center)

In the Field

Medical Problems Associated With Bulimia Nervosa

- Destroyed enamel and jagged edges on the teeth
- Irritated or bleeding gums
- Bleeding or rupture of the esophagus
- Irregular heartbeat or dysrhythmia
- Heart failure
- Peptic ulcers
- Pancreatitis
- Long-term constipation
- Death due to chemical imbalances and the loss of minerals

(*Source:* National Mental Health Information Center)

The assessment of the bulimic patient starts very much like that of the anorectic patient, in that you may be called by a loved one or family member. Based on historical information gathered, the emergency responder should inquire about the patient's normal eating habits and look at past patterns of eating. Has dieting and weight instability been prevalent in the past? Does the patient feel out of control when eating to a point of being uncomfortable? Does the patient eat in secret or hide food away?

During the physical examination, focus much of your time on the oral, facial, and GI regions. Be sure to take your time and thoroughly examine the teeth, gums, and salivary glands. Is there a decay of the tooth enamel or discoloration of the teeth? Is there a smell of vomit on the breath? Is there unusual swelling in their cheeks or jaw area? Although this may not be a commonly performed EMS assessment, it is very important for all patients with an eating disorder.

A common way to induce vomiting is to stick one's fingers down the throat and create a gag response. After many months or years of doing this, individuals will develop cuts, sores, or scar tissue across their knuckles. This is known as Russell's sign. Look at the hands for this indicator and also at the knees for bruises from bending over a commode to vomit.

Ask permission to examine the patient's abdomen, feeling for pain or discomfort. It is common for patients who abuse laxatives or diuretics to experience bloating, water retention, or swelling of the stomach. Ask if they routinely experience diarrhea or constipation, and if so, ask what they do about it. For patients with frequent diarrhea, a lack of potassium is common. This can result in cardiac dysrhythmias (irregular pulse), renal failure, or even death. Finding any of these conditions during your assessment warrants advanced life support (ALS) transport to a medical center for evaluation.

Binge-Eating Disorder

Binge-eating disorder (BED), or what is often called compulsive overeating, is one of the newest clinically recognized eating disorders, although the American Psychiatric Association has not officially accepted it as a stand-alone disorder. The last revision of the *DSM-IV-TR* in 2000 included it as an eating disorder NOS. However, since publication of the *DSM-IV-TR*, many governmental and scientific agencies have begun to report this condition as a true eating disorder or, in some cases, as an obesity disorder. BED is diagnosed when individuals have frequent episodes of compulsive or uncontrollable overeating. Unlike patients with bulimia nervosa, purging with vomiting or laxative use does not occur following the binge. Much like a drug addict, binge eaters are secretive with their eating. They often will eat alone and quickly, whether they are hungry or not, so as to hide their desire for food. As a result, body weight may vary from normal to severely or morbidly obese. Statistically, about 60% of people with BED are female.

BED is *not* the same as common obesity. Individuals with BED feel shame, distress, or guilt about their condition and their actions. As a result of their condition and possibly their appearance, patients often experience anxiety, depression, and loneliness. Patients are also known to hoard food, establish hiding places for food or wrappers, and eat throughout the day without planned mealtimes.

BED comes with many medical complications. Patients may experience a variety of cardiovascular and respiratory disorders such as shortness of breath, hypertension, high cholesterol level, and cardiac disease. The musculoskeletal system is stressed from the excess weight, so the patient may experience fatigue, joint pain, and difficulty walking. The GI and endocrine systems may be stressed because of high caloric intake, and patients will often end up with gallbladder disease or type II diabetes mellitus.

Often, prehospital response for a patient with this disorder will be due to a complication of the disorder, such as cardiac or respiratory disease, or because a patient has fallen and suffered an injury. It is important to recognize that in many cases, patients suffering from BED will be of normal or slightly above-normal weight. In other cases, patients will be morbidly obese.

For many individuals with BED, food is used as a means to relieve stress or to numb feelings of past events. Patients often have difficulty expressing their feelings and will be embarrassed and ashamed that you have been called. Remember that this is a condition that results in individuals becoming socially isolated, depressed, moody, or irritable. Assessing these patients will often require great patience on your behalf.

The prehospital provider should perform the initial and detailed survey as with any other patient. Extra time may be needed for the evaluation and treatment of comorbid conditions such as respiratory and cardiac illnesses. Dyspnea or chest pain may be common, requiring a thorough respiratory and cardiac workup and including 12-lead electrocardiography if it is available. Be prepared for the possibility that this patient could lapse into cardiac arrest if the condition is severe.

In the Field

Medical Problems Associated With BED

- Hypertension
- High cholesterol levels
- Fatigue
- Joint pain
- Difficulty walking
- Type II diabetes mellitus
- Gallbladder disease
- Respiratory distress
- Cardiac disease

(*Source:* National Mental Health Information Center)

Prehospital Management

When dealing with eating disorders, an empathetic approach is needed throughout the entire emergency call. The prehospital management of patients with eating disorders is usually not about treating the specific disorder; rather, management is about the side effects or sequelae of the disease process. Often, the hardest part for field providers is being persistent enough to get patients to go to the hospital for an evaluation and get help for their condition. In cases of anorexia and bulimia nervosa, treatment may focus on both the psychological component of denial and the management of life-threatening medical complications.

The emergency responder should be prepared to meet resistance from patients suffering from anorexia and bulimia nervosa. Use good interviewing skills to gain the patient's trust. With anorexia, you should be alert to a patient who may be frail, possibly with brittle bones, and who might have severe electrolyte, hormonal, or nutritional imbalances. These patients should receive a complete cardiac workup, and treatment will be based upon any specific abnormality found, often bradycardia. Oxygen should be administered, and IV therapy of lactated Ringer's or normal saline solution should be initiated if the patient is hypotensive and dehydrated, based on your local protocol. Because patients can be so chemically unstable, medical consultation may be recommended prior to initiating treatment. Remember that the severe loss of muscle mass and changes in metabolism may cause anorectics to be cold sensitive and even hypothermic, requiring blankets even in the summer (**Figure 17-4**).

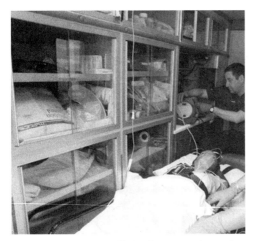

Figure 17-4 Patients suffering from anorexia may be cold sensitive and need blankets during transport, even in the summer time.

Bulimics often appear to be of normal size and stature. That does not mean that they do not have medical problems. As a responder, you should be prepared to acknowledge or treat pancreatitis, dehydration, electrolyte abnormalities, inflammation of the throat, or esophageal tears due to vigorous repeated vomiting. Because of the overuse of laxatives, patients may present with constipation or hemorrhoids, which may rupture and cause severe rectal bleeding. Your treatment should include oxygen, complete cardiac evaluation, and IV fluid therapy based on protocol for dehydration and possibly hemorrhage.

For patients with BED, management will tend to focus not on the disorder itself, but on the long-term effects of the disease process. The prehospital provider should always complete a thorough assessment of patients, with a particular focus on fluids and electrolyte imbalance, diabetes, hypertension, and cardiac disease. Many patients are severely or even morbidly obese, which will make moving the patient extremely difficult, if not dangerous. Extra people should be used for the safety of the patient and providers. Consider including the use of a special bariatric stretcher designed for the obese patient.

The patient's privacy should always be a priority in transport situations. In nearly all cases of eating disorders, self-esteem is a major issue. Every effort should be made to protect individuals and provide patient and professional care. In worst-case scenarios, the news media may show up when the fire department is removing a window or door in order to extricate a patient who may be in excess of 500 pounds. You have an ethical responsibility to be a patient advocate and to ask the media to remove itself from the scene, even if that means involving the police for support.

Long-Term Treatment

The EMS provider is not directly involved in long-term treatment of eating disorders; however, you should be aware that, as in many conditions involving mental disorders, treatment is often a lifelong battle. As a result, you may be called upon to respond to the same patient's home on multiple occasions over time.

Although long-term or life-treatment programs are different for each individual, there are similar approaches that are common. Your knowledge of these treatment plans can better prepare you to medically and psychologically respond to the patient with an eating disorder.

SAFER-R for Field Intervention With Eating Disorders

Stabilize: Present yourself in a professional manner, knowing that patients with eating disorders are often in denial about or embarrassed by their conditions. Be empathetic and supportive.

Acknowledge: Acknowledge that you are there to help and recognize that the patient may feel out of control of the current situation. Advise the patient that you will do your best to allow him or her to make appropriate choices during the EMS call.

Facilitate: Recognize that eating disorders affect not only the patient but family members as well. Facilitate the transfer of information from the patient and family to medical direction when possible.

Encourage: Constant reassurance is important for the patient with an eating disorder. Recognize that patients are very self-conscious about their situations and reiterate that you will do your best to protect their privacy.

Recovery: Be sure to discuss and reinforce your plan for getting the patient to the hospital, emphasizing that you are there to take care of his or her needs and that he or she is in good hands.

Referral: Suggest to family members that they seek out community resources or search the Internet for local and national information to help their loved one.

Common approaches to long-term treatment for eating disorders include:

- *Individual and group psychotherapy* helps teach people to recognize healthy versus unhealthy dietary habits. Strategies can also be developed in these settings to handle stressful situations, moods, and urges to return to previous behaviors. In situations involving children with eating disorders, family therapy should be considered.
- *There are no medications designed specifically for the treatment of eating disorders.* However, various antidepressant and anxiolytic medications can be used to stabilize the patient's mood and overall emotional state. Some antidepressants have a side effect of being an appetite suppressant and are being studied for use in patients with BED. Medications used for OCD may be used with some eating disorders.
- *Self-help tools* such as books, CDs, DVDs, and support groups can help many individuals with eating disorders. The focus of self-help strategies tends to be self-esteem and strategies for coping when urges occur.
- *Behavioral weight loss programs* are important for patients with BEDs. These programs are individually designed and implemented under medical supervision so that nutritional requirements are properly monitored. Programs should include psychotherapy, behavior modification, and exercise programs.

Pharmacologic Considerations

There are no medications that are specifically designed for prehospital treatment of eating disorders. As noted above, patients may be on many medications for other medical conditions or on antidepressants. The use of naloxone (Narcan®) or dextrose should be considered for the unresponsive patient should your local protocol suggest it.

Final Thoughts

Eating disorders represent two extremes of a continuum and many points along the way. Your patients will be people ranging from the frail and skinny to the morbidly obese. These individuals are potentially very sick and require your utmost care and compassion. Remember that the root of eating disorders is often poor self-esteem, so your psychological support is paramount. Your ability to be empathetic and obtain the patient's trust will allow you to complete a thorough assessment and provide exceptional care to your patient.

Selected References

American Psychiatric Association: *Diagnostic and Statistical Manual of Mental Disorders, Fourth Edition, Text Revision (DSM-IV-TR).* Washington, DC, American Psychiatric Press, 2000.

American Psychiatric Association Work Group on Eating Disorders: Practice guidelines for the treatment of patients with eating disorders (revision). *Am J Psychiatry,* 2000;1(suppl): 157.

Ebert MH, Loosen PT, Nurcombe B: *Current Diagnosis and Treatment in Psychiatry.* New York, NY, McGraw Hill Companies, 2000.

Free Health Encyclopedia. Available at: http://www.faqs.org/health/Healthy-Living-V3/Eating-Disorders.html. Accessed May 7, 2008.

Hersen M, Bellack AS: *Psychopathology in Adulthood,* ed 2. Needham Heights, MA, Allyn & Bacon, 2000.

Mayoclinic.com. Available at: http://www.mayoclinic.com/health/eating-disorders/DS00294/DSECTION=2. Accessed May 7, 2008.

National Eating Disorders Association Web site (2004). Available at: http://www.NationalEatingDisorders.org. Accessed April 24, 2008.

National Institute of Mental Health, National Institutes of Health Web site. Available at: http://www.nimh.nih.gov/. Accessed March 7, 2008.

National Mental Health Information Center. Available at: http://mentalhealth.samhsa.gov/publications/allpubs/ken98-0047/default.asp. Accessed May 7, 2008.

New York Times (retrieved January 8, 2008). Available at: http://health.nytimes.com/health/guides/disease/anorexia-nervosa/treatment-for-anorexia.html. Accessed May 7, 2007.

Office on Women's Health, US Department of Health and Human Services. Available at: www.4woman.gov. Accessed May 7, 2007.

Prep Kit

Ready for Review

- Eating disorders are conditions that are psychologically based and that result in serious physical changes in the body. In some cases, life-threatening emergencies can occur if the individual fails to receive prompt care.

- The National Eating Disorder Association outlines four factors that contribute to an eating disorder. The four factors are psychological, interpersonal, social, and biological.

- There are two types of anorexia nervosa. Restricting type anorexia is when the individual severely limits his or her caloric intake. Binge-eating/purging type anorexia occurs when the patient will eat food but regularly purges by using self-induced vomiting, laxatives, diuretics, or enemas.

- Bulimia nervosa involves the repeated process of binge eating, followed by the purging of consumed food to avoid gaining weight. These patients will usually appear of normal body weight.

- Binge-eating disorder is also commonly known as compulsive overeating. These individuals eat an excess amount of food, often over prolonged periods of time. As a result, these patients may be morbidly obese and present with severe, life-threatening complications such as respiratory, cardiac, or gastrointestinal diseases.

- The emergency responder should be prepared to contact an advanced life support EMS crew for treating and transporting patients with eating disorders. These patients will often present with severe medical complications that can lead to death if not promptly treated.

- In addition to the care needed for their associated medical complications, patients with eating disorders will need your empathy and psychological support. In most cases, they have been fighting a battle against food and self-esteem for many years.

Vital Vocabulary

amenorrhea The absence of menstrual cycles.

anorectic A person suffering from anorexia nervosa.

anorexia Lack of appetite.

anorexia nervosa An eating disorder in which the individual refuses to maintain a healthy body weight through the restriction of food intake or other means.

binge-eating disorder (BED) An eating disorder that involves the eating of large quantities of food during repetitive episodes in a restricted period of time over several months.

bingeing The process of eating an abnormally large amount of food over a short period of time.

bulimia nervosa An eating disorder characterized by a repeated cycle of bingeing and purging; it includes inappropriate ways to counteract the bingeing, such as forced vomiting or using laxatives.

bulimic A person suffering from bulimia nervosa.

eating disorder A psychological condition that focuses on the avoidance, excessive consumption, or purging of food.

lanugo Very fine hair, commonly found on newborn infants and anorectics, that grows over the body in an attempt to keep it warm when the body lacks enough fat or muscle to do so.

laxative A drug that induces the movement of fecal matter from the GI system.

purging A trait commonly seen in bulimia nervosa in which the person attempts to rid himself or herself of food by vomiting or using laxatives, diuretics, or enemas.

Russell's sign Calluses, cuts, and sores on the knuckles from repeated self-induced vomiting.

Assessment in Action

Answer key is located in the back of the book.

1. Patients with severe anorexia nervosa often grow soft, fine hair over their bodies because of the loss of fat and muscle tissue that normally keeps the body warm. This fine hair is known as _____.

Prep Kit | continued

A. anemia
B. lanugo
C. Russell's sign
D. amenorrhea

2. All of the following are long-term treatment options for patients with eating disorders EXCEPT:

A. individual and group psychotherapy
B. self-help materials such as CDs, DVDs, and support groups
C. electroconvulsive or electrical shock therapy
D. restoration to a healthy body weight and education about proper diet

3. Cardiac abnormalities or dysrhythmias are common in patients with eating disorders, primarily due to which of the following conditions?

A. Loss or imbalance of electrolytes
B. Hypothermia
C. Diminished muscle mass
D. Bleeding of the gastrointestinal tract or esophagus

4. The process of eating large amounts of food over a specific amount of time is known as _____.

A. bingeing
B. purging
C. addiction
D. anorexia

5. Which of the following eating disorders might cause a patient to present with poor oral hygiene, damaged tooth enamel, and bleeding gums?

A. Binge-eating disorder
B. Anorexia nervosa
C. Bulimia nervosa
D. All of the above

Chapter 18

Sleep Disorders

During your career you are unlikely to ever take an emergency call for a person who cannot sleep. However, if you conduct proper, thorough assessments, you are likely to find that many individuals requiring your assistance will have symptoms of sleep disturbance (**Figure 18-1**). Individuals with depression will often report that they want to sleep constantly, or patients with mania will tell you that they have not slept in 48 hours—if you ask.

Background

In order to understand abnormal sleep, you must first understand some facts about normal sleep. So what exactly is sleep? Sleep is a state of unconsciousness. During sleep, our brains are more responsive to internal stimuli than external stimuli. As we rest, our brain progresses through various cycles that move us from a level of being aware and conscious to one of restfulness and unconsciousness.

Normal sleep is divided into two categories: <u>non-rapid eye movement (NREM)</u> and <u>rapid eye movement (REM) sleep</u>. NREM sleep is further subdivided into four progressive stages known as stages I to IV. Stage I is light sleep and serves as a transition phase from wakefulness to the beginning of sleep, and makes up only about 5% of a full night's sleep. Stage II is the next level of deeper sleep during which approximately 50% of deep sleep occurs. An additional 10% to 20% of sleep occurs in stages III and IV, the deepest stages of sleep.

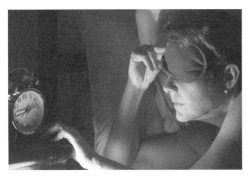

Figure 18-1 Sleep disorders can have extreme consequences for a person's health and well-being.

REM sleep occurs intermittently throughout the night and occurs for about 20% to 25% of the night on average. During this phase, the eyes move back and forth rapidly, giving the stage of sleep its name. Dreaming occurs during this phase. Individuals who fail to get "good" sleep or are constantly disrupted during sleep may not successfully get into REM sleep and often report that they do not dream.

Sleep changes with age. As we grow older, stage I sleep or wakefulness increases and in stages III and IV sleep (deep sleep) decreases. Age is a factor when evaluating for a sleep disorder and should be a consideration when assessing any patient complaining of sleep problems (**Figure 18-2**).

Circadian Rhythms and the Sleep-Wake Cycle

Each day we wake up, go to work, go home, watch television, and go to bed to sleep and prepare for the next day. This routine occurs over a 24-hour period in which we have a certain amount of time awake in the daylight and asleep in the dark. This is called the __sleep-wake cycle__, or what is commonly called __circadian rhythms__. During the daytime, a part of the brain known as the hypothalamus is exposed to light stimulation via the retina in the eye through a nerve pathway.

In the hypothalamus is the __suprachiasmatic nucleus (SCN)__. The SCN is responsible for signaling other parts of the brain to regulate hormone release, change body temperature, and make us feel sleepy or awake. It is the SCN that shuts us down at bedtime by lowering our body temperature and heart rate and making us sleepy. It also is responsible for controlling the release of a very important hormone called melatonin.

Melatonin

__Melatonin__ is a naturally occurring hormone produced by the pineal gland in the brain. The pineal gland is regulated by the amount of light that a person receives during the day. During daylight hours, the pineal gland shuts down and is inactive. However, once the evening arrives, the pineal gland is activated by the SCN. The gland then releases melatonin and individuals begin to feel sleepy. Melatonin remains elevated on average for about 12 hours, diminishing during the daylight hours. As you might suspect, people who work night shifts and need to sleep during the day often have difficulty either falling or staying asleep because of the lack of naturally occurring melatonin.

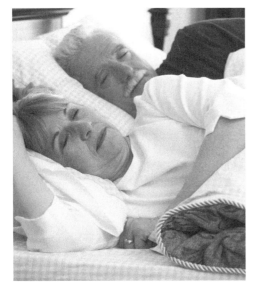

Figure 18-2 Age is a factor when evaluating for a sleep disorder.

Effects of Sleep Deprivation

Most studies show that the average person requires between 6 and 8 hours of good sleep per night. People who are unable to obtain good sleep for extended periods of time begin to experience physical and cognitive symptoms. Effects of sleep deprivation include:

- Decreased metabolic activity in the brain
- Decreased core body temperature
- Decreased immune system function, including changes in white cell count
- Decreased growth hormone
- Increased heart rate
- Diminished higher-level cognitive skills
- Inability to focus on complex tasks, such as driving a car
- Impaired judgment

What Is a Sleep Disorder?

Not everyone is fortunate enough to get 6 to 8 hours of regular sleep. Simply put, a sleep disorder is when a person does not regularly obtain sufficient and normal, healthy sleep. The *DSM-IV-TR* categorizes sleep disorders into primary sleep disorders, sleep disorders related to another mental disorder, and other sleep disorders. This chapter will focus on the primary sleep disorders, which are broken down into two categories, dyssomnias and parasomnias.

The *DSM-IV-TR* defines <u>dyssomnias</u> as "primary disorders of initiating and maintaining sleep or of excessive sleepiness that are characterized by a disturbance in the amount, quality, or timing of sleep." These disorders include:

- Primary insomnia
- Primary hypersomnia
- Narcolepsy
- Breathing-related sleep disorder
- Circadian rhythm sleep disorder

<u>Parasomnias</u> are defined by the *DSM-IV-TR* as "disorders characterized by abnormal behavioral or physiological events occurring in association with sleep, specific sleep stages, or sleep-wake transitions." Unlike the dyssomnias, parasomnias do not involve symptoms dealing with timing or wakefulness. These disorders include:

- Nightmare disorder
- Sleep terror disorder
- Sleepwalking disorder

Assessment

The assessment of the patient with a sleep disorder generally will focus on some other primary complaint, such as depression or a vehicle crash in which the driver fell asleep at the wheel. When questioning the patient, one normally would not go directly to a series of questions associated with a sleep disorder unless directed to do so by the individual or family member.

It is more common that your evaluation will be focused on those individuals with dyssomnias such as breathing-related sleep disorder or narcolepsy and less on adolescents with nightmare or sleep terror disorders. As with other disorders discussed in this book, consistent use of standardized questioning using SAMPLE, OPQRST, and the SEA-3 assessment will provide you with the information necessary for a thorough evaluation of the patient.

The Dyssomnias

Primary Insomnia

It is common for people to have problems sleeping every once in a while. Sometimes sleep disturbance is caused by stress. Other times it may be the side effects of medications or food or drink consumed prior to going to bed.

SAMPLE History for Sleep Disorders

Signs and symptoms: Depending upon the disorder, patients may present with extreme grogginess with hypersomnia, fatigue and exhaustion with insomnia, or sleep-related breathing disorders.

Allergies: Allergies can exist for any medication, many of which will cause signs or symptoms that can mimic sleeping disorders.

Medications: The most common medications will be those associated with insomnia. Do not forget that many over-the-counter medications exist for sleep problems. Patients with narcolepsy or hypersomnia may be using stimulants or antidepressants.

Past medical history: In most cases, individuals calling for assistance will have a history and diagnosis of some form of sleeping disorder. Family members and patients will provide you with needed information unless the patient happens to be alone when something occurs.

Last oral intake: Oral intake will not generally affect your assessment or treatment of these patients.

Events leading up to today's event: Assess to determine if emergency responders were called for an acute or chronic condition. The patient may or may not be able to recall the event. Most sleep disorder complaints will be about other medical or trauma emergencies.

OPQRST for Sleep Disorders

Onset: How long has the patient been diagnosed with this condition, and is it important to today's assessment?

Provocation: In most cases, the conditions presented in this chapter are not usually provoked by any specific event, although alcohol and some medications might exacerbate some of these disorders.

Quality: How pervasive is the condition in the person's life? Narcolepsy may inhibit a person from driving and create embarrassing moments in public or the workplace. Children with severe nightmares, sleep terrors, or sleepwalking may be afraid or embarrassed to participate in sleepovers at a friend's home or to attend summer camp.

Radiation: Does the disorder experienced by the patient radiate out to family members? Has it affected important components of the patient's life such as social life or employment?

Severity: Prehospital personnel can use a 1-10 scale to determine how much distress the disorder causes the patient. Has the condition become so invasive that other mental conditions such as depression or suicidal ideation have developed?

Time: Time is not as important in sleep disorders as with other mental conditions unless it involves some altered mental status. The length of time that a narcoleptic person is unresponsive is significant if it is outside of the patient's normal range.

SEA-3 Assessment for Sleep Disorders

Speech: The speech of an individual with a sleeping disorder will vary based upon the underlying cause of the event. Under most circumstances, normal speech patterns will be noted unless the patient is experiencing mania or another mental disorder. In cases of severe hypersomnia, the patient may be groggy and speech may be slightly slurred.

Emotion: Emotion is not generally affected by a specific sleep disorder. As with speech, emotional disturbances will more likely be related to other mental disorders such as depression, bipolar disorder, or psychosis.

Appearance: Appearance may be related to either the sleep disorder or another comorbid condition. For example, a patient with hypersomnia will be groggy, whereas a patient with insomnia will have dark circles under the eyes and appear fatigued.

Alertness: Patients are generally alert and oriented unless there is some comorbid disease process present, such as head injury or diabetes. Even patients with narcolepsy only lose consciousness for brief periods of time.

Activity: Most patients have learned how to cope with their sleep disorder and will be active upon your arrival. Patients with severe hypersomnia may be difficult to awaken or keep awake, but most other patients in this category respond to stimuli and will be able to respond to your requests.

Insomnia is a Latin word meaning "no sleep" and is the most common of all sleep complaints. It can be defined as a chronic condition that results in the inability to fall asleep or remain asleep for an adequate period of time. Research shows that insomnia is more common in women and more common as people grow older. Primary insomnia is sleeplessness that cannot be attributed to medical, psychiatric, or environmental causes such as substance abuse.

For a patient to receive a diagnosis of primary insomnia, the *DSM-IV-TR* notes that the patient must have difficulty initiating or maintaining sleep or must have suffered from nonrestorative sleep for a minimum period of one month. Additionally, the lack of sleep must cause significant distress in social, occupational, or other important areas of day-to-day functioning. Primary insomnia is not diagnosable for individuals in whom other disorders such as sleep apnea, narcolepsy, anxiety, depression, or substance abuse can be identified.

Epidemiologic studies have shown that primary insomnia can lead to an increase of morbidity and mortality. Individuals who live for years with this particular sleep disorder will often develop overall poor health, depression, anxiety, and substance abuse with nicotine, alcohol, illicit drugs, or prescription medications.

A variety of tools can help a person regain some control over the sleep cycle, from simple environmental changes in one's bedroom to prescription medications. The following is a list of suggestions for anyone who has insomnia or problems falling asleep.

- Attempt to go to bed at the same time each night.
- Be sure the temperature in the bedroom is comfortable for sleeping.
- Adjust outside or ambient light.
- Control outside noise or purchase a "white noise" machine.
- Be sure the bed is comfortable.
- Consider buying new pillows or a new mattress or pad if needed.
- Manage personal discomfort such as heartburn or joint pain.
- Take medications with side effects in the morning.
- Do not drink caffeinated beverages after noon.
- Do not exercise within 3 hours of bedtime.
- Do not nap during the day.

- If you smoke cigarettes, *quit;* nicotine is a stimulant.
- Learn to perform self-relaxation therapy.
- Absolutely do not lie in bed awake and toss and turn. Get up briefly, read a book, drink a glass of milk, and return to bed.

If a person is unable to regain control of proper sleep habits using the tips listed, over-the-counter or prescription sleep aids may be recommended. However, it is important to recognize that many individuals will become either psychologically or physically addicted to some medications. See **Table 18-1** for common medications used to treat insomnia.

Primary Hypersomnia

The *DSM-IV-TR* defines <u>primary hypersomnia</u> as "excessive sleepiness for at least one month as evidenced by prolonged sleep episodes or by daytime sleep episodes occurring almost daily." To be diagnosed, this disorder must be severe enough to cause significant problems in a person's social life, work life, or other important components of life.

Table 18-1 Pharmacotherapy for Insomnia		
Drug Classification	**Generic Name**	**Trade Name**
Hypnotic or benzodiazepine	lorazepam	Ativan®
	temazepam	Restoril®
	estazolam	ProSom®
	quazepam	Doral®
	flurazepam	Dalmane®
	oxazepam	Serax®
	triazolam	Halcion®
	clonazepam	Klonopin®
Nonbenzodiazepine hypnotic	zolpidem	Ambien®, Ambien CR®
	zaleplon	Sonata®
	eszopiclone	Lunesta®
Antidepressant	nefazodone	Serzone®
	trazodone	Desyrel®
Melatonin agonist	ramelteon	Rozerem®
Over-the-counter naturally occurring hormone	melatonin	
Antihistamine	diphenhydramine	Benadryl®
	doxylamine	Unisom®

The amount of time that individuals need for sleep varies. In this particular case, it is common for the person to sleep 8 to 12 hours and still not feel refreshed. Further, the process of awakening can be long and difficult, even to the point of mental confusion or ataxic gait (staggering) when walking. This particular form of ataxia is commonly called *sleep drunkenness.*

Characteristics of primary hypersomnia may include unintentional sleeping during the day (during periods of low stimulation) or actually lying down for prolonged naps lasting longer than one hour (**Figure 18-3**). It is possible that emergency personnel will be dispatched for a person who has fallen asleep at the wheel and crashed in the daytime hours. A good history on patients may provide you with information important for the receiving facility.

Many patients with primary hypersomnia remain untreated and adjust to their daily life with extended sleep. Treatment modalities vary. Some research is suggesting that prescribing medications in these cases only treats the symptoms. There is some evidence that the hypothalamus may be responsible for this disorder. The most common prescription medications are some form of stimulants or antidepressants. One specific new stimulant drug, modafinil or Provigil®, is being used for hypersomnia, narcolepsy, and shift work sleep disorder.

Narcolepsy

<u>Narcolepsy</u> is a disorder of sleep that results in the individual suddenly falling asleep without notice. The *DSM-IV-TR* outlines the

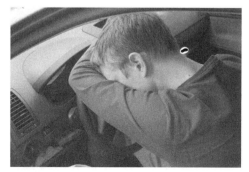

Figure 18-3 Hypersomnia may include unintentional sleeping during the day.

disorder as one that has "repeated irresistible attacks of refreshing sleep, cataplexy, and recurrent intrusions of REM sleep in the transition period between sleep and wakefulness." Narcoleptic episodes generally only last for a short period of time, usually from 30 seconds to 30 minutes.

During cataplexy, the patient experiences a loss of muscle tone or paralysis of voluntary muscles. The loss of tone can range from barely detectable to very dramatic in nature. A droopy jaw or eyelids and arms may not be noticed by those around the patient. At the other end of the continuum is a patient who may drop to the ground, having completely lost the muscular control required to maintain a standing position. Patients report that during cataplexy episodes, full consciousness and alertness is maintained.

Approximately 20–40% of individuals also report intense dream-like imagery or hallucinations. These hallucinations can occur just prior to falling asleep or just after awakening. Hallucinations may be kinetic, auditory, or visual in nature. Kinetic hallucinations are those in which the individual seems to be experiencing some form of motion, such as falling. Auditory hallucinations are hearing sounds, where as visual hallucinations occur when one sees things, such as moving objects in a room, that do not actually exist.

The prevalence of narcolepsy is only about 0.03% of the general population and is seen in both males and females. Onset can occur at any time during a person's life but is more commonly seen during one's teenage years. Experts estimate that between 30% and 57% of narcoleptic patients will experience depression, compared to approximately 8% of the general population.

Most patients control their narcolepsy through the use behavioral modification and medications. One simple way to decrease the number of episodes is with sleep behavior modification. Making sure that a full night sleep is obtained along with 2 or 3 scheduled naps during the day can help some patients control their disorder.

Other patients will require pharmacological intervention. Drugs such as amphetamines, antidepressants, and central nervous system stimulants (eg, modafinil) will assist the patient in staying awake during the daytime hours.

Patients are rarely transported to a hospital strictly for an evaluation because of narcolepsy. More commonly, you will be called because of some type of accident, vehicle crash, or work-related injury, or because someone was found asleep in an unusual place such as a car or lawn. There is no prehospital treatment for narcolepsy, so emergency care will focus on determining why you were called and ensuring that the patient is safe. In many situations, the patient will not need to be transported to the hospital once he or she awakens and is able to evaluate himself or herself.

Breathing-Related Sleep Disorder

Breathing-related sleep disorder (BRSD) is commonly called snoring or obstructive sleep apnea, but there are several types of disorders in this category. The *DSM-IV-TR* defines this disorder as one in which the patient has "sleep disruption, leading to excessive sleepiness or, less commonly, insomnia that is judged to be because of abnormalities of ventilation during sleep." Sleep anea can lead to pulmonary hypertension and heart failure. Patients often present with hypersomnolence due to lack of sleep. There are three types of BRSD: obstructive sleep apnea syndrome (OSAS), central sleep apnea syndrome (CSAS), and central alveolar hypoventilation syndrome. Each will be discussed.

Obstructive Sleep Apnea Syndrome

Obstructive sleep apnea syndrome (OSAS) is the most common type of BRSD. It is most prevalent in middle-aged, overweight males and prepubertal children with enlarged tonsils. Individuals present with repetitive episodes of upper-airway obstruction during the night. Commonly, periods of apnea (absence of breathing) and hypopnea (shallow, slow breathing) are present. Additionally, respiratory movements in the abdomen and chest are preserved. As a result, individuals characteristically have loud snoring or brief gasps for air that are followed by periods of silence that can last for 30 seconds or more. These periods of silence and apnea are actually caused by complete airway obstruction. In worst-case scenarios, individuals with severe OSAS can turn cyanotic at times during the night because of severe hypoxia.

Central Sleep Apnea Syndrome

Central sleep apnea syndrome (CSAS) is similar to OSAS except that apnea and hypopnea occurs without airway obstruction. In CSAS, ventilatory regulation by the central nervous system is altered and the patient has diminished respiratory effort, often because of chronic neurological or cardiac illness. This particular type of breathing disorder commonly develops between the ages of 40 and 60 years and is seen in the elderly, who report waking up at night. Individuals usually only have mild snoring.

Alveolar Hypoventilation Syndrome

The primary cause of alveolar hypoventilation syndrome is impairment in the regulation or function of the pateint's respiratory system that results in poor ventilation, particularly during sleep. As a result, patients have a normal respiratory system, but hypoventilate without the presence of apnea or hypopnea. This condition is most commonly found in severely obese patients where the weight of the chest impairs respiratory efforts during sleep. Central nervous system impairment of regulation may also cause hypoventilation. Additionally, hypoventilation may be due to neuromuscular diseases that result in severe weakness, such as myasthenia.

Presentation of Patients With Breathing-Related Sleep Disorders

Rarely will the prehospital provider be called to directly assist a patient with any form of breathing-related sleep disorder. Instead you will be called because the patient is complaining of some secondary symptom associated with the disorder.

Patients with BRSD will present with a variety of symptoms such as chest discomfort, choking, suffocation, and even stress-related events such as anxiety or near panic because of being afraid that they may stop breathing completely during sleep and not awaken. Individuals with these disorders may report fatigue, memory problems, poor concentration, problems staying awake, and, in worse cases, sleep drunkenness.

Patients under the care of a physician for sleep apnea will have a continuous positive airway pressure (CPAP) device at their bedside. To use the continuous positive airway pressure device, the patient wears a mask over the nose during sleep. Air is forced through the nasal mask to keep the nasopharynx open, reducing snoring and sleep apnea.

Circadian Rhythm Sleep Disorder

Circadian rhythm sleep disorder was previously known as sleep-wake schedule disorder. The *DSM-IV-TR* describes this disorder as a "persistent or recurrent pattern of sleep disruption that results from altered function of the circadian timing system or from a mismatch between the individual's endogenous circadian sleep-wake system and exogenous demands regarding the timing and duration of sleep." This disorder results in alterations in a person's sleep cycle because of internal changes or external stimuli such as travel or shift work. As with the other disorders in this chapter, these sleep conditions must affect a person's social life, work life, or other major component of daily life to be diagnosed. The majority of individuals with circadian rhythm sleep disorder do not seek medical attention, often rationalizing that it is simply part of the job. There are four subtypes of circadian rhythm sleep disorder: delayed sleep phase, jet lag, shift work, and unspecified.

1. *Delayed sleep phase disorder* is recognized as a "delay in circadian rhythms" that is often a response to societal needs or pressures. As a result, the internal biological clock gets moved, or delayed, and individuals tend to go to bed late at night and have great difficulty arising in the morning. It is common for this disorder to occur in college students and those individuals who stay up late and then try to go to work the next morning with minimal restorative sleep.

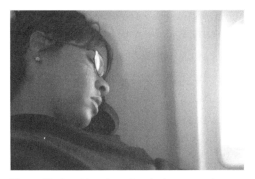

Figure 18-4 Jet lag sleep disorder is common in frequent travelers.

2. *Jet lag sleep disorder* is commonly seen in frequent travelers who find themselves crossing 8 or more time zones in a 24-hour period. As a result, the body becomes confused, quickly leaving the traveler fatigued. Traveling eastward is more difficult than traveling westward (**Figure 18-4**).

3. *Shift work sleep disorder* is common in individuals who are required to work during overnight hours when the body is prepared to sleep based on normal physiology. Unfortunately, the reality of the world is that some people must work night shifts, including fire, police, EMS, and other medical personnel, to mention a few.

People with shift work sleep disorder will find their body and mind wanting to go to bed in the evening when they are preparing to go to work. Research has shown that shift work comes with many physical and psychological hazards. Shift workers have 40% greater risk of cardiovascular disease than non-shift workers, as well as increased GI symptoms and psychiatric symptoms, including anxiety and depression.

Individuals report increased levels of stress because of difficulty meeting social and family demands. Shift work can be considered a risk factor for sleep-related injuries at the work site, motor vehicle accidents, alcohol and substance abuse, and family discord. **Table 18-2** provides some tools for surviving shift work.

Table 18-2 Tools for Surviving Shift Work
Bedtime Rituals
• Take a warm bath.
• Sleep in a cool environment.
• Don't stimulate your brain prior to going to bed.
Light
• Darken the bedroom and bathroom.
• Install light-blocking and sound-absorbing curtains.
• Wear eye shades.
Sound
• Wear ear plugs.
• Use a white noise machine or fan to block out noises.
• Install rugs, carpet, or drapes to absorb sounds.
• Unplug the telephone.
• Hang a "Do Not Disturb" sign on the door of your home.
Food
• Avoid caffeine at least 5 hours before bedtime.
• Don't drink alcohol before bedtime; although it is a depressant, it disturbs REM sleep.
• Eat a light snack prior to bedtime, especially turkey or milk that contains tryptophan.

Continued

Table 18-2 (Continued)

Balance Life and Work

- Sleep while family members are at work or school so you will be awake during evening hours.
- Schedule special time to spend with family.
- Realize that irritability, stress, and depression may be work-shift related. Do not blame your spouse or children for problems in family dynamics.

Exercise

- Do not exercise within 3 hours of sleep time, because exercise raises heart rate, temperature, and overall metabolism.

Napping

- Feeling fatigued, grouchy, or inattentive can often be fixed by a "power nap" of 20 to 30 minutes.
- Take a nap prior to departing for work so that you will be refreshed and alert.

The Ride Home

- If you are overly tired, driving with your windows open and car radio on does not always work, according to research. It is better to stop and get out for a short walk.
- If you are tired at the end of the work shift, arrange to take a 20- to 30-minute nap before getting behind the wheel.
- Carpool if possible, allowing the most alert person to drive.
- Take public transportation.
- If necessary, pull off for a quick nap in a secure, well-lit area. Be sure to notify family where you are located.
- Don't stop for a drink on the way home.

Manage Your Workplace

- Take short breaks throughout the work shift instead of fewer, longer ones.
- Try to work with someone who stimulates you.
- Exercise or walk during breaks.
- Try to eat healthy at work, avoiding fast food or foods that will cause gastric distress or heartburn.
- Talk to fellow workers and share ideas about how they cope with shift work.

Tips for the Employer

- Install bright lights in work areas.
- Provide sufficient breaks and days off.
- Provide vending machines with healthy choices.
- Develop a napping policy and provide short breaks, recognizing that naps can improve alertness, and judgment
- Be concerned about employee health and safety, including transportation, and family issues.

Seek Medical Attention

- Be aware of prolonged signs of sleep problems. Seek professional help if you suffer from insomnia, hypersomnia, or a breathing related sleep disorder.

Continued

Table 18-2 (Continued)

Operate Equipment Safely

- Be aware of fatigue or sleepiness, such as yawning, blinking, or dozing off. If you drive or provide health care, notify a supervisor that you need a break or opportunity to refresh yourself. Falling asleep behind the wheel of a vehicle is not acceptable!

(Information provided by the National Sleep Foundation; http://www.sleepfoundation.org/site/c.huIXKjMOIxF/b.2421189/k. DF93/Strategies_for_Shift_Workers.htm)

4. *Unspecified type* sleep disorder is a category used for those individuals who have severe sleep problems but do not meet the criteria for the previous three types. For example, individuals with advanced sleep phase or irregular sleep patterns would fall into this category. Another type is called non-24-hour sleep-wake pattern and is common in blind individuals whose perception of "daytime" is not based on daylight.

The Parasomnias

Nightmare Disorder

Nightmares are dreams that arouse feelings of extreme fear, horror, and distress and are a common occurrence in both children and adults. In order to be given the designation of nightmare disorder, they must occur repeatedly and awaken the individual from sleep. The nightmares must cause significant distress or result in "social or occupational dysfunction."

Nightmares can occur at any point during the night, as they develop during REM sleep. REM sleep occurs intermittently throughout the night. The event will cause extreme fear in most individuals, because they perceive that they are in physical danger or are being pursued. The majority of nightmares are based in non reality, but in some cases the nightmare can be a repetitive memory of a traumatic event that has happened to or was witnessed by the person.

In worst-case scenarios, some individuals will be so distraught about the potential for nightmares occurring that they will avoid sleep whenever possible. Individuals rapidly develop other symptoms such as fatigue, depression, anxiety, and diminished cognitive skills.

Sleep Terror Disorder

Sleep terror disorder is not to be confused with nightmare disorder. People with nightmare disorder will generally be able to wake up, become alert, and talk about the nightmare event. On the other hand, sleep terror disorder presents with an abrupt disturbance of deep (non-REM) sleep that usually begins with a panicky scream or cry. This event is accompanied by autonomic arousal and intense fear. During an episode of sleep terror, the individual is often unable to communicate. The individual will usually present with a frightened expression, sweating, anxiety, and confusion. In the unlikely event the person can be awakened, he or she generally will not remember the terror and will not recall the event the following morning.

Sleepwalking Disorder

It is not uncommon for people to sleepwalk on rare occasions, especially children. However, sleepwalking disorder is a clinical diagnosis when an individual has repeated episodes of complex motor behaviors that occur during sleep and include getting out of bed and walking about.

During these episodes, it may be difficult to awaken the individual. Contrary to popular belief, it is acceptable to attempt to awaken a person who is sleepwalking. As they walk about, you will notice a blank stare or flat affect along with diminished alertness. If the person can be awakened, individuals will generally reorient themselves after a few minutes of confusion.

It should be noted that in some cases, individuals with this disorder will walk around the house, go to the kitchen and fix food, and may even go outside. In some cases they return promptly, or in some situations, they will awaken in the morning to find themselves in a different location.

SAFER-R Field Intervention for Sleep Disorders

Stabilize: Create a calm environment by presenting yourself in a professional demeanor. Offer words of support that will make the patient and family feel safe.

Acknowledge: Assess and recognize the current situation by gathering information.

Facilitate: Understand the situation by determining if cognitive processes are intact or disturbed. Begin thinking about what type of help the patient and family need.

Encourage: Continue to build rapport with the patient and family by attempting to reorient the patient and move him or her toward transportation and definitive care.

Recovery: Reinforce the treatment and transportation plan with the patient.

Referral: Assist the family by suggesting community contacts such as local support groups.

Prehospital Management

The prehospital management of patients with the various sleep disorders will generally fall into the category of "supportive care." Patients who have extreme fatigue or other physical symptomatology may need a little extra time to make decisions or answer questions. Likewise, individuals with sleep problems secondary to medical conditions or substance abuse will present with special considerations during transport. Fatigue in particular makes it difficult for the patient to make rapid, rational decisions. Depending on the extent of the fatigue, the patient may even be confused and not competent to make health care-related decisions.

The other condition of concern for prehospital providers is patients with BRSD or severe sleep apnea. Patients with a history of sleep apnea are generally fatigued and may even be short tempered or moody. Being empathetic and listening carefully is the professional thing to do in these situations. With the exception of sleep apnea, few patients need anything more than minimal oxygen for their specific disorder and can be easily monitored with a pulse oximeter and cardiac monitor.

Pharmacologic Considerations

For the prehospital environment, it would be extremely unusual for EMS to pharmacologically treat a patient with a sleep disorder. Because the therapeutic drugs of choice for the dyssomnias generally are amphetamines and antidepressants, we do not normally give those medications in the field. In a rare case, there may be a patient who develops severe anxiety following an episode of night terrors or insomnia. In that situation, it would be wise to consult with medical direction and follow local protocols for an anxiolytic agent.

As part of your assessment, the emergency responder should always question the patient about the medications used to encourage sleep. With new medications coming onto the market regularly, more and more is being reported about severe side effects of sleep medications. Additionally, it is not unusual for severe insomniacs to take more than one kind of medication to assist them with sleep. Drug interactions such as respiratory depression, confusion, altered mental status, or amnesia may be witnessed. In some cases, severe drowsiness or side effects could result in injury or confusion.

Final Thoughts

How many times have you picked up a patient who fell asleep at the wheel and crashed his or her vehicle, or an injured factory employee who was not paying attention and ran his or her hand into a machine? How many times have you, as a health care provider who works shift work, gone to work or cared for a patient, and then realized that you were on auto pilot? Spend extra time reviewing the tools for surviving shift work. It might just save your life!

Selected References

American Psychiatric Association: *Diagnostic and Statistical Manual of Mental Disorders, Fourth Edition, Text Revision (DSM-IV-TR)*. Washington, DC, American Psychiatric Press, 2000.

Answers.com Web site (2008). Cataplexy. Available at: http://www.answers.com/topic/cataplexy?cat=health. Accessed May 23, 2008.

Bonds CL: Sleep disorders (2006). Available at: www.emedicine.com/med/topic609.htm. Accessed June 4, 2008.

Cataletto ME, Hertz G: Sleeplessness and circadian rhythm disorder (2005). Available at: www.emedicine.com/med/topic655.htm. Accessed June 4, 2008.

Helpguide.org Web site. Narcolepsy: symptoms, causes, diagnosis, and treatment (2007). Available at: http://www.helpguide.org/life/narcolepsy_symptom_causes_treatments.htm. Accessed May 7, 2008.

National Sleep Foundation: Topics from A to Zzzzs (2007). Available at: http://www.sleepfoundation.org. Accessed May 7, 2008.

Ranjan A, Gentili A: Primary insomnia (2005). Available at: http://www.eMedicine.com. Accessed June 4, 2008.

Russo MB: Normal sleep, sleep physiology, and sleep deprivation: general principles (2005). Available at: http://www.emedicine.com/med/topic444.htm. Accessed May 7, 2008.

Prep Kit

Ready for Review

- Normal sleep is divided into two categories: rapid eye movement (REM) and non-rapid eye movement (NREM).
- Research shows that our bodies need between 6 and 8 hours of good sleep each night. The effects of sleep deprivation are many, including decreased metabolic activity in the brain, decreased immune function, diminished cognitive skills, impaired judgment, and inability to multitask, to mention a few.
- Dyssomnias are those conditions that disturb the amount, quality, or timing of our sleep.
- Parasomnias are abnormal or physiological events that occur with sleep, sleep stages, or sleep-wake cycles.
- Emergency responders should always be cognizant that any patient with a history of sleep disorder who presents altered mental status or confusion may be under the influence of one or more medications to treat his or her specific condition.

Vital Vocabulary

alveolar hypoventilation syndrome A type of disorder, commonly seen in very obese patients, which presents because of some impairment in the patient's respiratory system that affects breathing efforts, particularly during sleep.

apnea Absence of breathing.

breathing-related sleep disorder (BRSD) Sleep disruption leading to excessive sleepiness or, less commonly, insomnia that is judged to be because of abnormalities of ventilation during sleep.

cataplexy A sudden loss of muscle tone and strength, usually caused by an extreme emotional stimulus or narcolepsy.

central sleep apnea syndrome (CSAS) A type of breathing-related sleep disorder that is prevalent in those older than 40 years who present with apnea and hypopnea, without airway obstruction.

circadian rhythm Also known as the sleep-wake cycle. The routine sleep-wake cycle experienced by humans is over a 24-hour period of time.

circadian rhythm sleep disorder A persistent or recurrent pattern of sleep disruption that results from altered function of the circadian timing system or from a mismatch between the individual's endogenous circadian sleep-wake system and exogenous demands regarding the timing and duration of sleep.

continuous positive airway pressure (CPAP) An airway system in which a patient sleeps with a mask device over the nose that continually forces air into the airway in order to keep the nasopharynx open, hence reducing snoring and sleep apnea episodes.

dyssomnia Any of a group of primary sleep disorders of initiating and maintaining sleep or of excessive sleepiness that are characterized by a disturbance in the amount, quality, or timing of sleep.

hypopnea Shallow, slow breathing.

insomnia A chronic condition that results in the inability to fall asleep or remain asleep for an adequate period of time.

melatonin Naturally occurring hormone produced by the pineal gland in the brain that assists in falling asleep.

narcolepsy A disorder that has repeated irresistible attacks of refreshing sleep, cataplexy, and recurrent intrusions of REM sleep in the transition period between sleep and wakefulness.

nightmare A dream that arouses feelings of extreme fear, horror, and distress.

nightmare disorder Repeated occurrence of frightening dreams that lead to awakenings from sleep and result in social or occupational dysfunction.

non-rapid eye movement (NREM) sleep The majority of time spent sleeping throughout the night in which REM does not occur. It is divided into four stages.

obstructive sleep apnea syndrome (OSAS) A type of breathing-related sleep disorder that is prevalent in middle-aged, overweight men and children with enlarged tonsils. These individuals commonly present with repetitive episodes of upper-airway obstruction during the night, along with periods of apnea and hypopnea. Frequently presents with hypersommolence during the day.

parasomnia Any of a group of primary sleep disorders characterized by abnormal behavioral or physiological events occurring in association with sleep, specific sleep stages, or sleep-wake transitions.

primary hypersomnia A condition designated in the *DSM-IV-TR* as excessive sleepiness for at least one month as evidenced by prolonged sleep episodes or by daytime sleep episodes occurring almost daily.

primary insomnia Difficulty initiating or maintaining sleep or nonrestorative sleep.

rapid eye movement (REM) sleep The stage of sleep that occurs intermittently throughout the night in which dreaming occurs. It is named such because of the back-and-forth movement made by the eyes during this phase.

sleep terror disorder A condition resulting in abrupt awakenings from sleep, usually beginning with a panicky scream or cry, and accompanied by autonomic arousal and behavioral manifestations of intense fear.

sleep-wake cycle See circadian rhythm.

sleepwalking disorder A condition in which repeated episodes of complex motor behavior are initiated during sleep, including rising from bed and walking about.

suprachiasmatic nucleus (SCN) Part of the hypothalamus that is responsible for signaling other parts of the brain to regulate hormone release, change body temperature, and make us feel sleepy or awake.

Assessment in Action

Answer key is located in the back of the book.

1. The most common type of breathing-related sleep disorder is _____.

   A. central sleep apnea syndrome
   B. central alveolar hypoventilation syndrome
   C. obstructive sleep apnea syndrome
   D. circadian rhythm sleep disorder

2. Shallow, slow breathing best defines which of the following terms?

   A. Hyperpnea
   B. Hypopnea
   C. Apnea
   D. Tachypnea

3. The administrative assistant at your place of employment recently has been diagnosed with a sleeping disorder in which she has repeated irresistible attacks of refreshing sleep and cataplexy. This morning, you walked into her office and found her slumped in her chair asleep. You suspect that she is diagnosed with which sleep disorder?

   A. Obstructive sleep apnea syndrome
   B. Pickwickian syndrome
   C. Narcolepsy
   D. Sleep terror disorder

4. From the following list, select the disorder that would most benefit from the use of continuous positive airway pressure.

   A. Obstructive sleep apnea syndrome
   B. Nightmare disorder
   C. Jet lag disorder
   D. Advanced sleep phase disorder

5. The stage of sleep in which dreaming occurs is _____.

   A. Non-rapid eye movement (NREM), Phase I
   B. Non-rapid eye movement (NREM), Phase III
   C. Non-rapid eye movement (NREM), Phase IV
   D. Rapid eye movement (REM)

Personality Disorders

Your personality, or how you present yourself, is often the first thing that someone remembers about you. The *DSM-IV-TR* defines personality traits as "enduring patterns of perceiving, relating to, and thinking about the environment and oneself that are exhibited in a wide range of social and personal contexts." It further states that "only when personality traits are inflexible and maladaptive and cause significant functional impairment or subjective distress do they constitute Personality Disorders."

Personality disorders are pervasive and inflexible alterations of one's traits that lead to distress or impairment. These disorders are considered to be some of the more difficult psychological disorders to diagnose and treat because they affect every facet of an individual's life (**Figure 19-1**). Diagnosis is complicated because of the high comorbidity rates among people with these disorders. Comorbidity is defined as having multiple psychological or medical conditions occurring simultaneously within one individual. Personality disorders are often compounded by depression, making it difficult to classify a person's underlying personality disorder.

The subjectivity of the clinician may also affect this diagnosis. EMTs, paramedics, and mental health professionals often interpret symptoms differently, as many symptoms of personality disorders ambiguously overlap one another. Additionally, symptoms tend to change over the years, making it difficult to fit an individual into a diagnostic category.

The *DSM-IV-TR* identifies 10 distinct categories of personality disorders that are divided into three clusters. Cluster A includes individuals

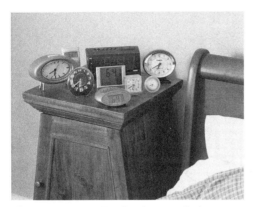
Figure 19-1 Personality disorders can affect every aspect of a person's life.

who possess odd and eccentric characteristics. Cluster B includes individuals who demonstrate overdramatic and emotional characteristics. Lastly, cluster C patients present with anxious and fearful character traits.

Conditions that will be discussed in this chapter:

Cluster A
- Paranoid personality disorder
- Schizoid personality disorder
- Schizotypal personality disorder

Cluster B
- Antisocial personality disorder
- Borderline personality disorder
- Histrionic personality disorder
- Narcissistic personality disorder

Cluster C
- Avoidant personality disorder
- Dependent personality disorder
- Obsessive-compulsive personality disorder

Background

Personality disorders as a group generally manifest in the adolescent period of development. The period of development, from the ages of 15 to 18 years, is when individuals tend to start living with more responsibility and stress. Stress is a common factor that can cause the emergence of a personality trait that can then develop into a full disorder.

If a particular impairment has been persistent since childhood, it is likely to be diagnosed as a personality disorder. An individual who wins the state EMS competition and then brags about the win would not be considered as having a personality disorder. However, if this individual demonstrated a pattern of boasting, bragging, and needing to be the center of attention throughout his lifetime (to the point of intrusiveness), then he most likely would be diagnosed as being <u>histrionic</u>, or someone who seeks to be at the center of attention.

The exact cause of most personality disorders is not known. Current research shows that most are genetically linked and may include several other causes. Evidence connects the presence of <u>dopamine</u>, a naturally occurring CNS neurotransmitter, or in some cases evidence of degradation of <u>dopaminergic</u> function to personality disorders. In some cases there is reason to believe that actual physical changes within brain tissue itself occur. Specifically, heredity appears to be a direct link in patients experiencing those conditions known as schizotypal, schizoid, and paranoid personality disorders.

Other theorists suspect that environmental situations that occur during childhood can trigger the development of personality disorders. This particular argument is commonly made with individuals who develop conditions such as *dependent personality disorder (DPD)*, in which individuals develop a pattern of submissive and clinging behavior with loved ones on whom they are overly dependent. They have difficulty making decisions and often require parents or spouses to decide where they should live and work or who to befriend. It is unknown whether a traumatic event might be the catalyst to this illness.

Other conditions, such as *borderline personality disorder (BPD)*, present with a pattern of instability in interpersonal relationships, self-image, affect, and marked impulsivity. BPD is recognized as having sexual abuse as a common risk factor in young individuals, especially those younger than 13 years. The causes of some types of personality disorders are not understood yet. Specifically, narcissistic, histrionic, and avoidant personality disorders have been minimally researched and little evidence exists to explain why they occur.

> ### SEA-3 Assessment for Personality Disorders
>
> **Speech:** Patients are able to speak with a range of speech patterns from quiet to confrontational.
>
> **Emotion:** Most patients with personality disorders are under the control of their emotions, although paranoia, flat affect, or shyness may be exhibited in some cases.
>
> **Appearance:** Patients with personality disorders are generally well kempt and groomed. Although some may be withdrawn, they tend to be dressed appropriately.
>
> **Alertness:** Unless there is some other medical condition present, these patients should be alert and oriented.
>
> **Activity:** Activity will vary according to cluster diagnosis.

Assessment

Because of the extreme range of individuals classified in this category of mental disorder, the prehospital provider cannot go into a situation with a preset agenda. Emergency responders may be called to the scene of a residence for someone demonstrating the odd characteristics associated with schizotypal personality disorder or to a bar fight where a narcissistic agitated patron was beaten with a pool stick when he insulted his opponent's ability at the game.

People with personality disorders are generally known by their family, friends, and neighbors as being "a little different." The key to approaching individuals suffering from personality disorders is calmness and patience (**Figure 19-2**). Conflict and instability are common in their lives. Only time, good questioning, and structure will get you the answers that you need. The SAMPLE history and OPQRST will be helpful in these situations. Even though you may not have been called for a behavioral emergency call, the SEA-3 assessment tool may be very beneficial in completing a thorough survey.

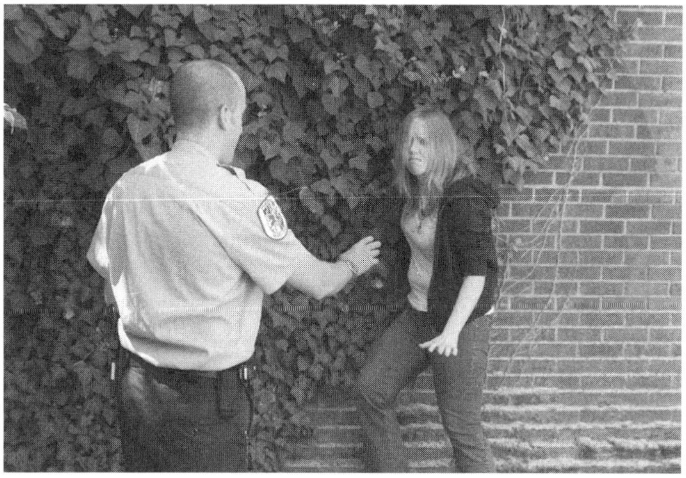

Figure 19-2 Remain composed and attempt to keep patients calm during calls related to personality disorders.

Cluster A

Paranoid Personality Disorder

<u>Paranoid personality disorder</u> is a pattern of distrust and suspiciousness such that others' motives are interpreted as malevolent. The primary paranoid personality disorder characteristic is <u>paranoia</u>, or the suspicion that others will harm or deceive an individual, in the absence of a psychotic event.

An individual fearful of death in a wartime environment would not be diagnosed with paranoid personality disorder. However, an individual who is fearful of death in a nonthreatening environment

> ### In the Field
>
> In conducting the interview, remember that cluster A individuals are odd and eccentric, cluster B individuals are dramatic and emotional, and cluster C patients are anxious and fearful.

for no apparent reason would likely fall into this category. Individuals view a helping hand as a personal attack and may become very defensive and hostile, especially when receiving criticism. Unjustified grudges and jealousy are common, as is placing blame on others for personal shortcomings.

Schizoid Personality Disorder

Schizoid personality disorder is defined as an indifference to interpersonal and sexual relationships accompanied by a lack of emotional expression. This disorder usually develops or becomes apparent during early adulthood and can have a variety of presentations. Individuals avoid close relationships of any kind, including family relationships, and are seemingly uninterested in being accepted or loved. Individuals are rarely interested in romantic relationships or sexual activity, infrequently marry, and are viewed by others as unsociable, reclusive, and cold. As a result, people with schizoid personality disorder commonly withdraw to solitary lifestyles, often in a single room, avoiding social contact of any kind.

Schizoid personality disorder is often associated with schizophrenia. Schizoid personality disorder involves schizophrenia-like qualities, but is not as disabling as schizophrenia, because it does not incorporate hallucinations, delusions, or the complete disconnection with reality.

Schizotypal Personality Disorder

Schizotypal personality disorder is similar to schizoid personality disorder in that it involves a pattern of difficulty with social and interpersonal relationships. Individuals diagnosed with schizotypal personality disorder exhibit an eccentric, distorted way of thinking often accompanied by very unusual behavior. They have unusual beliefs, superstitions, or magical thoughts that may include belief in telepathy or psychic phenomena. They may have perceptual experiences in the form of illusions and believe that unrelated events are related to them in an important and personal way.

At first glance this disorder may appear benign or harmless. However, individuals living with this disorder are unable to truly enjoy life or experience pleasure. Schizotypal personality disorder is more closely related to schizophrenia than schizoid personality disorder. There is evidence that both have similar biological abnormalities such as memory deficits, eye movement abnormalities, and enlarged brain ventricles.

Cluster B

Antisocial Personality Disorder

Antisocial personality disorder is a personality disorder that classically presents in combination with criminal activity. The *DSM-IV-TR* states that individuals with antisocial disorder will display a frank disregard to the rules and norms of the society in which they live, as well as the disassociation of right from wrong. Antisocial behavior can lead to patterns of disregard for laws with repeated criminal offenses. Individuals with antisocial personality disorder use lying and deception as a form of communication and interaction because of candid distrust of others. People who develop antisocial personality disorder will commonly have unstable family and personal relationships primarily caused by the blatant disregard for others. Irresponsibility is demonstrated by history of inconsistent work patterns, frequent relocation, and the inability to plan ahead.

Sometimes referred to as sociopaths, antisocial personalities are very difficult to manage because of the distrust and lack of comprehension of societal norms and laws. The inability of these persons to conform to the rules and norms of society tends to further alienate them from society, perpetuating the disorder. Antisocial personality disorders can also manifest in physical aggression and anger. A history of physical assault may be common.

Family history may be an important assessment item in those suffering from antisocial personality disorder. In many cases, individuals have a history of various childhood traumas such as an abusive or chaotic home life or a severely abusive alcoholic parent.

Histrionic Personality Disorder

Histrionic personality disorder (HPD) is classified in the *DSM-IV-TR* as someone with attention-seeking behavioral patterns and frequent and rapid shifts in emotion and mood. Simply put, histrionics need to be the center of attention.

Histrionic individuals are usually seen as dramatic and theatrical because of their excessive reactions and mannerisms. They may demonstrate lack of inhibition regarding sexual behavior and appear seductive, flirtatious, and promiscuous. It is common for histrionic individuals to develop rapid emotional attachments to partners.

It is also common for persons with HPD to use suicidal threats as a means of getting attention. HPD often makes it difficult for individuals to maintain personal relationships. Histrionic personalities do not tend to be self-destructive, but can progress into depression or other degenerating conditions because of the rapid transition of moods or feelings.

HPD generally begins and develops in adolescence. Males and females have certain characteristics of HPD that are distinct to each gender. Males demonstrate lack of impulse control and immaturity, and can have antisocial tendencies. Females demonstrate an intense dependency on others as well as self-indulgence and lack of judgment with sexual partners. Although histrionics generally maintain a good social status and good work habits, they often suffer in their personal lives.

Narcissistic Personality Disorder

The *DSM-IV-TR* provides a wide range of personality characteristics used to classify someone with narcissistic personality disorder. Of nine traits listed, the individual must meet at least five of them to be diagnosed. Traits include having a grandiose sense of self-importance, a pre-occupation with fantasies of unlimited success or power, a belief that he or she is special or unique, requiring excessive admiration, and a sense of entitlement. Additional characteristics include having behaviors that are interpersonally exploitative (taking advantage of others to make achievements for themselves), lacking empathy, acting envious of others, and showing arrogance or haughty behavior.

Narcissists feel as if they are too great compared to the average person and that they are unable to be understood by "the common man." They often do not have empathy for other people. This is draining on any interpersonal relationships in which the individual may be involved and can result in short relationships and some degree of isolation.

Narcissism is found commonly with a history of reckless behavior and substance abuse. As with any personality disorder, drugs and alcohol only further inhibit the brain from working through thoughts logically and can fuel the disorder.

Borderline Personality Disorder

Borderline personality disorder (BPD) is one of the most commonly overdiagnosed disorders in the *DSM-IV-TR*. Individuals experiencing BPD will struggle with maintaining interpersonal relationships because of a fear of abandonment. People with this diagnosis often have been damaged at some point in their bonding processes, and will see almost every action and statement from others as a clue to abandonment. An inverse relationship for love and trust is often created; the more they love someone, the more they are going to fear and imagine abandonment from this person. Borderlines, as they are commonly called, are often near delusional about the "clues" and reasons for thinking abandonment is imminent.

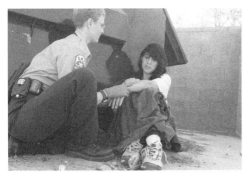

Figure 19-3 Substance abuse and alcoholism are commonly associated with BPD.

Impulsiveness is commonly seen with this condition and can contribute to further destructive behaviors and addictions. Gambling, substance abuse, sexual deviance, and alcoholism are associated problems that occur with BPD (**Figure 19-3**). When impulsivity and inability to trust people are combined, many individuals suffer from a "short fuse" and are easily agitated and upset.

Cluster C

Avoidant Personality Disorder

Avoidant personality disorder is classified in the *DSV-IV-TR* as a "pervasive pattern of social inhibition, feelings of inadequacy, and hypersensitivity to negative evaluation, beginning by early adulthood and present in a variety of contexts." Individuals feel that they are not equal to other people and thus shy away from almost all social interaction in fear of rejection and criticism. It is important to note that these individuals might be on a football team or the lead singer in a band. They might be very good at something but feel as though they are inadequate.

Avoidant personality disorder shares certain commonalities with antisocial personality disorder. Both disorders result in frank distrust for other individuals, making it difficult or impossible to communicate or develop relationships with people. However, whereas antisocial personalities do not understand how they fit into society or its norms, avoidant personalities know how they should fit into society, but are paralyzed out of fear of rejection.

Dependent Personality Disorder

Dependent personality disorder usually develops during early adulthood and is marked by an anxiety about making or an inability to make independent decisions. This behavior is often accompanied by separation anxiety, clinginess, and submissiveness. Individuals require excessive advice to make a very small decision, such as what color shirt to wear, and avoid responsibility for major life decisions such as job choices.

Seeking approval or support leads to excessive agreement with other people's decisions as well as going to excessive lengths to gain that approval. When a relationship fails, the need to fill that void with a new relationship becomes paramount. People with this disorder tend to feel helpless, inadequate, and lost when alone, in addition to having low self-esteem and a perpetual fear of abandonment.

Obsessive-Compulsive Personality Disorder

Obsessive-compulsive personality disorder, one of the more common personality disorders, is marked by a person's obsession for perfection, neatness, and control, as well as the inability to make a decision. This disorder often develops during early adulthood. Individuals are focused primarily on schedules, rules, lists, and details, to the point of losing perspective on what is truly important. This in turn leads to an inability to complete certain tasks as they strive for unattainable, self-defeating perfection. The need for perfection is present in all aspects of daily life. Individuals are often excessively devoted to work, creating a lifestyle incompatible with friends, family, or hobbies. Obsessive work habits are not accounted for by an extreme need for money, but rather by a desire to hoard money and even worthless objects in the event that they may be required in the future.

Individuals with obsessive-compulsive personality disorder have difficulty forming relationships because they are extremely inflexible and unable to compromise when a disagreement may arise. Relationships in the workplace are usually poor, and individuals have difficulty delegating authority unless others agree to accomplish the task precisely how the person desires it to be done.

Although hardworking, organized, task-oriented people are often accused of having OCD, a distinction must be made between the two. Although the two categories of people share similar characteristics, individuals with obsessive-compulsive personality disorder are generally unproductive, whereas the former are usually very productive and efficient.

Prehospital Management

Personality disorders are not the type of disorder you can throw a pill at and cure. Personality disorders describe *who the person is,* rather than *something the person suffers from* on an occasional basis. Individuals who deal with a personality disorder often do not even know that there is anything different about them. Normally, the only people who receive help for personality disorders are individuals who suffer from some side effect of the given disorder. Depression is a major secondary effect that many people with personality disorders experience. Many cases of personality disorders are only identified after the person meets with a professional about depression or suicidal thoughts.

As the emergency responder, you generally will not be providing any type of treatment specific to the personality disorder except for compassionate, reassuring care. The SAFER-R model presents a good guideline for you to use in this situation. It is important to recognize that a person with a personality disorder is not necessarily a danger to the prehospital provider. With this particular group of mental disorders, more can be accomplished with sugar than with vinegar. Kind words, compassion, and understanding go a long way. Proper communication with the individual in a respectful manner will usually allow you to have safe and peaceful transport to the hospital.

SAFER-R Field Intervention for Personality Disorders

Stabilize: Create a calm environment by presenting yourself with a professional demeanor. Offer words of support that will make the patient and family feel safe.

Acknowledge: Assess and recognize the current situation by gathering information.

Facilitate: Understand the situation by determining if cognitive processes are intact or disturbed. Begin thinking about what type of help the patient and family need.

Encourage: Continue to build rapport with the patient and family by attempting to reassure the patient that you are there to help. Tell the patient why you need to move him or her toward transportation and definitive care.

Recovery: Reinforce the treatment and transportation plan with the patient.

Referral: Assist the family by suggesting community contacts such as the department of social services or local mental health authority.

Pharmacologic Considerations

Along with therapy, some personality disorders require medication to control some impulses and symptoms. Antianxiety and antidepressant medications are commonly prescribed for personality disorders. Although these drugs do not cure the underlying personality disorder, they can help alleviate some of the negative aspects.

Depression is a common problem for many people who suffer from severe and advanced personality disorders. Depression can cause physical symptoms as well as psychological ones. Therapy will not be nearly as effective if the individual is severely depressed or anxious about the sessions. Some of the common antidepressants are sertraline (Zoloft®), fluoxetine (Prozac®), citalopram (Lexapro®), mirtazapine (Remeron®), and nefazodone (Serzone®). These are all medications that are taken orally and need to be taken consistently.

Other medication types used are drugs such as valproic acid (Depakote®), which is an anticonvulsant. Depakote® is the most commonly prescribed anticonvulsant and is used because it generally helps to inhibit impulsivity associated with personality disorders. Depakote® is also used with bipolar disorder.

Prehospital providers should be warned against encouraging patients with personality disorders to take their own medications until they have been evaluated by a physician. It is not uncommon for individuals suffering from a personality disorder to be less than truthful during the assessment interview. Further, it may be common for the patient to have distortions in thoughts or perspectives and, for whatever reason, feel the need not to take his or her medications. In some situations, the individual may have forgotten that he or she has taken prescribed medication, thus risking an overdose. The best bet is to always err on the side of a conservative pharmacologic approach and allow the patient to be thoroughly assessed at the emergency department.

Final Thoughts

As an emergency responder, you will probably deal with many of these personality types at some point or another over your career. The major reason you may be called to be involved with a patient with a personality disorder is not because the patient is avoidant and shy, but because the patient is severely depressed and has not eaten in a week. Likewise, providers may deal with antisocial or narcissistic personalities because of an assault or dispute.

Prehospital personnel should treat these patients with two simple steps. Step one is to reduce the stimuli. If patients are agitated, be calm, speak clearly, and explain everything as an option before it is a command. If patients are depressed, let them know they can trust you to provide good care and transport. Step two is listening to what individuals have to say and responding in a nonjudgmental way. The time you have with these patients is limited and so it should be focused on making the transition from the home to help at a hospital setting as quickly and with as little trauma as possible.

Selected References

American Psychiatric Association: *Diagnostic and Statistical Manual of Mental Disorders, Fourth Edition, Text Revision (DSM-IV-TR)*. Washington, DC, American Psychiatric Press, 2000.

Anderson (ed): *Mosby's Medical, Nursing, and Allied Health Dictionary*, ed 4. St Louis, MO, Elsevier Publishing, 1994.

Bienenfeld D: eMedicine: personality disorders. Available at: http://www.emedicine.com/med/topic3472.htm. Accessed May 14, 2008.

Frances A, First MB, Pincus HA: *DSM-IV Guidebook*. Washington, DC, American Psychiatric Press, 1995.

Halgin RP, Whitbourne SK: *Abnormal Psychology: Clinical Perspectives on Psychological Disorders,* ed 4 updated. New York, NY, McGraw Hill; 2005.

Helen's World of BPD Resources Web site. Diagnostic criteria for borderline personality disorder. Available at: http://www.bpdresources.com/diagnostic.html#DSM. Accessed July 7, 2008.

Long, PW: Internet mental health: paranoid, schizoid, schizotypal, dependent, obsessive-compulsive personality disorders. Available at: http://www.mentalhealth.com. Accessed May 14, 2008.

MayoClinic.com Web site. Available at: http://www.MayoClinic.com.

National Institute of Mental Health: Borderline personality disorder: raising questions, finding answers. Available at: http://www.nimh.nih.gov/publicat/bpd.cfm. Accessed July 7, 2008.

National Institute of Mental Health Web site. Available at: http://www.nimh.nih.gov/nimhhome/index.cfm. Accessed May 14, 2008.

Paranoid, schizoid, schizotypal, dependent, obsessive-compulsive personality disorders. Available at: http://psychologytoday.com.

PsychCentral. Paranoid, schizoid, schizotypal, dependent, obsessive-compulsive personality disorders. Available at: http://psychcentral.com. Accessed May 14, 2008.

Prep Kit

Ready for Review

- Personality disorders are pervasive and inflexible alterations of one's traits that lead to distress or impairment. They are often considered to be some of the more difficult psychological disorders to diagnose and treat because they affect every facet of an individual's life.

- The rate of comorbidity is high in those with personality disorders, including medical conditions and depression.

- The personality disorders are divided in the *DSM-IV-TR* into three clusters or groups based on their common characteristics. Cluster A individuals are odd and eccentric, cluster B individuals are dramatic and emotional, and cluster C patients are anxious and fearful.

- There is no specific prehospital care for these individuals, because you cannot treat a patient's personality. However, by reducing the stimuli and using good active listening skills, you should be able to efficiently and professionally get care for those individuals in need.

Vital Vocabulary

antisocial personality disorder (cluster B) A pattern of disregard for, and violation of, the rights of others.

avoidant personality disorder (cluster C) A pervasive pattern of social inhibition, feelings of inadequacy, and hypersensitivity to negative evaluation.

borderline personality disorder (BPD) (cluster B) A pattern of instability in interpersonal relationships, self-image, and affect, and marked impulsivity.

comorbidity Multiple psychological or medical conditions occurring simultaneously within one individual.

dependent personality disorder (DPD) (cluster C) A pattern of submissive and clinging behavior related to an excessive need to be taken care of by another.

dopamine A naturally occurring central nervous system neurotransmitter that transmits signals between cells; it has been linked with many functions such as mood, sexual pleasure, muscle movement, and balance.

dopaminergic Having the effect of dopamine.

histrionic One who seeks to be the center of attention.

histrionic personality disorder (HPD) (cluster B) A pattern of excessive emotionality and attention seeking.

illusion A false interpretation of an external sensory stimulus, commonly auditory or visual in nature.

narcissistic personality disorder (cluster B) A pattern of grandiosity, need for admiration, and lack of empathy.

obsessive-compulsive personality disorder (cluster C) A pattern of preoccupation with orderliness, perfectionism, and control.

paranoia A psychological condition exemplified by extreme suspiciousness, usually focused on one central theme. It often includes delusions of grandeur or persecution.

paranoid personality disorder (cluster A) A pattern of distrust and suspicion such that others' motives are interpreted as malevolent.

personality disorder Pervasive and inflexible alteration of one's traits that leads to distress or impairment.

schizoid personality disorder (cluster A) A pattern of detachment from social relationships and a restricted range of emotional expression.

schizotypal personality disorder (cluster A) A pattern of acute discomfort in close relationships, cognitive or perceptual distortions, and eccentricities of behavior.

Assessment in Action

Answer key is located in the back of the book.

1. A concerned neighbor calls EMS to an apartment complex for a 56-year-old woman who reportedly has been "acting strange" over the past few months. Police advise you that they have been at her place several times prior to this. During the interview, she appears to be alert and oriented; however, she seems preoccupied with telling you about her neighbor, whom she no longer trusts. The patient tells you that her neighbor has been watching her and wants to get her kicked out

of her apartment. She states that the neighbor is always "too friendly" in an effort to trick her into thinking that they are friends. Based on the case presentation, you suspect which personality disorder?

A. Schizoid
B. Schizotypal
C. Paranoid
D. Antisocial

2. EMS is dispatched to the local jail where a 20-year-old man has been arrested for destruction of property. During the arrest, he was chased by the police canine unit and was bitten in the arm. Officers inform you that he is a repeat offender and has a long criminal record for fighting and cruelty to animals since adolescence. Over the past few years, he has been unable to maintain employment, so he has resorted to being a professional criminal. His crimes have become more aggressive, and he appears to have no regard to his or anyone else's safety. Based on the case presentation, you suspect which personality disorder?

A. Borderline
B. Antisocial
C. Schizotypal
D. Narcissistic

3. Upon reporting to work one morning, you find that a new EMT has been assigned to your station. For the first several shifts, all appears to be going well and the person is willing to listen and learn. However, after about two weeks, things begin to change with this individual and a "new side" is presented. You notice that the top buttons of the uniform shirt are now often left unbuttoned and the person has become somewhat flirtatious and inappropriately sexually provocative toward several other crew members. Additionally, when entering the lounge area, there is always a dramatic, theatrical-style entrance. Based on the case presentation, you suspect which personality disorder?

A. Narcissistic
B. Dependent
C. Histrionic
D. Borderline

4. Over the past few months, a close friend has been sharing details about one of the "characters" who works at her office. She simply describes him as "creepy and strange." Upon questioning, she tells you that the guy is a loner who comes in to work and does not interact with the others in their section. He tends to eat alone in the corner of the cafeteria where he works on the crossword puzzle each day. He appears to have a flat affect and seems indifferent even when the supervisor gave him a "Job Well Done" certificate. Based on the case presentation, you suspect which personality disorder?

A. Schizoid
B. Paranoid
C. Antisocial
D. Schizotypal

5. EMS is dispatched to an office for a 37-year-old woman who became angry and smashed her hand into a wall after finding out that someone in the office drank the bottle of water that she had stored in the snack room refrigerator. On examination, it appears that the hand is obviously broken because it is swollen and painful to touch. One of the coworkers takes you to the side and informs you that things like this are common. Apparently, the patient has a history of poor interpersonal relationships and comments on how everyone she dates abandons her. Coworkers have been worried about her because she has made several suicidal comments over the past two years. In fact, last week, one coworker saw what appeared to be two or three cuts across her right wrist. Based on the case presentation, you suspect which personality disorder?

A. Dependent
B. Histrionic
C. Obsessive-compulsive
D. Borderline

Chapter 20

Sustaining Staff

No matter how well trained, experienced, and sophisticated emergency services and crisis intervention workers may be, they need a support system to sustain them or they will cease to function effectively. Crisis work is tough. Those who do it expose themselves to powerful and potentially destructive stressors that can have a significant negative impact on their work and their personal lives (**Figure 20-1**). A common-sense stress management system can do much to alleviate distress in crisis intervention personnel and to help maintain organizations.

What Works

There are many approaches to staff support associated with work-related traumatic crises, but most include the following important characteristics.

First, every successful crisis-oriented staff support program is *comprehensive*. That is, it has elements that address actions before, during, and after traumatic events, and the program is broad based and an integral part of the everyday operations of the department. Administration must accept a support program and build it into the fabric of the organization. Staff support programs must communicate, coordinate, and link their efforts with professionals in human resources, psychological services, and employee assistance programs. Staff support programs work best when the program recognizes the differences between support and therapy. Staff support

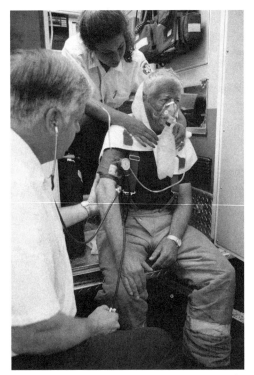

Figure 20-1 Crisis is tough on emergency personnel as well as the patients they assist.

services function at peak performance when they function separately under the umbrella of operations support. A crisis intervention program for staff is a support function, not a psychotherapeutic function.

Second, well-developed staff support programs designed to manage crises are *integrated*. All of the elements of a program are interrelated and blended with one another. The combined effects of an integrated program—that is, a crisis support program in which all of the parts are interlocked and blended—are far more powerful than any single element.

Third, staff members are best sustained by a *systematic* program, or a support package that has phases, segments, or logical steps. Staff support programs should, therefore, take a few simple steps, such as resting personnel and talking with them on an individual basis, before increasing the complexity, number, and duration of the available staff support functions after a distressing event. The order of support services usually cycles through individual support, immediate small-group support, then more individual support followed by a Critical Incident Stress Debriefing, family support, follow-up services, and closure of the interventions or referrals for additional services.

Finally, effective crisis staff support programs must be *multi-tactic* in approach. Many different types of support services must be available, as every person will have a somewhat different response to a highly stressful event. Some will benefit from group crisis support; others need individual support services. Some will need a referral for professional care. Each person will have different requirements to help recover from the stress of an experience or incident.

Linkage to a wide range of resources is another key characteristic of any staff support program. The magnitude of some events can be so severe and the personal reactions of some individuals may be so intense that additional assistance may be necessary. A staff support program must have mental health resources or other types of services within easy reach for people who need more help beyond crisis intervention. Among emergency services organizations, including EMS agencies, fire services, and police departments, crisis support teams are most effective when they are run and staffed by peer support personnel and backed up by both mental health professionals and chaplains who are trained in Critical Incident Stress Management.

In the Field

Support Services

- Individual support
- Immediate Small-Group Support
- Additional individual support
- Critical Incident Stress Debriefing (CISD)
- Family support
- Follow-up services
- Closure of the intervention with referrals as needed

In the Field

Elements of a Successful Crisis-Oriented Staff Support Program (CISM)

- Comprehensive
- Integrated
- Systematic
- Multi-tactic

The Well-Organized Staff Support Program

CISM team members go through extensive, multi-course training programs before engaging in CISM work. A typical training program has five central modules that include training for 1) assisting individuals in crisis, 2) working with large and small groups, 3) suicide prevention, intervention, and recovery, 4) advanced crisis intervention tactics, and 5) strategic planning. These five programs require a minimum of 10 days of crisis intervention training, and there are many specialty courses that enhance staff support services. The International Critical Incident Stress Foundation can provide additional information on Critical Incident Stress Management team development and training.

Comprehensive Staff Support

An effective crisis-oriented staff support program should be able to provide at least the following general categories of services:

- Assessment of the situation and of the reactions of personnel
- Strategic planning to provide the right help at the best time under the most advantageous circumstances
- Crisis intervention services designed for individuals
- Crisis intervention services for large groups
- Crisis intervention services for small groups
- Follow-up and referral services

Those six categories are considered the core competencies of any good staff support program. If a program cannot effectively deliver at least these six services, it should either accept additional training or cease to function as a crisis response team.

Important issues for the management of crises in a staff support program are spread over three general periods: pre-event, during the event, and post-event.

Pre-Event

Before operations personnel are exposed to traumatic events, their organizations should make provisions for a Critical Incident Stress Management (CISM) program. Leadership should be placed in the hands of a committed and dedicated person who has sufficient time to devote to support services. The program should be well organized and appropriately staffed by adequately trained peer support personnel, mental health professionals, and other resource personnel, such as clergy. Organizational policies must be developed to provide appropriate resources to the staff members. Finally, an education and training program for stress management should be built into the organization's structure; this program can be presented well in advance of traumatic events. Continuing education classes are excellent opportunities to educate personnel about reactions to stress and stress management.

During the Event

Once an event is underway, personnel must be supported by information and, when necessary, individual crisis intervention and other services. Shelter from the elements, food, fluids, and other necessities should never be overlooked (**Figure 20-2**). Common CISM services provided during an emergency situation include large-group services such as Rest, Information and Transition Sessions and Crisis Management Briefings.

Crisis Management Briefings (CMB) are large-group information sessions that may be used for virtually any size group of people who have experienced the same traumatic or distressing event. The group process remains in the cognitive (thinking) domain and avoids or limits

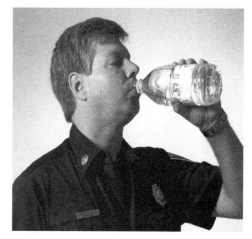

Figure 20-2 Shelter from the elements, food, fluids, and other necessities should never be overlooked during a crisis.

discussions in the affective (emotions) domain. The emphasis during the CMB group meeting is on practical information that can help to reduce anxiety and distress. Rest, Information and Transition Sessions (RITS) is a technique similar to the Crisis Management Briefing, except it does not contain a question-and-answer period, and the session is aimed at staff personnel who have just completed their first shift of work at a large-scale incident. CISM team members are also available to support and provide consultations to command and supervisory staff.

Post-Event

There are many support services that are helpful when an emergency situation ends. They include, but are not limited to, individual crisis intervention, Immediate Small Group Support (ISGS) or defusing services followed later by Powerful Event Group Support (PEGS), which is also known as Critical Incident Stress Debriefing (CISD). It is also important to have in place support services for family and significant others, chaplain services, post-incident education, follow-up services, and referrals for additional care if that becomes necessary.

A Package of Interventions

Crisis intervention tactics must be blended and combined into a sensible support package. It is not effective to simply choose one or even a few tactics if those interventions are used in isolation from each other; the best support programs are those that appropriately utilize all of the tools at the team's disposal.

Integrated Staff Support

No single staff support tactic or crisis intervention process should be considered a stand-alone procedure. Every procedure must be carefully blended and combined with other support services in a logical, sensible manner. For example, the CISD, which is an excellent small-group support process, should be incorporated into a package of other services, including individual support and follow-up services. The CISD is often preceded by a small-group 'defusing' and followed by individual contacts. Other services such as significant-other support, chaplain services, telephone calls, and station visits are blended into the support package as the specific needs of the individuals or group suggest.

Systematic Staff Support

Some tactics in a comprehensive and integrated staff support program are time or phase sensitive. Tactics may need to be applied within certain periods of time and/or in a specific order. Steps one, two, and three in a program, for example, are applied before steps four, five, and six. Crisis response teams should be trained to plan support services strategically so that they can be arranged in an appropriate order and applied under circumstances that enhance the support services. For example, in a case in which a small group of emergency personnel are exposed to a horrific auto accident involving the death of two small children, it is best to provide the Immediate Small Group Support service (defusing) within 8 hours (**Figure 20-3**). Individuals having the most difficulties are identified by the crisis support team, and those individuals receive one-on-one support. A more formal group discussion, the Powerful Event Group Support (also known as the Critical Incident Stress Debriefing) process is then held about 4 or 5 days after the incident. The Immediate Small Group Support process usually helps the Powerful Event Group Support process to be more effective by opening the paths to communication.

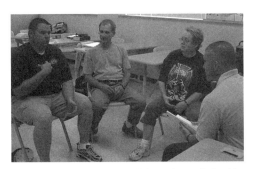

Figure 20-3 Immediate Small Group Support should be provided within 8 hours of a traumatic event.

Multitactic Staff Support

Crisis intervention has many tools, tactics, or procedures for different purposes to help people struggling through a crisis. Helpful procedures are limited only by the people selecting them and by the circumstances under which they are applied. **Table 20-1** catalogs some of the many support services that trained CISM personnel may utilize. Circumstance, specific needs, availability of trained and experienced resources, and administrative endorsement will all limit or enhance the development and application of a range of crisis intervention services.

Preincident Preparation

Preincident preparation includes every activity that educates people about crises, prepares a team to respond to a critical incident, or establishes policies and procedures to manage a psychological

Table 20-1 Summary of Commonly Used Crisis Intervention Tactics

Intervention	Timing	Target Group	Potential Goals
Pre-event planning/preparation	Pre-event	Anticipated target/victim population	Anticipatory guidance, foster resistance, resilience
Surveillance and assessment	Pre-intervention	Those directly and indirectly affected	Determine need for intervention(s)
Strategic planning	Pre-event, during the event, and after the event	Anticipated exposed and victim populations	Improve overall crisis response
Individual crisis intervention (including "psychological first aid") and SAFER-R	As needed	Individuals as needed	Assessment, screening, education normalization, reduction of acute distress, triage, and facilitation of continued support
Large-group crisis intervention			
• Rest, Information, and Transition Session (RITS) (formerly known as "demobilization")	Shift disengagement, end of deployment	Emergency personnel, large groups	Decompression, ease transition from intense to less intense work, screening, triage, education, and meet basis needs
• Respite center	Ongoing, large-scale events as needed	Usually emergency personnel	Respite, refreshment, screening, triage, and support
• Crisis Management Briefing (CMB) and provide large-group "psychological first aid"	On-going and post-event; may be repeated as needed	Heterogeneous large groups	Inform, control rumors, increase cohesion

Continued

Table 20-1 (Continued)

Small-group crisis intervention

• Small-group Crisis Management Briefing (CMB)	Ongoing events and post-events	Small groups seeking information and resources	Inform, control rumors, reduce acute distress, increase cohesion, facilitate resilience, screening, and triage
• Immediate Small-Group Support (also known as defusing), and a form of small-group "psychological first aid"	12 hours or less post-event:	Small homogeneous groups	Stabilization, ventilation, reduce acute distress, screening, information
• Group debriefing (Powerful Event Group Support (PEGS) {also known as Critical Incident Stress Debriefing (CISD)}	1-10 days for acute incidents; may be 3-4 weeks or even longer if group is in postdisaster recovery phases	Small homogeneous groups with equal trauma exposure (eg, work groups, emergency service, and military)	Increase cohesion, ventilation, information normalization, reduce acute distress, facilitate resilience, screening, and triage; follow-up is essential
Family crisis intervention	Pre-event; as needed	Families	Wide range of interventions (eg, pre-event preparation, individual crisis intervention, CMB, PEGS (CISD), or other group process)
Organization/Community Intervention, Consultation	Pre-event; as needed	Organizations affected by trauma or disaster	Improve organizational preparedness and response; leadership consultation
Pastoral Crisis Intervention	As needed	Individuals, small groups, large groups, congregations, and communities who desire faith-based presence/crisis intervention	Faith-based support
Follow-up and/or referral; facilitate access to continued care	As needed	Intervention recipients and exposed individuals	Ensure continuity of care

Adapted, with permission, from: Everly GS, Mitchell JT: *Integrative Crisis Intervention & Disaster Mental Health.* Ellicott City, MD, Chevron Publishing Corporation, 2008.

crisis. CISM teams work hard to train their members and to plan for emergencies in which their services might be required. In down times between callouts, the CISM team reviews and improves its policies and procedures. Administrators must be informed of the policies and procedures that guide the team. They should also know the team's capabilities and the activities of the team on previous callouts. Before emergencies, the team should identify potential referral resources and learn of their services. When a referral is required, the referral source is ready to assist an emergency services person. The preincident preparation process includes the following:

a) Planning

b) Policy development

c) Education/training

d) Administrative briefings

e) Critical Incident Stress Management team development

f) Protocol and procedures development

g) Identification of referral resources

Assessment

A key element in a CISM program is the ability to properly assess the magnitude of the event and the intensity of the impact on the personnel. The elements of the assessment are situation assessment, reactions of personnel, determination of immediate needs, and availability and suitability of resources. The situation assessment describes what has happened, its duration, unusual circumstances, and any factors that might have a psychological impact on emergency services personnel. The reactions of personnel are gauged by whether or not they are able to function, whether they miss time from work, and whether they have suffered personal responses such as dreams, nightmares, or emotional distress. A CISM team must determine the best course of action quickly and assist distressed emergency personnel with their immediate needs. During the support process, a CISM team also must determine if anyone requires a special resource to recover from the traumatic event.

Strategic Planning

The application of crisis intervention tactics to assist emergency personnel must make sense in the context of the assessment of the situation and the effects on the personnel. The best formula to make a strategic plan includes the five Ts: target, type, timing, theme, and team. That is, the plan should include:

a) Identifying appropriate *targets* for support

b) Selecting the best *types* of interventions

c) *Timing* interventions for best effects

d) Considering all the *themes* or circumstances, concerns, and issues and working through them to ensure maximum benefit of the support services

e) Choosing the best *team* to deliver the support services

Individual Crisis Intervention

The most common type of CISM intervention is individual crisis intervention. It occurs approximately 100 times as often as the small-group crisis intervention process known as Critical Incident Stress Debriefing (CISD). Individual support is given by a trained CISM team member, typically a peer support person, to an individual needing assistance. The SAFER-R crisis intervention model is the most common tool utilized in the one-on-one support process. CISM team members are trained to use this tool to assist emergency personnel and others in recovering rapidly from a traumatic experience. No one should assume that everything is just fine after a single contact. In crisis intervention, some form of brief follow-up is always required. That may be accomplished by a phone call or by a brief visit to the workplace. In a small percentage of personnel, a referral to professional assistance may be necessary to help a person fully recover after exposure to a traumatic event. The features of an individual crisis intervention program are:

a) Individual support by trained peer support personnel

b) Use of the SAFER-R model for individual crisis intervention

c) Follow-up services until recovery is evident (telephone calls, home visits, and worksite visits)

d) Referrals to the proper resources for those needing additional services

e) Ongoing assessment and adjustment to the needs of the individual

Large-Group Informational Sessions

Large-scale events like disasters, wildland fires, and searches for missing people may generate enough distress to require large-group crisis intervention procedures. Large-group crisis intervention tactics include RITS and CMBs. For the staff working a disaster for instance, the Rest, Information, and Transition Session provides exactly what the title describes. It is a period of rest after emergency crews have worked their first shift at a disaster. During this rest period, crisis intervention staff share information about stress control tactics with emergency crew personnel. Personnel are then fed and either released to get sleep or are assigned to more routine duties away from the disaster.

The Crisis Management Briefing is a more versatile large-group crisis intervention process. It is used to brief people about a situation before they are exposed to it, and it is used to help guide and direct them after they have had an exposure to a traumatic event. The Crisis Management Briefing contains a question-and-answer period to help people obtain the most information they can about a situation and the accompanying stress reactions. Stress reactions are normalized and specific practical advice is given.

Small-Group Services

When a homogeneous (same) group of operations, personnel is stressed by the same event, they can benefit from the support provided in a group session by their trained crisis support colleagues. There are two main small-group, crisis intervention processes. They are Immediate Small Group Support (also known as *defusing*) immediately after a disturbing event, and Powerful Event Group Support (PEGS), also known as Critical Incident Stress Debriefing (CISD), a few days after the event.

The Immediate Small Group Support (ISGS) process is designed for immediate use after a homogeneous group has been exposed to a disturbing traumatic event. Most often the process is provided within a very short time of the incident. After about 8 to 12 hours, the process loses its effectiveness, because people tend to shut down their response to a bad experience. ISGS is led by two members of a trained CISM team. The team members introduce themselves and go over a few guidelines for the ISGS service. This process is also known as a defusing, and it was developed to take the edge off the bad experience. In the second phase of the process, the group members are asked to briefly review the incident they just experienced. The information they provide helps the CISM team members provide the most helpful information to the group. The final stage of the ISGS process is a stress information presentation by the team members. They provide practical advice on the proper foods to eat, resting, exercising, avoiding alcohol, and being in contact with people they trust. The entire session is usually complete within 30 to 45 minutes.

The second main small-group crisis intervention process is known as the Critical Incident Stress Debriefing (CISD). The United Nations has adopted alternative terminology. They call the process Powerful Event Group Support (PEGS). It is a guided group discussion of a traumatic event. The process may take between one and three hours, depending on both the nature of the incident and the number of people attending. Between two and four members of a trained CISM team conduct the CISD. There are three criteria for the use of the CISD: the small group must be a *homogeneous* group; the situation is over or the *mission is complete*; and the small group must have had more or less *equal exposure to the event.*

The team leads the group through seven phases in the CISD. The steps in the process are:

1. Introduction and guidelines for the CISD
2. A brief situation review
3. A discussion of the group members' first impressions
4. A discussion of the part of the incident that caused the greatest personal impact for the group members
5. A discussion of the signals of distress encountered by the group members
6. Stress information and guidelines for stress management from the CISD team
7. A summary of the discussion and a question-and-answer period

The primary objectives of the process are to mitigate distress, enhance group cohesion, and restore individuals and the group as a whole to effective performance. In addition, the session provides the opportunity to identify individual members of a group who might require additional assistance and to ensure proper referrals for those individuals.

Under no circumstances should the interventions provided by a CISM team be viewed as psychotherapy or a substitute for psychotherapy. Every effort made by a CISM team is a support service, not a therapy.

Family and Significant Other Support Programs

Emergency personnel live among family and friends. They are not in isolation. An effective CISM program must address the needs of the workers' family and friends. Significant others have many needs, not the least of which is accurate information about what has happened to their loved ones and what can be done about it. The following list shines a spotlight on some of the things that a CISM team should be able to provide to the families and friends of emergency personnel.

a) Information
b) Resource identification
c) Family/significant other liaison
d) Family-oriented group support
e) Referrals
f) Chaplain services
g) Direct assistance in daily life issues (child care, lawn care, and shopping) during the crisis period

Chaplain Support Services

In many organizations, a chaplain program is an integral part of the support services for emergency personnel. Chaplains help to keep operations personnel healthy and motivated in their work. They provide many services, including funerals, sick visits, follow-up services, counseling, referrals, locating and obtaining resources, and participation in CISM support services.

Organizational Support

Command and supervisory personnel need guidance and support from CISM teams. They sometimes do not see the ramifications of their decisions. CISM team members have been helpful in providing consultations with command and supervisors, crisis intervention advice, assistance with

In the Field

Peer support can be helpful in the following ways:

- Providing one-on-one support to their fellow workers.
- Reducing stimuli. By cutting auditory, visual, and olfactory stimuli in the early stages of a traumatic event, they have already done good crisis intervention.
- Assessing a situation and the impact on the personnel.
- Providing information and stress management guidelines.
- Calling in additional resources from a CISM team.
- Consulting with supervisors and administration regarding stress reactions.
- Advocating for stress support on behalf of their fellow workers.
- Participating in large- and small-group support services.
- Providing family and significant other support services.
- Providing many different follow-up services for emergency personnel.

public information announcements, and guidance for policy and protocol development.

Follow-up Services

The assumption that personnel are completely over a traumatic event after just one contact is a flawed belief. It is not unusual for two or three contacts to be made before CISM team members can be assured that the personnel have recovered from the shock of a traumatic event. Procedures used to provide follow-up services include telephone calls, home visits, work site visits, individual support, and other assistance as required.

The vast majority of emergency personnel will not need formal professional services after they have been exposed to a traumatic event. Most recover and accomplish that recovery fairly quickly. Sometimes the magnitude of the event or the impact on a few of the personnel is so great that recovery becomes difficult. In such cases a referral to a professional may be helpful. There are many sources of professional support, including employee assistance programs, medical services, psychological services, legal services, human resources, counseling services, and other referrals as identified.

When an incident ends and all of the support services are completed, there is still work to be done. There are many lessons to be learned and incorporated into the knowledge base of the organization. In some cases, improvements to procedures can be made on the basis of previous experience. Key issues for CISM teams after an incident include incident reviews and education and incorporation of lessons learned into staff support programs. The members of a CISM team are specially trained and should know when and how to use the appropriate support services and crisis intervention procedures. They also should be able to learn from experience and incorporate what they learn into the services they offer.

Peer Support

Peer support encompasses a wide range of support services provided by trained peer support personnel on a CISM team. Peers do the bulk of the individual support services and the follow-up services. Peers also encourage their colleagues to accept professional support when it is necessary, and may actually drive a colleague to an appointment and sit through the first session to get the colleague through the transition to someone else's care. Peers have been known to go to a police officer's or a paramedic's home in the middle of the night to prevent a suicide.

Experience indicates that peer support personnel are quite remarkable in their ability to care for others within their profession. They are efficient and effective. Good training combined with a caring personality is an unbeatable combination.

Final Thoughts

Well-developed CISM programs have been credited with significant reductions in sick time utilization, premature retirements, and disability claims against employers. They are instrumental in the maintenance of healthy personal relationships and in the prevention of suicides among emergency personnel. The overall health of an emergency organization is improved when a staff support program is in place.

Selected References

Bohl N: The effectiveness of brief psychological interventions in police officers after critical incidents, in Reese JT, Horn J, Dunning C (eds): *Critical Incidents in Policing, Revised.* Washington, DC, Department of Justice, 1991, pp 31–38.

Bohl N: Measuring the effectiveness of CISD. *Fire Engineering,* 1995, 125–126.

Bordow S, Porritt D: An experimental evaluation of crisis intervention. *Soc Sci Med,* 1979;13:251–256.

Boscarino JA, Adams RE, Figley CR: A prospective cohort study of the effectiveness of employer sponsored crisis intervention after a major disaster. *Int J Emerg Ment Health,* 2005;7:31–44.

Bunn T, Clarke A: Crisis intervention. *Brit J Med Psychology,* 1979;52:191–195.

Campfield K, Hills A: Effect of timing of critical incident stress debriefing (CISD) on posttraumatic symptoms. *J Trauma Stress,* 2001;14:327–340.

Chemtob C, Tomas S, Law W, Cremniter D: Post disaster psychosocial intervention. *Am J Psychiatry,* 1997;134:415–417.

Deahl M, Srinivasan M, Jones N, Thomas J, Neblett C, Jolly A: Preventing psychological trauma in soldiers: the role of operational stress training and psychological debriefing. *Brit J Med Psychiatry,* 2000;73:77–85.

Dyregrov A: The process in critical incident stress debriefings. *J Trauma Stress,* 1997;10:589–605.

Dyregrov A: Psychological debriefing: an effective method? *Traumatology,* 1998;4:1.

Eid J, Johnsen BH, Weisaeth L: The effects of group psychological debriefing on acute stress reactions following a traffic accident: a quasi-experimental approach. *Int J Emerg Ment Health,* 2001;3:145–154.

Everly GS, Flannery RB, Eyler V, Mitchell JT: Sufficiency analysis of an integrated multi-component approach to crisis intervention: critical incident stress management. *Adv Mind-Body Med.* 2001;17:174–183.

Everly GS, Flannery R, Mitchell JT: Critical incident stress management (CISM): a review of the literature. *Aggression Violent Behav Rev J,* 2000;5:23–40.

Everly GS, Mitchell JT: *Integrative Crisis Intervention.* Ellicott City, MD, Chevron Publishing Corporation, 2008.

Flannery RB: *The Assaulted Staff Action Program: Coping With the Psychological Aftermath of Violence.* Ellicott City, MD, Chevron Publishing, 1998.

Flannery RB: Assaulted Staff Action Program (ASAP): ten years of empirical support for critical incident stress management (CISM). *Int J Emerg Ment Health.* 2001;3:5–10.

Hiley-Young B, Gerrity ET: Critical incident stress debriefing (CISD): value and limitations in disaster response. *NCP Clin Q.* 1994;4:17–19.

Jenkins SR: Social support and debriefing efficacy among emergency medical workers after a mass shooting incident. *J Soc Behav Per,* 1996;11:447–492.

Leeman-Conley M: After a violent robbery. *Criminology Australia.* 1990;April/May:4–6.

Mitchell JT: *Group Crisis Support: Why It Works, When and How to Provide It.* Ellicott City, MD, Chevron Publishing, 2007.

Mitchell JT: *Critical Incident Stress Management (CISM): A Defense of the Field.* Ellicott City, MD, International Critical Incident Stress Foundation, 2004.

Mitchell JT: *Critical Incident Stress Management (CISM): Group Crisis Intervention,* ed 4. Ellicott City, MD, International Critical Incident Stress Foundation, 2006.

Mitchell JT: Characteristics of successful early intervention programs. *Int J Emerg Ment Health,* 2004;6:175–184.

Mitchell JT: *Crisis Intervention and Critical Incident Stress Management: A Research Summary.* Ellicott City, MD, International Critical Incident Stress Foundation, 2003.

Mitchell JT, Bray G: *Emergency Services Stress.* Englewood Cliffs, NJ, Prentice Hall, 1990.

Nurmi L: The sinking of the Estonia: the effects of critical incident stress debriefing on rescuers. *Int J Emerg Ment Health,* 1999;1:23–32.

Richards D: A field study of critical incident stress debriefing versus critical incident stress management. *J Ment Health,* 2001;10:351–362.

Robinson RC, Mitchell JT: Evaluation of psychological debriefings. *J Traumatic Stress,* 1993;6:367–382.

Swanson WC, Carbon JB: Crisis intervention: theory and technique, in Task Force Report of the American Psychiatric Association: *Treatments of Psychiatric Disorders.* Washington, DC, APA Press, 1989.

Wee DF, Mills DM, Koelher G (1999): The effects of critical incident stress debriefing on emergency medical services personnel following the Los Angeles civil disturbance. *Int J Emerg Ment Health.* 1999;1:33–38.

Western Management Consultants: *The Medical Services Branch CISM Evaluation Report.* Vancouver, BC, Western Management Consultants, 1996.

Prep Kit

Ready for Review

- Supporting one's staff is a critical component to surviving work-related trauma. A good organization will have a program that is comprehensive, integrated, systematic, and multi-tactic.
- A well-organized staff support program requires that CISM team members go through extensive training. CISM responders must be versed in prevention, management, and intervention tactics for both individuals and groups of various sizes.
- Preincident preparation includes every activity that educates people about crises, prepares a team to respond to a critical incident, or establishes policies and procedures to manage a psychological crisis in staff.
- A comprehensive program recognizes that the family members are also part of the team.

Vital Vocabulary

Critical Incident Stress Debriefing (CISD) A group support meeting for a small group that works together and has experienced a disturbing traumatic event together. The CISD is a specific, seven-phase process that takes place typically within a few days of the traumatic event. It is not psychotherapy, nor is it a substitute for psychotherapy. CISD aims at group support during a period of distress, and its primary goal is the enhancement of unit cohesion and unit performance.

Crisis Management Briefing (CMB) A meeting to present stress management information, typically to a large, mixed group of people who experienced a traumatic event. The CMB emphasizes practical, immediately useful information to manage the crisis situation. The CMB focuses on a cognitive discussion instead of an exploration of emotions. It is useful in reducing anxiety and distress in the group members.

Immediate Small Group Support (ISGS) New and improved descriptive terminology for the small-group defusing process. ISGS takes place as soon as possible after the traumatic event, allows for a very brief discussion of the

traumatic event, and stresses survival information to assist the members of the small group with managing their distress until additional support can be rendered by means of a PEGS or other support services.

Rest, Information and Transition Session (RITS) A technique similar to the crisis management briefing except it does not contain a question-and-answer period and the session is aimed at staff personnel who just completed their first shift of work at a large-scale incident like a disaster.

Powerful Event Group Support (PEGS) New and improved descriptive terminology approved by the United Nations to describe the Critical Incident Stress Debriefing process. The PEGS is a small-group process for primary groups who are known to each other, have a history together, and have worked together on the same traumatic event.

Assessment in Action

Answer key is located in the back of the book.

1. In order for a crisis support program to work effectively, it must have the backing of which of the following?

   A. The administrative officers at the top of the organization
   B. EMS providers within the organization
   C. In-the-field supervisory personnel
   D. All of the above

2. Research has shown that following severe critical incidents, prehospital providers benefit greatly from the support that they receive from their own peer group.

   A. True
   B. False

3. Well-developed staff support programs designed to manage crises are composed of four basic elements. From the following list, select the one that is NOT an element of the program.

A. Integrated and interrelated
B. Composed only of external personnel
C. Multitactic
D. Systematic

4. The effective crisis-oriented staff support program should be able to provide all of the following services EXCEPT:

A. crisis intervention to small groups of individuals
B. assessment of personnel following a traumatic incident
C. follow-up and referrals for individuals needing more assistance
D. long-term counseling

5. Key components of preincident preparation are planning, policy development, education, and CISM team development.

A. True
B. False

Note: As a result of extensive work with the United Nations in 2007, alternatives to the terms 'defusing' and 'Critical Incident Stress Debriefing' have been developed to reflect improvements and clarifications in those two group crisis intervention processes. Defusing may also be called "Immediate Small Group Support" ISGS) and the Critical Incident Stress Debriefing (CISD) may also be called "Powerful Event Group Support" (PEGS). These alternative terms more accurately describe what is actually done within the defusing and CISD processes.

Glossary

abuse Abuse occurs when an individual continues the use of a substance despite significant impairment or distress caused during or shortly after the use of the substance.

acrophobia Irrational fear of heights.

active phase The second phase of schizophrenia. During this phase, the person is completely detached from reality and the surrounding environment, often resulting in isolation. The individual believes and lives in a confabulated or made-up world and commonly experiences increased mental pain and suffering.

actual consent Direct verbal or written agreement by the patient to accept a medical intervention.

acute stress disorder An anxiety disorder that develops after a traumatic event, with symptoms such as depersonalization, numbing, dissociative amnesia, intense anxiety, hypervigilance, and impairment of everyday functioning that last for less than one month after a stressor.

adaptive functioning A measure of how effectively the person can perform everyday tasks. Skills involved in adaptive functioning include, but are not limited to, communication and social interaction abilities, fine motor skills, and occupational skills.

affect The observable emotion or feeling, tone, and mood attached to a thought; one's emotional presentation to the evaluator.

affective disorder See mood disorder.

affective flattening Exhibiting decreased emotions, facial expression, and responsiveness to one's surrounding environment.

agnosia The inability to identify or recognize common people or objects that would normally be familiar.

agnosia The inability to identify or recognize familiar people or objects.

agoraphobia The intense fear of being trapped, stranded, or embarrassed in a situation without help if a panic attack were to occur; also the fear of open spaces.

akathisia A feeling of restlessness, having to constantly move or leave.

alignment A crisis intervention technique in which the person attempting to help expresses understanding of the person's situation and feelings.

alogia The inability to speak because of a medical or psychological reason.

alveolar hypoventilation syndrome A type of disorder, commonly seen in very obese patients, which presents because of some impairment in the patient's respiratory system that affects breathing efforts, particularly during sleep.

Alzheimer's disease (AD) A disease process that results from a loss of nerve cells in specialized areas of the brain that deal with cognitive functions, especially with those cells that release the neurotransmitter, acetylcholine. It is the most common form of dementia among older patients.

amenorrhea The absence of menstrual cycles.

amnesia A pathological absence, impairment, or loss of memory.

amnestic apraxia A condition in which patients cannot perform a function simply because they cannot remember how to accomplish the task.

amphetamine derivative Drugs that are chemically similar or that produce similar effects to that of amphetamines. These drugs stimulate the central nervous system, resulting in elevated blood pressure, heart rate, and other metabolic functions.

anhedonia The inability to experience pleasure.

anorectic A person suffering from anorexia nervosa.

anorexia Lack of appetite.

anorexia nervosa An eating disorder in which the individual refuses to maintain a healthy body weight through the restriction of food intake or other means.

anterograde amnesia A condition in which the individual is unable to retain new memories or to learn new bits of information.

anticipatory grief Actively processing thoughts and feelings related to the loss of a person before the death has occured.

antisocial personality disorder (cluster B) A pattern of disregard for, and violation of, the rights of others.

anxiety The sense of fear, apprehension, or worrying about something terrible happening in the near or distant future.

anxiety disorder A class of mental health disorders characterized by irrational fear and intense anxiety that leads to significant detriment to an individual's quality of life.

anxiolytic Classification of a group of medications given to reduce anxiety.

apathetic Condition in which a patient exhibits a lack of emotion; indifferent.

aphasia The inability to produce or comprehend language.

apnea Absence of breathing.

apraxia An inability to perform useful tasks or conduct object manipulation even though the patient is not paralyzed.

Asperger's syndrome A developmental disorder, usually diagnosed in childhood, characterized by impairments in social interactions and repetitive behavior patterns.

attention-deficit/hyperactivity disorder (ADHD) A condition characterized by an impaired ability to regulate activity level (hyperactivity), attend to tasks (inattention), and inhibit behavior (impulsivity).

autism A disorder that typically affects a person's ability to communicate, form relationships with others, and respond appropriately to the environment. Some people with autism have few problems with speech and intelligence and are able to function relatively well in society. Others are mentally retarded or mute or have serious language delays. Autism makes some people seem closed off and shut down; others seem locked into repetitive behaviors and rigid patterns of thinking.

aversion Normal response of discomfort or dislike to a particular object or situation.

avoidance A type of intrusive symptom commonly seen in PTSD in which the traumatic event is so distressing that the individual attempts to avoid contact with those things or people that may trigger memories of the event.

avoidant personality disorder (cluster C) A pervasive pattern of social inhibition, feelings of inadequacy, and hypersensitivity to negative evaluation.

avolition An unwillingness to respond or act.

axis A domain of behaviors or a set of signs and symptoms aligned in such a manner that they lead to certain conclusions about the person. Axes include: clinical disorders, personality disorders, mental retardation, general medical conditions, psychosocial and environmental problems, and the GAF.

behavior Any organism's activities and reactions in response to either internal or external stimuli.

bereavement A more generalized state of loss, sadness, grief, and mourning following the loss of a loved one.

binge-eating disorder (BED) An eating disorder that involves the eating of large quantities of food during repetitive episodes in a restricted period of time over several months.

bingeing The process of eating an abnormally large amount of food over a short period of time.

bipolar disorder A major mental disorder characterized by episodes of mania, depression, or mixed mood.

borderline personality disorder (BPD) (clusterB) A pattern of instability in interpersonal relationships, self-image, and affect, and marked impulsivity.

bradycardia Slow heart rate.

breathing-related sleep disorder (BRSD) Sleep disruption leading to excessive sleepiness or, less commonly, insomnia that is judged to be because of abnormalities of ventilation during sleep.

brief psychotic disorder A condition lasting less than one month in which an individual presents with a sudden onset of the symptoms of psychosis such as delusions, hallucinations, or gross disorganization as the result of a stressful or traumatic event.

buccofacial apraxia The inability to perform skilled movements involving the tongue, lips, and mouth (in the absence of paralysis).

bulimia nervosa An eating disorder characterized by a repeated cycle of bingeing and purging; it includes inappropriate ways to counteract the bingeing, such as forced vomiting or using laxatives.

bulimic A person suffering from bulimia nervosa.

cataplexy A sudden loss of muscle tone and strength, usually caused by an extreme emotional stimulus or narcolepsy.

catatonia A state of psychologically induced immobility with muscular rigidity; can be interrupted with agitation.

catatonic type schizophrenia A type of schizophrenia with marked psychomotor disturbances that may involve motor immobility, excessive motor activity, extreme negativism, mutism, peculiarities of voluntary movement, echolalia, or echopraxia.

central sleep apnea syndrome (CSAS) A type of breathing-related sleep disorder that is prevalent in those older than 40 years who present with apnea and hypopnea, without airway obstruction.

childhood disintegrative disorder A condition occurring in young children that is characterized by normal development in the first several years of life, followed by a marked developmental regression (a child who previously had been speaking in sentences becomes totally mute); various autistic features develop. Also known as dementia infantilis or Heller's syndrome.

circadian rhythm Also known as the sleep-wake cycle. The routine sleep-wake cycle experienced by humans is over a 24-hour period of time.

circadian rhythm sleep disorder A persistent or recurrent pattern of sleep disruption that results from altered function of the circadian timing system or from a mismatch between the individual's endogenous circadian sleep-wake system and exogenous demands regarding the timing and duration of sleep.

claustrophobia The fear of being in small or confined spaces.

cognition The mental process of gaining knowledge and comprehension, including aspects such as awareness, remembering, perception, reasoning, judgment, and problem solving.

combined type A form of ADHD in which the individual exhibits signs of both the predominantly inattentive and hyperactive-impulsive types of ADHD. The individual will present with the inability to pay attention and hyperactivity-impulsiveness.

commission A form of negligence that occurs when the EMS provider with a duty to act performs assessments or procedures that in turn harm or create injury to the patient.

comorbidity Multiple psychological or medical conditions occurring simultaneously within one individual.

compulsion Repetitive behaviors, either observable or mental, that are intended to reduce the anxiety engendered by obsessions.

conduct disorder A personality disorder of children and adolescents involving persistent antisocial behavior. Individuals with conduct disorder frequently participate in activities such as stealing, lying, truancy, vandalism, and substance abuse.

confabulation The fabrication of events, facts, or experiences to fill in gaps in memory.

contagion theory Crowds exert tremendous influence on individuals, causing those individuals to act quite differently in the crowd than they would as individuals; also known as mob rule.

continuous amnesia A form of dissociative amnesia in which the individual cannot recall anything following a traumatic incident and becomes unable to learn new information, often resulting in impairment in the person's school, work or social life.

continuous positive airway pressure (CPAP) An airway system in which a patient sleeps with a mask device over the nose that continually forces air into the airway in order to keep the nasopharynx open, hence reducing snoring and sleep apnea episodes.

convergence theory Like-minded people come together and form a crowd that ultimately acts on similar goals held by the individuals who make up the crowd.

craving A strong drive to use a substance, often seen as a common sign of substance dependence.

crisis An acute emotional reaction to a powerful stimulus (plural: crises).

crisis intervention A temporary, active, and supportive entry into the life situation of a person or a group during a period of acute distress.

Crisis Management Briefing (CMB) A meeting to present stress management information, typically to a large, mixed group of people who experienced a traumatic event. The CMB emphasizes practical, immediately useful information to manage the crisis situation. The CMB focuses on a cognitive discussion instead of an exploration of emotions. It is useful in reducing anxiety and distress in the group members.

critical incident Significant, severe events that can overwhelm a person's or even a group's ability to cope; these events disrupt normal functions.

Critical Incident Stress Debriefing (CISD) A group support meeting for a small group that works together and has experienced a disturbing traumatic event together. The CISD is a specific, seven-phase process that takes place typically within a few days of the traumatic event. It is not psychotherapy, nor is it a substitute for psychotherapy. CISD aims at group support during a period of distress, and its primary goal is the enhancement of unit cohesion and unit performance.

cyclothymia (or cyclothymic disorder) A disorder of mood wherein the essential feature is a chronic mood disturbance of at least 2 years' duration, involving numerous periods of mild depression and hypomania.

delirium A disturbance of consciousness and a change in cognition that develop over a short period of time.

delirium tremens (DTs) A syndrome resulting from the withdrawal of alcohol.

delusion False beliefs that significantly hinder a person's ability to function.

delusional disorder A condition in which the individual has a firm belief based on something that is not true. Delusional disorders are classified according to the prominent delusional theme as erotomanic, grandiose, jealous, persecutory, or somatic.

dementia A condition with multiple cognitive deficits that include impairment in memory.

dementia infantilis See childhood disintegrative disorder.

dependence When an individual continues to use a substance despite adverse physiological changes and negative life events.

dependent personality disorder (DPD) (cluster C) A pattern of submissive and clinging behavior related to an excessive need to be taken care of by another.

depersonalization A state in which someone loses the feeling of his or her own identity in relation to others in the family or peer group or loses the feeling of his or her own reality.

depersonalization disorder Condition characterized by a persistent or recurrent feeling of being detached from one's mental processes or body that is accompanied by intact reality testing.

depression A syndrome in which a depressed mood is accompanied by several other symptoms, such as fatigue, loss of energy, difficulty in sleeping, and changes in appetite.

derealization An internal perception that an individual is living through a dream or in a movie, or that one is outside of oneself and looking on as a spectator to their own experience.

Diagnostic and Statistical Manual of Mental Disorders, Fourth Edition, Text Revision (DSM-IV-TR) A guidebook published by the American Psychiatric Association that sets forth diagnostic criteria, descriptions, and other information regarding the classification and diagnosis of mental disorders.

diplopia Double vision.

disassociation An unconscious separation of a group of mental processes from the rest, resulting in an independent functioning of these processes and a loss of the usual associations.

disaster Any event that overwhelms the available emergency resources of a particular jurisdiction or community and causes them to function at a less than an optimal level of performance.

disorganized type schizophrenia Considered to be the most severe and debilitating form of schizophrenia, with a presentation that includes disorganized speech, thought, and actions, along with extremely bizarre behavior.

dissociate To cease associating with or to separate.

dissociative amnesia Condition characterized by an inability to recall important personal information, usually of a traumatic or stressful nature, that is too extensive to be explained by ordinary forgetfulness.

dissociative disorder not otherwise specified (NOS) Condition in which the predominant feature is a dissociative symptom, but does not meet the criteria for any specific dissociative disorder.

dissociative fugue Condition characterized by sudden, unexpected travel away from home or one's customary place of work, accompanied by an inability to recall one's past and confusion about personal identity or the assumption of a new identity.

dissociative identity disorder (DID) Condition characterized by the presence of two or more distinct identities or personality states that recurrently take control of the individual's behavior, accompanied by an inability to recall important personal information; the condition is too extensive to be explained by ordinary forgetfulness. It is a disorder characterized by identity fragmentation rather than a proliferation of separate personalities.

dissociative trance disorder A rarely seen condition where a person enters a trace-like state for the purpose of sharpening one's awareness to their immediate surroundings, often taking on a new identity during the trace; commonly seen in religious or spiritual ceremonies.

domestic violence See family violence.

dopamine A naturally occurring central nervous system neurotransmitter that transmits signals between cells; it has been linked with many functions such as mood, sexual pleasure, muscle movement, and balance.

dopaminergic Having the effect of dopamine.

dysphoria A disorder of affect characterized by depression and anguish.

dyssomnia Any of a group of primary sleep disorders of initiating and maintaining sleep or of excessive sleepiness that are characterized by a disturbance in the amount, quality, or timing of sleep.

dysthymia (or dysthymic disorder) A chronic mild depressive condition that has been present for greater than two years, in which the patient exhibits at least two of the following six symptoms: poor appetite or overeating, insomnia or hypersomnia, low energy or fatigue, low self-esteem, poor concentration or difficulty making decisions, and feelings of hopelessness.

eating disorder A psychological condition that focuses on the avoidance, excessive consumption, or purging of food.

echolalia An involuntary parrot-like repetition of a word or phrase that another individual has just spoken.

echopraxia The repetitive imitation of movements of others.

egomania Extreme self-centeredness, self-appreciation, or self-content.

emergency A life-threatening situation that requires an immediate response.

emergent-norm theory Theory that combines factors from both the contagion and convergence theories; similar interests draw people together, and then certain behaviors emerge from the crowd itself.

emotional shock An acute and severe emotional condition that can produce immediate physiological reactions that can jeopardize a person's physical well-being.

episode A time-limited period during which specific, intense symptoms of a disorder are evident.

euphoria An exaggerated or abnormal sense of physical and emotional well-being that is usually not based on reality or truth and is inappropriate for the situation and disproportionate to its cause.

excited delirium A term used by medical examiners to explain why people—often high on drugs or alcohol—die suddenly while in police custody. Symptoms are said to include extreme agitation, aggressive, violent behavior, and incoherence.

family violence Includes physical, sexual, or psychological abuse of a spouse, partner, or child and neglect of family members. It can involve incest, murder, and suicide.

flashback A symptom commonly seen in PTSD in which the individual re-experiences or relives a traumatic event as though he or she were actually there.

Ganser's syndrome An unusual condition in which the patient gives answers that appear deliberately false.

generalized amnesia A form of dissociative amnesia in which the individual cannot remember any personal information such as name or address or other personal identifying information.

generalized anxiety disorder (GAD) An anxiety disorder characterized by anxiety that is not associated with a particular object, situation, or event but seems to be a constant feature of a person's day-to-day existence.

germophobia See mysophobia.

global assessment of functioning (GAF) Scale A tool outlined in the DSM-IV-TR that is used to give a numeric value to a person's overall daily function.

grief The intense sorrow or mental anguish that occurs with one's death, which may include physical, social, behavioral, or cognitive aspects.

hallucination False perceptions that relate to any of the five senses.

haplessness Deserving or inciting pity because bad things just keep happening to the person.

Heller's syndrome See childhood disintegrative disorder.

helplessness Powerlessness, as revealed by an inability to act; a feeling of being unable to manage.

heterogeneous group A group made up of "mixed" members who do not have the same background, perceptions, or objectives surrounding an event.

histrionic One who seeks to be the center of attention.

histrionic personality disorder (HPD) (cluster B) A pattern of excessive emotionality and attention seeking.

homogeneous group A group made up of similar members with similar backgrounds, such as police, EMS, or military personnel. A homogeneous group should also have similar experiences, goals, and objectives.

hopelessness The despair one feels when he or she has abandoned hope of comfort or success.

hospice A multi-disciplinary service program for the dying person and his or her family, which provides the support needed to keep the dying person comfortable and free from pain until the time of death.

hyperactive-impulsive type A form of ADHD in which the individual exhibits excessive uncontrollable physical movements and impatience.

hyperarousal A condition of unusual and intense nervousness due to persistent stimulation of the autonomic nervous system; commonly seen as a sign of PTSD.

hyperventilation syndrome An episodic disorder wherein the individual breathes faster than normal.

hypnotic A class of drug that induces sleep.

hypochondria A morbid concern about one's own health and exaggerated attention to any unusual bodily or mental sensation.

hypomania An episode of increased energy that is not sufficiently severe to qualify as a full-blown manic episode.

hypopnea Shallow, slow breathing.

ideational apraxia An impairment that results from a loss of the understanding of how to use a familiar object or to perform a task.

ideomotor apraxia A form of apraxia in which one is unable to respond and perform a requested task.

idiopathic Arising from an unknown cause.

illusion A false interpretation of an external sensory stimulus, commonly auditory or visual in nature.

Immediate Small Group Support (ISGS) New and improved descriptive terminology for the small-group defusing process. ISGS takes place as soon as possible after the traumatic event, allows for a very brief discussion of the traumatic event, and stresses survival information to assist the members of the small group with managing their distress until additional support can be rendered by means of a PEGS or other support services.

implied consent An assumption that a person who is unconscious or otherwise unable to communicate actual permission for treatment would agree to treatment if he or she were capable of communicating such permission.

information gap An uncomfortable feeling that arises when some people have information and others do not.

information push The process of providing information and direction to a crowd aiming to answer questions such as who, what, when, where, and sometimes why. This information is given in an effort to avoid stimulating additional unwanted emotional responses in the crowd members.

insomnia A chronic condition that results in the inability to fall asleep or remain asleep for an adequate period of time.

intoxication Being under the influence of a drug, possibly causing a loss of senses.

intrusion A condition caused by traumatic events where unpleasant thoughts or memories cannot be ignored or supressed.

kinetic apraxia A condition in which the patient is unable to perform skilled movements with the extremities (in the absence of paralysis).

labile mood Unstable, unsteady, not fixed; denotes free and uncontrolled moods or behaviors expressing emotions.

lacrimation Increased tear production.

lanugo Very fine hair, commonly found on newborn infants and anorectics, that grows over the body in an attempt to keep it warm when the body lacks enough fat or muscle to do so.

laxative A drug that induces the movement of fecal matter from the GI system.

limb apraxia See kinetic apraxia.

localized amnesia A most common form of dissociative amnesia in which the individual cannot recall the specific time and period in which a stressful or traumatic event occurred.

major depressive disorder Also known as major depression or unipolar depression; a disorder characterized by a pervasive low mood, loss of interest in a person's usual activities, and diminished ability to experience pleasure.

mania A disturbance in mood characterized by such symptoms as elation, inflated self-esteem, hyperactivity, and accelerated speaking and thinking; an exaggerated feeling of physical and emotional well-being.

maturational crises Crises that occur as part of the growth process.

melatonin Naturally occurring hormone produced by the pineal gland in the brain that assists in falling asleep.

mental retardation A condition in which a person has an IQ that is below average and that affects an individual's learning, behavior, and development. This condition is present from birth.

mental status examination (MSE) A tool used by mental health professionals to evaluate the state of a person's mind. MSEs vary in length and look at various characteristics of one's behavior, mood, affect, thought process, judgment, and memory.

mood The pervasive feeling, tone, and internal emotional state of a person; how one feels.

mood disorder Disorders in which a disturbance in mood is the predominant feature, such as depression, mania, or hypomania.

mood episode The presentation of a mood disturbance such as depression or mania that appears for a short period of time, lasting only days or a few weeks.

mood stabilizer A psychiatric medication used to treat mood disorders, particularly bipolar disorder, in which patients experience wide-ranging mood swings from mania to depression.

mourning The process in which one adapts to the loss of an individual or loved one. Mourning is often affected by cultural customs, norms, and rituals.

multi-axial assessment An approach used in assessing the overall status of a patient.

multi-infarct dementia See vascular dementia.

mysophobia The irrational fear of harmful pathogens such as viruses and bacteria.

narcissistic personality disorder (cluster B) A pattern of grandiosity, need for admiration, and lack of empathy.

narcolepsy A disorder that has repeated irresistible attacks of refreshing sleep, cataplexy, and recurrent intrusions of REM sleep in the transition period between sleep and wakefulness.

negligence Professional action or inaction on the part of the EMS provider that does not meet the standard of care expected of similarly trained and prudent health care professionals and that results in injury to the patient.

nightmare A dream that arouses feelings of extreme fear, horror, and distress.

nightmare disorder Repeated occurrence of frightening dreams that lead to awakenings from sleep and result in social or occupational dysfunction.

non-rapid eye movement (NREM) sleep The majority of time spent sleeping throughout the night in which REM does not occur. It is divided into four stages.

numbing Insensitivity to outside stimulation.

nystagmus Rapidly oscillating eye movement.

obsession Intrusive, recurrent, unwanted ideas, thoughts, or impulses that are difficult to dismiss, despite their disturbing nature.

obsessive-compulsive disorder (OCD) An anxiety disorder characterized by recurrent obsessions or compulsions that are inordinately time-consuming or that cause significant distress or impairment.

obsessive-compulsive personality disorder (cluster C) A pattern of preoccupation with orderliness, perfectionism, and control.

obstructive sleep apnea syndrome (OSAS) A type of breathing-related sleep disorder that is prevalent in middle-aged, overweight men and children with enlarged tonsils. These individuals commonly present with repetitive episodes of upper-airway obstruction during the night, along with periods of apnea and hypopnea. Frequently presents with hypersommolence during the day.

omission A form of negligence that occurs when the EMS provider with a duty to act fails to perform assessments or procedures and this failure in turn harms or creates injury to the patient.

oppositional defiant disorder A disruptive pattern of behavior of children and adolescents that is characterized by defiant, disobedient, and hostile behaviors directed toward adults in positions of authority, lasting at least 6 months.

panic attacks Periods of time marked by intense fear, opposition, and physical discomfort in which an individual feels helpless or as if he or she is about to lose control or even die.

panic disorder An anxiety disorder in which an individual has recurrent panic attacks or has apprehension about the possibility of future attacks.

paranoia A psychological condition exemplified by extreme suspiciousness, usually focused on one central theme. It often includes delusions of grandeur or persecution.

paranoia A psychological condition exemplified by extreme suspiciousness, usually focused on one central theme. It often includes delusions of grandeur or persecution.

paranoid personality disorder (cluster A) A pattern of distrust and suspicion such that others' motives are interpreted as malevolent.

paranoid type schizophrenia A type of schizophrenia distinguished by the presence of delusions and hallucinations in the form of visions or voices often aimed against a governmental figure or agency.

parasomnia Any of a group of primary sleep disorders characterized by abnormal behavioral or physiological events occurring in association with sleep, specific sleep stages, or sleep-wake transitions.

Parkinson's disease A condition in which the part of the brain that controls muscle movement fails because of a breakdown of the dopamine-producing neurons. Patients will present with trembling of the hands, arms, legs, jaw, and face, stiffness of the joints, slow muscle movement, and poor balance and coordination.

personality disorder Pervasive and inflexible alteration of one's traits that leads to distress or impairment.

pervasive developmental disorder (PDD) A group of disorders seen in children characterized by delays in the development of socialization and communication skills.

piloerection When one's hair stands on end; commonly called *goose bumps*.

polysubstance abuse Abuse of more than one substance.

post traumatic stress disorder (PTSD) An anxiety disorder in which the individual experiences several distressing symptoms for more than a month following a traumatic event, such as re-experiencing the traumatic event, avoiding reminders of the trauma, numbing of general responsiveness, and increasing arousal.

Post-Action Staff Support A program of support for CISM personnel who have assisted others in the aftermath of a traumatic event such as a disaster.

Powerful Event Group Support (PEGS) New and improved descriptive terminology approved by the United Nations to describe the Critical Incident Stress Debriefing process. The PEGS is a small-group process for primary groups who are known to each other, have a history together, and have worked together on the same traumatic event.

predominantly inattentive type A form of ADHD in which the person's mind easily wanders and the person pays little or no attention to his or her surroundings.

primary hypersomnia A condition designated in the *DSM-IV-TR* as excessive sleepiness for at least one month as evidenced by prolonged sleep episodes or by daytime sleep episodes occurring almost daily.

primary insomnia Difficulty initiating or maintaining sleep or nonrestorative sleep.

prodromal phase The initial phase of schizophrenia in which the individual begins to withdraw from society, interpersonal and work place relationships begin to deteriorate, and productivity declines markedly. The individual may also experience thought and perception disturbances such as visual hallucinations, hearing voices (usually two voices talking about the person), and incoherent muttering.

psychological toxicity A term used to describe when people lose hope and self-confidence, become anxious and depressed, feel hopeless, and wish to give up.

psychomotor agitation Excessive motor activity, such as pacing or wringing of the hands; often seen as unintentional and purposeless and commonly caused by inner tension.

psychomotor retardation An abnormal slowing of movement, physical reaction, or speech that is directly related to brain activity.

psychosis Mental disorder with the presence of delusions or hallucinations.

psychotic disorder due to a general medical condition The presentation of psychotic symptoms such as hallucinations and delusions that are directly linked to the physiological effects of some medical condition and not better described by another mental disorder.

purging A trait commonly seen in bulimia nervosa in which the person attempts to rid himself or herself of food by vomiting or using laxatives, diuretics, or enemas.

rapid cycling Changing from one mood to the other and back again at short intervals, sometimes several times a day and even several times an hour, commonly between depression and elation.

rapid eye movement (REM) sleep The stage of sleep that occurs intermittently throughout the night in which dreaming occurs. It is named such because of the back-and-forth movement made by the eyes during this phase.

rapport A feeling of relationship, especially when characterized by emotional affinity or bonding.

reactive attachment disorder A mental health disorder in which a child is unable to form healthy social relationships, particularly with a primary caregiver.

residual phase The third phase of schizophrenia that marks the end of the active phase. Individuals may be listless, have trouble concentrating, and be withdrawn, as well as experience thought and perception disturbances like those present in the initial prodromal phase.

residual type schizophrenia A type of schizophrenia in which patients who have recovered from prominent symptoms such as delusions, hallucinations, or disorganized behavior still show some mild evidence of the continuing disease process, such as a flat affect or poverty of speech.

Rest, Information and Transition Session (RITS) A technique similar to the crisis management briefing except it does not contain a question-and-answer period and the session is aimed at staff personnel who just completed their first shift of work at a large-scale incident like a disaster.

retrograde amnesia A condition in which the individual is unable to recall parts of the past.

Rett's syndrome An inherited developmental disorder observed only in females that is characterized by a short period of normal development, followed by loss of developmental skills (particularly purposeful hand movements) and marked psychomotor retardation.

reversible dementia Specific types of dementia that can be reversed if they are diagnosed and treated in a timely manner.

rhabdomyolysis A condition in which skeletal muscle cells break down, releasing myoglobin, which carries oxygen in the muscle, along with enzymes and electrolytes from inside the muscle cells. Two major risks with this condition are the continuing breakdown of the muscle, and, because myoglobin is toxic to the kidneys, renal failure.

rhinorrhea Nasal discharge; a runny nose.

Russell's sign Calluses, cuts, and sores on the knuckles from repeated self-induced vomiting.

schizoaffective disorder A condition that is actually a combination of two disorders: the active phase of schizophrenia and severe mood disorder, which must be either preceded or followed by at least two weeks of delusions or hallucinations (without prominent mood symptoms). The mood disorder can be a major depressive, manic, or mixed episode.

schizoid personality disorder (cluster A) A pattern of detachment from social relationships and a restricted range of emotional expression.

schizophrenia A persistent, often chronic disorder that involves disturbances in content of thought, form of thought, perception, affect, sense of self, motivation, behavior, and interpersonal functioning. Thinking may be disconnected and illogical, and present with delusions or hallucinations. Peculiar behaviors may be associated with social withdrawal and disinterest.

schizophreniform disorder A condition in which the individual shows the same psychotic symptoms attributed to schizophrenia, but lacks the required duration. Symptoms typically last between 1 and 6 months and may not precipitate social and occupational deterioration or dysfunction.

schizotypal personality disorder (cluster A) A pattern of acute discomfort in close relationships, cognitive or perceptual distortions, and eccentricities of behavior.

school violence Any form of violence that occurs within the school system, including elementary, middle, or high schools and colleges or universities. The violent acts can include threats to murder, bullying, Internet crimes, vandalism, property damage, sexual harassment, assault, gang violence, attacks on faculty and staff, and suicide.

SEA-3 assessment tool A brief, five-component tool used for a quick evaluation of the person in crisis. It is used to evaluate a patient's speech, emotion, appearance, alertness, and activity.

selective amnesia A form of dissociative amnesia in which the individual can recall a traumatic event however is unable to remember specific parts of the trauma that are particularly disturbing.

separation anxiety disorder A child's apprehension associated with separation from a parent or other caregiver.

septal erosion Wearing away of the wall of the nasal septum, commonly seen as the result of repeated inhalation of drugs such as cocaine or inhalants.

shared psychotic disorder A condition, commonly called folie a deux, in which an otherwise mentally healthy individual develops delusions while in a close relationship with someone who has an actual psychotic disorder.

situational bound (cued) panic attack A form of panic attack that occurs immediately following the exposure to, or anticipation of, some event, trigger, or situational stimulus.

situational crises Crises that are associated with events or circumstances such as accidents, illness, financial losses, marital problems, and being exposed to a disaster.

situationally predisposed panic attack A form of panic attack that is similar to situationally bound panic attacks but does not occur every time the individual is exposed to a trigger.

sleep terror disorder A condition resulting in abrupt awakenings from sleep, usually beginning with a panicky scream or cry, and accompanied by autonomic arousal and behavioral manifestations of intense fear.

sleep-wake cycle See circadian rhythm.

sleepwalking disorder A condition in which repeated episodes of complex motor behavior are initiated during sleep, including rising from bed and walking about.

social phobia Anxiety disorder characterized by an irrational and constant fear of being scrutinized by one's peers or strangers, causing the individual to feel extreme embarrassment in social situations.

specific phobia An irrational and unabating fear of a particular object, activity, or situation.

street violence Any form of violence that occurs outside of homes, workplaces, organizations, or social areas. The violent acts can include arson, assaults, threats with a weapon, sexual assault, vandalism, armed robbery, home invasions, drug violence, kidnapping, gang violence, carjacking, and murder.

substance-induced psychotic disorder The development of psychotic symptoms such as prominent hallucinations or delusions that are judged to be due to the direct physiological effects of a substance such as drug abuse, prescribed medication, or toxic exposure.

suicidal attempts The act of trying to take one's own life through the use of deliberate, potentially lethal actions.

suicidal completion The act of dying as a result of one's suicide attempt.

suicidal gestures Actions that indicate that one is considering suicide.

suicidal ideation The process of having general or unfocused ideas toward harming oneself.

suicidal thoughts See suicidal ideation.

suicide The act of causing one's own death.

suprachiasmatic nucleus (SCN) Part of the hypothalamus that is responsible for signaling other parts of the brain to regulate hormone release, change body temperature, and make us feel sleepy or awake.

sympathomimetic Substances that mimic epinephrine (adrenalin) or norepinephrine.

systematized amnesia A form of dissociative amnesia in which the individual cannot recall all of the information about one specific aspect of their life such as work, family or personal relationships.

tachycardia Fast heart rate.

technological disaster A disaster that results secondarily because of something that humans have created.

tolerance When a higher amount of substance is required in order to produce the effect previously induced by a lower dose of substance.

toxidrome A group of clinical signs that suggest a specific type of overdose or poisoning.

traumatic experience Any event that has disastrous psychological and/or physical consequences for the person involved; it may include witnessing others' distress.

trypanophobia The fear of medical procedures or medical injections.

undifferentiated type schizophrenia A category of schizophrenia in which individuals show very complex signs and symptoms of the disease but do not meet specific *DSM-IV-TR* criteria to be diagnosed as paranoid, disorganized, or catatonic type.

unexpected (uncued) panic attack A form of panic attack that occurs suddenly and without warning and is not associated with an internal or external situational trigger.

unipolar mood disorder A type of mood disorder in which the person only experiences episodes of depression.

validation The process or statements used in crisis intervention that acknowledge that the person's feelings or reactions are being heard and are acceptable given the current situation.

vascular dementia A degenerative cerebrovascular disease that leads to a progressive decline in memory and cognitive functioning.

vein sclerosis A scarring, hardening, or thickening of the venous tissue secondary to repeated needle injections; commonly seen in intravenous drug users.

vicarious traumatization Vicarious trauma is a term used to describe the thoughts, feelings, and behaviors that can result from repeated exposure to the trauma of others.

violence associated with organized crime, terrorism, or war Any form of violence involving organized crime groups, acts of terrorism, or war. The acts of violence can include identity theft, arson, assault on members of certain ethnic groups, gang violence, murder, genocide, sexual assault as a terror tactic, bombs, hostage takings, torture, attacks against environmental targets, assassinations, trafficking in humans, nuclear, biological, or chemical attacks, slavery, or narco-terrorism.

withdrawal A series of symptoms experienced by the individual when the substance is no longer taken.

workplace violence Any form of violence or threat of violence that occurs in the setting of someone's place of employment is classified as workplace violence, such as intimidation, harassment, assaults, thefts, robbery, stalking, Internet crimes, vandalism, suicide, or murder.

worthlessness Feelings that one's life has no value.

Answer Key

CHAPTER 1 Vital Views: The Importance of Crisis and Behavioral Emergencies Training

1. A
2. C
3. D
4. C
5. B

CHAPTER 2 Crisis Intervention Principles for Prehospital Personnel

1. B
2. B
3. A
4. C
5. B

CHAPTER 3 Assessment in the Prehospital Environment

1. A
2. A
3. C
4. B
5. C

CHAPTER 4 Responding to the Emotional Crisis
1. C
2. B
3. D
4. A
5. D

CHAPTER 5 Assisting Large Groups
1. B
2. A
3. B
4. A
5. D

CHAPTER 6 Emergency Response to Violent Events
1. A
2. D
3. D
4. A
5. B

CHAPTER 7 Suicide: An Extraordinary Case of Violence
1. B
2. C
3. A
4. B
5. A

CHAPTER 8 Supporting Victims of Death-Related Crises
1. A
2. D
3. C
4. D
5. B

CHAPTER 9 Crisis Intervention in Disasters and Other Large-Scale Incidents
1. C
2. A
3. A
4. C
5. D

CHAPTER 10 Developmental Disorders Diagnosed in Infancy, Childhood, and Adolescence
1. B
2. C
3. A
4. B
5. D

CHAPTER 11 Delirium, Dementia, and Amnesic Disorders
1. D
2. A
3. D
4. A
5. C

CHAPTER 12 Substance-Related Disorders
1. D
2. B
3. D
4. A
5. A

CHAPTER 13 Psychosis and Schizophrenia
1. A
2. D
3. B
4. C
5. B

CHAPTER 14 Mood Episodes and Disorders
1. D
2. B
3. A
4. D
5. C

CHAPTER 15 Anxiety Disorders
1. C
2. D
3. B
4. B
5. D

CHAPTER 16 Dissociative Disorders
1. D
2. A
3. D
4. B
5. C

CHAPTER 17 Eating Disorders
1. B
2. C
3. A
4. A
5. C

CHAPTER 18 Sleep Disorders
1. C
2. B
3. C
4. A
5. D

CHAPTER 19 Personality Disorders
1. C
2. B
3. C
4. A
5. D

CHAPTER 20 Sustaining Staff
1. D
2. A
3. B
4. D
5. A

Index

Credits

Chapter 1
1-1 © Mark C. Ide; 1-3 © Steven Townsend/Code 3 Images; 1-4 © Stockbyte/Creatas

Chapter 2
2-1 Courtesy of Michael Rieger/FEMA; 2-2 © National Library of Medicine; 2-3 © Sean O'Brien/Custom Medical Stock Photo; 2-4A © David Buffington/Photodisc/Getty Images; 2-5 © Keith Cullom

Chapter 3
3-2 © LM Oteror/AP Photos

Chapter 4
4-1 © Mikael Karlsson/Alamy Images; 4-3 © ThinkStock/age fotostock; 4-5 © Jack Dagley Photography/ShutterStock, Inc.; 4-6 Courtesy of the U.S. Department of Health and Human Services

Chapter 5
5-1 © Ryan Gardner/AP Photos; 5-2 © Bob Daemmrich/PhotoEdit, Inc.; 5-3 Courtesy of Leif Skoogfors/FEMA; 5-4 © Alexandru Axon/ShutterStock, Inc.; 5-5 © Andrew F. Kazmierski/ShutterStock, Inc.; 5-6 Courtesy of Petty Officer 2nd Class Kyle Niemi, U.S. Coast Guard/U.S. Army

Chapter 6
6-3 © ShutterStock, Inc.; 6-4 © Glen E. Ellman

Chapter 7
7-1 © Craig Jackson/IntheDarkPhotography.com; 7-3 © LM Otero/AP Photos; 7-4 © Bill Fritsch/age fotostock

Chapter 8
8-2 © StockByte/age fotostock; 8-3 © ImageState/age fotostock; 8-4 © Mark C. Ide

Chapter 9
9-1A © Jerry Sharp/ShutterStock, Inc.; 9-1B © Hugh Threlfall/Alamy Images; 9-2 Courtesy of Todd Swain/FEMA; 9-3 Courtesy of Win Henderson/FEMA; 9-4 Courtesy of Jocelyn Augustino/FEMA; 9-5 © Mark C. Ide; 9-6 Courtesy of James Tourtellotte/U.S. Customs and Border Protection

Chapter 10
10-2 Used with permission of the American Academy of Pediatrics, *Pediatric Education for Prehospital Professionals,* © American Academy of Pediatrics, 2000;

Chapter 11
11-2 © Anne Kitzman/ShutterStock, Inc.; 11-3 © Mark C. Ide

Chapter 12
12-1 © Tiburon Studios/ShutterStock, Inc.; 12-2A © AbleStock; 12-2B © Laurin Rinder/ShutterStock, Inc.; 12-2C © Stockbyte/Creatas

Chapter 13
13-2 © Glen E. Ellman

Chapter 14
14-1 © Glen E. Ellman; 14-2 SuperStock/Alamy Images; 14-3 © Mark C. Ide

Chapter 15
15-1 © Cecilia Lim H M/ShutterStock, Inc.; 15-2 © Glen E. Ellman; 15-4 © Jeu/Dreamstime.com; 15-5 © Robert Lahser/*The Charlotte Observer*/AP Photos

Chapter 16
16-1 © Mikael Karlsson/Alamy Images; 16-2 © *The Express Times*/AP Photos; 16-4 Courtesy of DEA

Chapter 17
17-1 © Lauren Greenfield/VII/AP Photos; 17-2 © Phanie/Photo Researchers, Inc.

Chapter 18
18-1 © Karen Winton/ShutterStock, Inc.; 18-2 © Photos.com; 18-3 © semenovp/ShutterStock, Inc.; 18-4 © Kirk Pearl Professional Imaging/ShutterStock, Inc.

Chapter 19
19-1 © Peter Dazeley/Alamy Images

Chapter 20
20-1 © Photodisc

Unless otherwise indicated, all photographs and illustrations are under copyright of Jones and Bartlett Publishers, LLC, and photographed by Maryland Institute of Emergency Medical Services Systems.